...

COMPREHENSIVE APPLICATIONS

OF

SHAOLIN CHIN NA

(Qin Na)

...

The Practical Defense of Chinese Seizing Arts
For All Martial Arts Styles

擒 拿 匯 宗

YMAA Publication Center
Main Office:
  4354 Washington Street
  Roslindale, Massachusetts, 02131
  1-800-669-8892   www.ymaa.com   ymaa@aol.com

15   14   13

ISBN: 0-940-871-36-X

Publisher's Cataloging in Publication
(Prepared by Quality Books Inc.)

  Yang, Jwing-Ming, 1946-
    Comprehensive applications of Shaolin chin na / by Yang
Jwing-Ming
      p. cm.
      Includes index
      ISBN 0-940871-36-X

    1. Martial arts–China–Handbooks, manuals, etc. I. Title.

  GV1100.7.A2Y36 1995   796.8'0951
                                       QBI94-2334

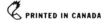 **PRINTED IN CANADA**

Disclaimer:
The author and publisher of this material are NOT RESPONSIBLE in any
manner whatsoever for any injury which may occur through reading or following the instructions in this manual.
The activities, physical or otherwise, described in this material may be too
strenuous or dangerous for some people, and the reader(s) should consult a
physician before engaging in them.

This book is bound
"Otabind" to lay
flat when opened.

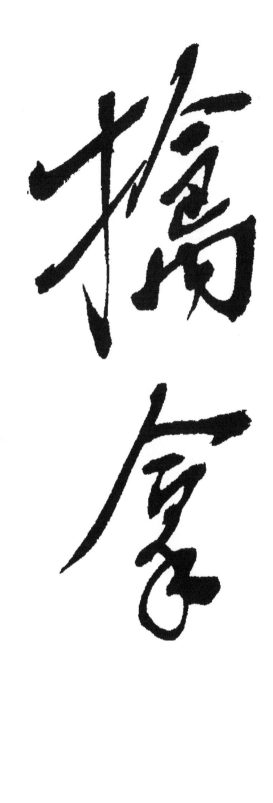

To My

White Crane Master Cheng Gin-Gsao

and

Long Fist Master Li Mao-Ching

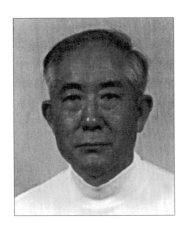
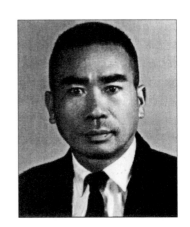

謹奉獻給
曾金灶師父
與
李茂清老師

PROVERBS:

"The Taller the Bamboo Grows, the Lower it Bows."

———————

*"A True Humble-One Always Knows Others and
Does Not Care If Other People Know Him."*

———————

*"Those Who Have to Criticize Others are
Those Whose Minds are Void."*

———————

"The Yin Side of Dignity is False Pride and Self-Spite."

———————

*"Those Who Despise Themselves are Always
Concerned With Their Dignity."*

ACKNOWLEDGMENTS

Thanks to Tim Comrie for his photography, Jerry Leake for design and layout and James B. Philips for the cover drawing. Thanks also to Yang Mei-Ling, Ramel Rones, and Craig McConnell for general help, to Andrew Murray, Jeffrey Pratt, David Ripianzi, Sean Hessman and many other YMAA members for proofing the manuscript and for contributing many valuable suggestions and discussions. Special thanks to James O'Leary for his editing. And a very special thanks to Liang Dexing (Jeffrey D. S, Liang) for his beautiful calligraphy on the front pages of this volume.

ABOUT THE AUTHOR

DR. YANG JWING-MING, PH.D.

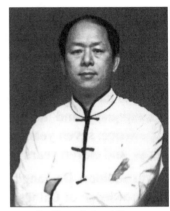

Dr. Yang Jwing-Ming

Dr. Yang Jwing-Ming was born on August 11th, 1946, in Xinzhu Xian, Taiwan, Republic of China. He started his Wushu (Gongfu or Kung Fu) training at the age of fifteen under the Shaolin White Crane (Bai He) Master Cheng Gin-Gsao. Master Cheng originally learned Taizuquan from his grandfather when he was a child. When Master Cheng was fifteen years old, he started learning White Crane from Master Jin Shao-Feng, and he followed him for twenty-three years until Master Jin's death.

In thirteen years of study (1961-1974 A.D.) under Master Cheng, Dr. Yang became an expert in the White Crane style of Chinese martial arts, which includes both the use of barehands and of various weapons such as saber, staff, spear, trident, two short rods, and many other weapons. With the same master he also studied White Crane Qin Na (or Chin Na), Tui Na and Dian Xue massages, and herbal treatment.

At the age of sixteen, Dr. Yang began the study of Taijiquan (Yang Style) under Master Kao Tao. After learning from Master Kao, Dr. Yang continued his study and research of Taijiquan with several masters and senior practitioners such as Master Li Mao-Ching and Mr. Wilson Chen in Taipei. Master Li learned his Taijiquan from the well-known Master Han Ching-Tan, and Mr. Chen learned his Taijiquan from Master Chang Xiang-San. Dr. Yang has mastered the Taiji barehand sequence, pushing hands, the two-man fighting sequence, Taiji sword, Taiji saber, and Taiji Qigong.

When Dr. Yang was eighteen years old he entered Tamkang College in Taipei Xian to study Physics. In college he began the study of traditional Shaolin Long Fist (Changquan or Chang Chuan) with Master Li Mao-Ching at the Tamkang College Guoshu Club (1964-1968 A.D.), and eventually became an assistant instructor under Master Li. In 1971 he completed his M.S. degree in Physics at the National Taiwan University, and then served in the Chinese Air Force from 1971 to 1972. In the service, Dr. Yang taught Physics at the Junior Academy of the Chinese Air Force while also teaching Wushu. After being honorably discharged in 1972, he returned to Tamkang College to teach Physics and resume study under Master Li Mao-Ching. From Master Li, Dr. Yang learned Northern style Wushu, which includes both barehand (especially kicking) techniques and numerous weapons.

In 1974, Dr. Yang came to the United States to study Mechanical Engineering at Purdue University. At the request of a few students, Dr. Yang began to teach Gongfu (Kung Fu), which resulted in the foundation of the Purdue University Chinese Kung Fu Research Club in the spring of 1975. While at Purdue, Dr. Yang also taught college-credited courses in Taijiquan. In May of 1978 he was awarded a Ph.D. in Mechanical Engineering by Purdue.

In 1980, Dr. Yang moved to Houston to work for Texas Instruments. While in Houston he founded Yang's Shaolin Kung Fu Academy, which was eventually taken over by his student Mr. Jeffery Bolt after he moved to Boston in 1982. Dr. Yang founded Yang's Martial Arts Academy (YMAA) in Boston on October 1, 1982.

In January of 1984 he gave up his engineering career to devote more time to research, writing, and teaching. In March of 1986 he purchased property in the Jamaica Plain area of Boston to be used as the headquarters of the new organization, Yang's Martial Arts Association. The organization has continued to expand, and, as of July 1st 1989, YMAA has become just one division of Yang's Oriental Arts Association, Inc. (YOAA, Inc).

In summary, Dr. Yang has been involved in Chinese Wushu since 1961. During this time, he has spent thirteen years learning Shaolin White Crane (Bai He), Shaolin Long Fist (Changquan), and Taijiquan. Dr. Yang has more than twenty-five years of instructional experience: seven years in Taiwan, five years at Purdue University, two years in Houston, Texas, and eleven years in Boston, Massachusetts.

In addition, Dr. Yang has also been invited to offer seminars around the world to share his knowledge of Chinese martial arts and Qigong. The countries he has visited include Canada, Mexico, France, Italy, Poland, England, Ireland, Portugal, Switzerland, Germany, Latvia, and Saudi Arabia.

Dr. Yang has published eighteen other volumes on the martial arts and Qigong:

1. *Shaolin Chin Na*; Unique Publications, Inc., 1980.
2. *Shaolin Long Fist Kung Fu*; Unique Publications, Inc., 1981.
3. *Yang Style Tai Chi Chuan*; Unique Publications, Inc., 1981.
4. *Introduction to Ancient Chinese Weapons*; Unique Publications, Inc., 1985.
5. *Chi Kung - Health and Martial Arts*; YMAA Publication Center, 1985.
6. *Northern Shaolin Sword*; YMAA Publication Center, 1985.
7. *Advanced Yang Style Tai Chi Chuan*, Vol.1, Tai Chi Theory and Tai Chi Jing; YMAA Publication Center, 1986.
8. *Advanced Yang Style Tai Chi Chuan*, Vol.2, Martial Applications; YMAA Publication Center, 1986.
9. *Analysis of Shaolin Chin Na*; YMAA Publication Center, 1987.
10. *The Eight Pieces of Brocade*; YMAA Publication Center, 1988.
11. *The Root of Chinese Chi Kung - The Secrets of Chi Kung Training*; YMAA Publication Center, 1989.
12. *Muscle/Tendon Changing and Marrow/Brain Washing Chi Kung - The Secret of Youth*; YMAA Publication Center, 1989.
13. *Hsing Yi Chuan - Theory and Applications*; YMAA Publication Center, 1990.

14. *The Essence of Tai Chi Chi Kung - Health and Martial Arts*; YMAA Publication Center, 1990.
15. *Qigong for Arthritis*; YMAA Publication Center, 1991.
16. *Chinese Qigong Massage - General Massage*; YMAA Publication Center, 1992.
17. *How to Defend Yourself*; YMAA Publication Center, 1992.
18. *Baguazhang - Emei Baguazhang*; YMAA Publication Center, 1994.

Dr. Yang has also produced the following videotapes:

1. *Yang Style Tai Chi Chuan and Its Applications*; YMAA Publication Center, 1984.
2. *Shaolin Long Fist Kung Fu - Lien Bu Chuan and Its Applications*; YMAA Publication Center, 1985.
3. *Shaolin Long Fist Kung Fu - Gung Li Chuan and Its Applications*; YMAA Publication Center, 1986.
4. *Shaolin Chin Na*; YMAA Publication Center, 1987.
5. *Wai Dan Chi Kung, Vol. 1 — The Eight Pieces of Brocade*; YMAA Publication Center, 1987.
6. *Chi Kung for Tai Chi Chuan*; YMAA Publication Center, 1990.
7. *Qigong for Arthritis*; YMAA Publication Center, 1991.
8. *Qigong Massage - Self Massage*; YMAA Publication Center, 1992.
9. *Qigong Massage - With a Partner*; YMAA Publication Center, 1992.
10. *Defend Yourself 1 - Unarmed Attack*; YMAA Publication Center, 1992.
11. *Defend Yourself 2 - Knife Attack*; YMAA Publication Center, 1992.

FOREWORD

GRANDMASTER LI MAO-CHING

Dr. Yang Jwing-Ming, a master of Gongfu, currently resides in the United States of America to continue the spread of Chinese culture to the western world. Since his childhood, he has received the twin gifts of education and moral cultivation from his family. He is wise and intelligent. When he was teenager, he admired and loved Chinese Wuyi (martial arts)(武藝), and he traveled many miles every night to the mountain near his hometown to learn from a renowned southern style martial arts teacher, Grandmaster Cheng Gin-Gsao. After thirteen years of study under Grandmaster Cheng, he ascertained the essence of southern Chinese martial arts.

Later, he left his hometown and went to Taipei for his undergraduate and graduate study (bachelor's degree in physics at Tamkang University and Master's degree in Physics at Taiwan University). He then began to study northern Long Fist styles of Chinese martial arts and their theories.

In 1974, Dr. Yang journeyed to the United States of America for his Doctorate degree in Mechanical Engineering; he obtained his Ph.D. from Purdue University in 1978.

During this period, although he was so busy with his studies, he never forgot to study and practice Chinese Wuyi. He can be considered a determined martial arts scholar of very deliberate purpose.

Presently, he concentrated all of his effort on researching and studying Chinese culture, especially Chinese self-defense techniques (called Chinese Gongfu), which have been passed down for thousands of years. From his study and research, he has written twenty books related to Chinese martial arts and Qigong practice. When he teaches or writes, he always uses the scientific method and logical judgment in analyzing the arts. From this scientific approach, the learners or readers are able to understand and absorb **much** knowledge much more thoroughly then they would otherwise. In my opinion, he is the foremost contributor to the spread of Chinese culture to western society. This is especially valuable and unique, since Dr. Yang possesses both southern and northern martial skills. In addition, he is also a scholar of the west and east.

After he obtained his doctorate in Mechanical Engineering, he enjoyed his dream of developing and introducing Chinese Wuyi. Moreover, he still respects his teachers (*Qin Shi*, 親師) and appreciates the origin of his learning (*Zhui Yuan*, 追源). When his southern style master passed away, he traveled thousands miles to mourn and showed respect at his master's grave. This manner of "Humble Study and Respecting One's Teacher" (*Bo Xue Jing Shi*, 博學敬師) has especially earned my respect and praise. Whenever he comes home, he always shows his great feelings of love and respect to his parents (*Shi Qin Zhi Xiao*,侍親至孝). When he is around his relatives and friends, he is known as very "Humble and Polite"(*Qian Cheng Li Rang*, 謙誠禮讓). All of these qualities have been praised by the people around him.

After more than thirty years of study and practice, he has accumulated much experience in Qin Na. Now, he has again completed this new book on Qin Na, entitled *Comprehensive Applications of Shaolin Chin Na.*

Last week, as I was home with my wife, I received his telephone call from America inviting me to write this foreword. The time was urgent and his sincerity was so real that, even though I do not have a deep scholarship in writing that will help him to promote his book, I am still very happy to write for him from what I have learned from my Master, Han Ching-Tang.

If we study the history of Qin Na, we find that it used to be called "Locking Hands (techniques)" (*Kou Zhi Shou*, 扣子手), "Dividing Tendon Hands (techniques)" (*Fen Jin Shou*, 分筋手), or "Misplacing the Bone Hands (techniques)"(*Cuo Gu Shou*, 錯骨手), among other names. All of these techniques were developed from the skills developed from the Chinese martial arts sequences. These key techniques are: Hooking (*Diao*, 刁), Grabbing (*Na*, 拿), Locking (*Suo*, 鎖), Wrapping (*Kou*, 扣), Plucking (*Cai*, 採), and Pulling (*Le*, 将). The six techniques are used by all of the Chinese martial arts styles and exist in almost all of the sequences. Among them, hooking, grabbing, plucking, and pulling are commonly used in hand techniques, and locking and wrapping are often executed in two hands techniques.

In 1928, the Chinese government established the "Nanking Central Guoshu Institute." The first student of the first generation to graduate was Grandmaster Han Ching-Tang. Right after his graduation, he was sent to Zhejiang province police academy to teach martial arts, including Qin Na, wrestling, striking, and kicking. At this time, he also cooperated with his martial brother, Grandmaster Liu Jin-Sheng, to study and research together the techniques of "Dividing the Muscle/Tendon and Misplacing the Bone" Chin Na. They compiled this knowledge into a sequence and named it *Qin Na Shu* (Qin Na Techniques) (擒拿術). Since then, these techniques have become a required course in all Chinese police academies. Each technique was given a name, and a standardized training system has been established.

Later, during World War II, the Chinese government moved to Chongqing City, Sichuan province. Grandmaster Han was assigned to be a martial arts teacher for the special police unit. Before long, the Chinese government moved to Taiwan to escape the Chinese communists. Again, Grandmaster Han was recommended as the chief martial arts coach for the Taiwanese Police Academy. At that time, he wrote a book: *The Applications of Police Qin Na Techniques* (*Jing Cha Qin Na Ying Yong Shu*, 警察擒拿應用術). Although this book was used as a text by the Chinese police, it was not published to the general public. During this time, he also created several "Qin Na" matching sequences which helped to preserve many Qin Na techniques. Some of the names in the sequence are: 1. Bend the Finger to Count (*Qu Zhi Yi Suan*, 曲指一算); 2. Old Mule Holds Its feet (*Lao Lu E Ti*, 老驢扼蹄); 3. Federal Lord Invites for Dinner (*Ba Wang Qing Ke*, 霸王請客); 4. Yellow Eagle Pulls Its Wings (*Huang Ying Che Chi*, 黃鷹掣翅); 5. The Boat Man Pushes His Oar (*Chuan Fu Cheng Gao*, 船夫撐篙); 6. Single Wrapping Wrist (*Dan Chan Si Wan*, 單纏絲腕); 7. Double Wrapping Wrist (*Shuang Chan Si Wan*, 雙纏絲腕); 8. Black Tiger Digs the Heart (*Hei Hu Tao Xin*, 黑虎掏心); 9. The Hero Carries the Tiger (*Zhuang Shi Bei Hu*, 壯士背虎), and many others. This is only a partial list of the sequences for your reference. I hope these names will reveal to you some of the knowledge that inspired this book: Comprehensive Applications of Shaolin Chin Na.

I respect Doctor Yang's personality and the manner with which he treats others. I have even greater admiration for his hard work in developing Chinese martial arts. Therefore, I am very delighted to write this foreword for him.

Li Mao-Ching, September 3rd, 1994
Research Member
Guoshu Promoting Committee Republic of China

FOREWORD

MASTER LIANG SHOU-YU

Chinese martial arts have a rich, long history. Consequently, thousands of styles or schools have developed. Each of these styles or schools has its own unique characteristics and special emphases. Nevertheless, all the martial techniques developed in any of them can be generally classified into four categories: kicking (*Ti*), striking (*Da*), wrestling (*Shuai Jiao*), and grabbing-controlling (*Qin Na*). From this, you can see that Qin Na techniques have played an important role in Chinese martial arts, and are commonly mixed with other categories of techniques in sequence training. Qin Na is also an important part of barehand sparring.

Qin Na includes: **Dividing the Muscle/Tendons** (*Fen Jin*, 分筋), **Misplacing the Bones** (*Cuo Gu*, 錯骨), **Cavity Press** (*Dian Xue*, 點穴), **Grabbing Artery/Qi Channels** (*Na Mai*, 拿脈), **Grabbing Tendons** (*Zhua Jin*, 抓筋), and **Seal the Breath** (*Bi Qi*,閉氣). The theories and principles of Qin Na are, from the arrangement of the mutual relative positions and angles, to immobilize the opponent's joint movements and control his vital areas. This must be done with correct shifting of weight, footwork, and body postures. In actual combat conditions, the variations on the techniques are many, and the timing for executing them is very short. If you only know a few Qin Na movements or techniques, you may be unable to handle the situation. You must be familiar with and have comprehended the essence of techniques covering a wide range of situations. Furthermore, you must have mastered the techniques with accuracy of angle, sharp power (*Jin*), and the right timing. Only then will you be able to use them effectively.

I have practiced Chinese martial arts for more than forty years, and I am very fond of Qin Na techniques. I have known many martial artists and friends, both in Chinese and western martial arts societies. I have also had opportunities to visit many high level Qin Na martial artists. Almost every Gongfu style or school has told me that they know Qin Na, and have memorized and mastered the names and the techniques skillfully. They were able to perform them or talk about them wonderfully and attractively. When I was young, in order to comprehend the real essence of Wugong (武功) (martial Gongfu), I liked these discussions, and researched various areas of Chinese martial arts with other Chinese martial artists. However, very few of them were able to apply their Qin Na techniques on me. After I came to America, I also discussed and researched Qin Na with many martial artists. What I would do was only use a single hand to grab them. However, no matter which styles (道)(*Dao*) or what degree they were (段位), these martial artists were unable to apply their Qin Na techniques on me. Because of this, many good Qin Na martial artists called me "High Hands" (高手)(i.e., high level artist) and invited me to teach them Qin Na.

I have many martial arts friends who studied and researched Qin Na with me when I was still in mainland China. For nearly forty years in China, I found only a couple of good Qin Na experts to really appraise and admire. They could not only talk about the theory of Qin Na, but could also really apply them in Qin Na circles, and not just outside that circle.

I became acquainted with Dr. Yang Jwing-Ming eight years ago. We meet each other a few times each year, and study from and practice with each other. Of all the Qin Na experts I have met in the past, he is the Great Qin Na Teacher (擒拿大師), who has really comprehended Qin Na to the deepest level, and his techniques cover the widest range. In the last thirty years he has learned, pondered, and researched different Qin Na styles or schools, Chinese or non-Chinese, ancient or modern. In addition, he has adopted the scientific method, and studied the body's anatomical structure, mechanical dynamics, and psychological analysis, mixing them with traditional theory and training, and has established a new independent system. Though he has written two popular Qin Na books, *Shaolin Chin Na* and *Analysis of Shaolin Chin Na*, he still feels unsatisfied and tries to deepen his understanding even more. I admire his spirit of research very much. It is also this spirit which has led to his Qin Na reaching the stage of "Applying the Techniques as a Wish" (隨心所欲) and "Consummation of Skill" (爐火純青).

Many Qin Na books have been published both in China and the west in the last few decades. However, none of them has reached so deep and so wide. The title of this book: *Qin Na Essence Gathering (Comprehensive Applications of Shaolin Qin Na)* (*Qin Na Hui Zong*) (擒拿匯宗) was suggested by me. At the beginning, Dr. Yang felt that this book could not be good enough to be titled "Essence Gathering" (匯宗). Later, after comparing many other Qin Na books, he finally accepted my title. This book can really be called the "Gathering" of the "Essence" of Qin Na from every style.

Dr. Yang's Qin Na is reached through real Gongfu (energy-time) (功夫), and is the real art. In American martial arts society, the origin or the teacher of a martial artist is very important. If your teacher is a famous Chinese master, then it does not matter if the student is good or not, he has the opportunity to be chosen and his photo can be used on the cover of some martial arts magazine. The magazine can serve as an advertisement for them. If you have a good and famous teacher, it is your luck. But it is said in Chinese martial arts society: "Sifu leads you into the door, the cultivation depends on oneself."[1] In China, it is very different now. You must have real Gongfu and contribute a great deal in Chinese martial arts society before you will be respected.

Though Dr. Yang had several good teachers when he was young, his Gongfu was really obtained from his past thirty years of pondering and research, learning and studying humbly, absorbing the best from all styles and schools, in addition to his own comprehension and understanding. Consequently, he has reached an incredibly refined and detailed stage in every Qin Na technique. That is why people call him the "King of Qin Na" (擒拿王) in America.

Though I have studied Qin Na for many years, and I believe that I have reached a deeply profound level, after I knew Dr. Yang, I realized how accomplished he was and realized that there were many things I must learn from him. The International San Shou Dao Association has decided to use his Qin Na as part of its requirements. I believe that this book will bring those people interested in Qin Na a great help. I would also like to congratulate him for this new contribution to the world martial arts society.

Liang Shou-Yu
March 23, 1994

1. 師父領進門，修行在自身。

PREFACE

DR. YANG JWING-MING

Even though Qin Na (Chin Na) has been popularly practiced in Chinese martial arts for hundreds of years, it was not until the 1982 publication of my first Qin Na book, *Shaolin Chin Na*, by Unique Publications, that these secret techniques of the Chinese martial arts were widely revealed to the western world. Since then, this art has grown so rapidly that my book has been translated into several different languages, making its way all over the world in less than ten years.

Later, due to the tremendous number of requests, I decided to write another volume, covering Qin Na theory and techniques in a more in-depth manner. This second volume, *Analysis of Shaolin Chin Na - Instructor's Manual* was published in 1987. I am truly stunned that, less than fifteen years after my first book, this art has become so popular that I must travel to more than twelve countries around the world, at least twice a year, to teach this art. I believe that the main reason for this is simply because this art can be adapted easily by almost any martial arts style, and blended into its own techniques. Moreover, Qin Na has proven one of the most effective defense systems, and can be learned easily even by the martial arts beginner.

From my experience teaching seminars, I realized that the hardest part of the art is not learning the techniques themselves, but applying those techniques to dynamic situations. Usually, a practitioner can pick up a technique easily and make it effective, but only when his partner is cooperative. However, as we already know, when you encounter an enemy in real life, his cooperation is unlikely. Any success in executing a technique depends on how **accurate**, **fast**, **natural**, and **automatic** your reactions are, and the only way to develop skills in these areas is in your practice. For this reason, I decide to write this book *Comprehensive Chin Na Applications*, making this "**seizing and controlling**" art more complete.

The main differences between this book and the earlier two books is that first, more techniques will be introduced, second, all of the techniques are laid out according to actual combat scenarios, and third, some of the tendon grabbing, cavity press, and taking down Qin Na will also be introduced in different combat situations. From this perspective, you may find it easier to adapt the techniques which are most suitable to various situations.

In China, there probably exist more than seven hundred Qin Na techniques. In this book, I will introduce only those Qin Na techniques with which I am familiar. These techniques include about 60% White Crane and Tiger Claw Qin Na from my first master, Cheng Gin-Gsao, and 20% Northern Long Fist Qin Na (mainly from Eagle Claw, Praying Mantis, and Cha Chuan styles) from my third master, Li Mao-Ching. The remaining 20% I developed myself, through more than thirty years of martial arts experience.

Though one can learn a great portion of basic Qin Na techniques from books and videotapes, very often one needs a qualified master to lead to the deep, advanced levels. Books can offer you the theory of the techniques while the videotapes can offer you the continuous movements of the techniques. However, neither offers the correct **"feeling"** of the locking, nor a clear concept of **"how an angle is set up."** If you are sincere in your desire to become a proficient Qin Na expert, you should also participate in seminars offered by qualified Qin Na masters. Very often, only a few minutes in a Qin Na seminar can clear the confusion which, without such instruction, would have bogged your training down for months or even years.

Other than reading this book, the interested reader should also refer to the book Shaolin Chin Na, published by Unique Publications, and also *Analysis of Shaolin Chin Na - Instructor's Manual*, published by YMAA, both of which are available from YMAA. These two books will help you build a firm foundation, both in theory and routine practice, before you begin the advanced training in this book. In addition, these two books - especially the second one - will teach you how to train the power required for Qin Na techniques, and also the theory and methods for treating common injuries. In the Appendix of the second volume, some secret herbal prescriptions for injury, passed down to me by my White Crane master, are also included. In order to avoid replication, I will not repeat these subjects in this volume.

I am very pleased to see that there are currently more Qin Na books on the market, published by other martial artists. Naturally, because of this, I must make this new book more complete, comprehensive and as near to perfect as I am able. As I pointed out earlier, there are probably more than 700 Qin Na techniques available. Therefore, if you also refer to these other books, you will increase your knowledge beyond what I know in my books. To preserve and continue to promote Qin Na art to a higher level, I sincerely hope these other Qin Na experts can open their minds and share their knowledge with the general public.

Finally, you may noticed that all of the Chinese pronunciations are spelled according to the Pinyin system of translation. The reason for this is simply that the Pinyin system has become more popular than any other system in the last fifteen years. I have been told that this system will become the only system in the next few decades.

Dr. Yang Jwing-Ming
Jeddah, Saudi Arabia
January 28th, 1993

CONTENTS

CHAPTER 1. GENERAL CONCEPTS

CHAPTER 2. QIN NA AGAINST BAREHAND ATTACKS

CHAPTER 3. QIN NA AGAINST BLOCKING

CHAPTER 4. QIN NA AGAINST KICKING

· Chapter 1 ·

GENERAL CONCEPTS

1-1. Introduction

What is Qin Na:

"Qin" (Chin) in Chinese means "To seize or catch," in the way an eagle seizes a rabbit or a policeman catches a murderer (Qin Xiong). "Na" means "To hold and control." Therefore, Qin Na can be translated as "seize and control."

Generally speaking, in order to have effective and efficient fighting capability, almost all Chinese martial styles include three categories of techniques. The first category includes the techniques of striking, punching, pushing, pressing, kicking, etc. In these techniques, the contact time between you and your opponent is very short. and the power for attacking is usually explosive and harmful. The second category is called "Shuai Jiao" (wrestling), and contains the skills of destroying the opponent's root and balance, consequently throwing him down. These techniques can be leg sweeps or trips, body swings or even throws. The last category is Qin Na, containing grabbing techniques which specialize in controlling or locking the opponent's joints, muscles, or tendons.

However, you should understand an important fact. In a combat situation, the above three categories are often applied together, and cannot really be separated. For example, while one of your hands is grabbing and controlling your opponent, the other hand is used to strike a vital cavity. Another example of this is that often, you use grabbing to lock your opponent's joints while throwing him down for further attack. Because of this, sometimes it is very difficult to discriminate clearly between them in a real situation. As matter of fact, many Chinese martial artists believe that since there are many other non-grabbing techniques, such as pressing or striking the cavities or nerves, which can make the opponent numb in part of the body (or even render him unconscious), consequently providing control of the opponent, these techniques should also be included as Qin Na. You can see that, as long as the techniques are able to immobilize the opponent, it does not matter if the cause is a joint lock, numbness, or unconsciousness - all of them should be classified as Qin Na.

In summary, grabbing Qin Na techniques control and lock the opponent's joints or muscle/tendon so he cannot move, thus neutralizing his fighting ability. Pressing Qin Na techniques are used to numb the opponent's limbs, causing him to lose consciousness, or even to kill him. Pressing Qin Na is usually applied to the Qi cavities to affect the normal Qi circulation to the organs or the brain. Pressing techniques are also frequently used on nerve endings to cause extreme pain and unconsciousness. Qin Na striking techniques are applied to vital points, and can be very deadly. Cavities on the Qi channels can be attacked, or certain vital areas struck to rupture arteries. All of these techniques serve to "seize and control" the opponent. Therefore, Qin Na techniques can be generally categorized as:[1]

1. "Fen Jin" (dividing the muscle/tendon) 分筋
2. "Cuo Gu" (misplacing the bone) 錯骨
3. "Bi Qi" (sealing the breath) 閉氣
4. "Dian Mai" (Dim Mak, in Cantonese)(pressing a vein/artery) or "Duan Mai" (sealing or blocking the vein/artery)[2] 點脈，斷脈
5. "Dian Xue" (cavity press) or "Dian Mai" (Dim Mak, in Cantonese)(pressing a primary Qi channel)[3] 點穴，點脈

Within these categories, Fen Jin also includes "Zhua Jin" (grabbing the muscle/tendon) and Dian Xue also includes "Na Xue" (grabbing or pressing the cavities).

Generally, dividing the muscle/tendon, misplacing the bone, and some techniques of sealing the breath are relatively easy to learn, and the theory behind them is easy to understand. They usually require only muscular strength and practice to make the control effective. When these same techniques are used to break bones or injure joints or tendons, you usually need to use Jin (martial power). (For a discussion of Jin, see the author's book *Advanced Yang Style Tai Chi Chuan, Vol. 1, Tai Chi Theory and Tai Chi Jing*). Sealing the vein/artery and pressing the cavities requires detailed knowledge of the location, depth, and timing of the cavities, development of Yi (mind), Qi (internal energy), and Jin (martial power), and special hand forms and techniques. This usually requires formal instruction by a qualified master, not only because the knowledge is deep, but also because most of the techniques are learned from sensing and feeling. Many of the techniques can easily cause death, and for this reason a master will normally only pass this knowledge down to students who are moral and trustworthy.

Qin Na in Chinese Martial Arts:

Nobody can tell exactly when Qin Na was first used. It probably began the first time one person grabbed another with the intention of controlling him. Grabbing the oppo-

---

1. Throwing down Qin Na is often also classified as a part of the Chinese wrestling (Shuai Jiao).
2. "Mai" here means "Xue Mai" and translates to "Blood vessels."
3. "Mai" here means "Qi Mai" and translates to "Primary Qi channels."

nent's limbs or weapon is one of the most basic and instinctive ways to immobilize him or control his actions.

Because of their practicality, Qin Na techniques have been trained right along with other fighting techniques since the beginning of Chinese martial arts, many thousands of years ago. Although no system has sprung up which practices only Qin Na, almost every martial style has Qin Na mixed in with its other techniques. Even in Japan, Korea, and other oriental countries which have been significantly influenced by Chinese culture, the indigenous martial styles have Qin Na techniques mixed in to some degree.

Generally speaking, since martial styles in southern China specialize in hand techniques and close range fighting, they tend to have better developed Qin Na techniques, and they tend to rely more upon them than do the northern styles. Also, because southern martial styles emphasize hand conditioning more than the northern styles, they tend to use more muscles for grabbing and cavity press. Southern styles' emphasis on short range fighting causes them to train more for sticking and adhering. The techniques are usually applied with a circular motion, which can set the opponent up for a Qin Na control without his feeling the preparation. Footwork is also considered a very important part of Qin Na training for a southern martial artist. Remember that these statements are only generalizations; there are northern styles which also emphasize these things.

In Chinese internal styles such as Taiji and Liu He Ba Fa, neutralization is usually done with a circular motion, and so the Qin Na techniques tend to be smooth and round. Often the opponent will be controlled before he realizes that a technique is being applied. In coordination with circular stepping, circular Qin Na can be used to pull the opponent's root and throw him away.

Japanese Jujitsu and Aikido are based on the same principles as Qin Na and Taiji. Since these countries were significantly influenced by Chinese culture, it seems probable that Chinese Qin Na also influenced their indigenous martial arts.

Since fundamental Qin Na techniques can be used to seize and control a criminal without injuring or killing him, they have been an important part of training for constables, government officers, and modern policemen. Around 527 A.D., the Shaolin temple became heavily involved in the martial arts. Since many non-lethal Qin Na techniques are very effective, the martial artists at the temple extensively researched, developed, and trained them. In the late Qing dynasty in the 19th century, Shaolin techniques were taught to people in the general population, and Qin Na techniques were passed down along with the different martial styles which were developed in the Shaolin temple. Many Qin Na techniques were also developed for use with weapons specially designed to seize the opponent's weapon. If your opponent is disarmed, he is automatically in a disadvantageous situation. For example, the hook of the hook sword or the hand guard of a Chai (Sai) were designed for this purpose.

1-2. Qin Na Categories and Theory

Although Qin Na techniques from one Gongfu style may seem quite different from the techniques of another style, the theories and principles of application remain the same. These theories and principles form the root of all Qin Na techniques. If you adhere to these roots, your Qin Na will continue to grow and improve, but if you ignore these roots, your Qin Na will always remain undeveloped. In this section we will discuss these general theories and principles.

Before we discuss each Qin Na category, you should understand that there is no technique which is perfect for all situations. What you do depends upon what your opponent does, and since your opponent will not stand still and just let you control him, you must be able to adapt your Qin Na to fit the circumstances. Like all martial arts techniques, your **Qin Na must respond to and follow the situation**; techniques must be **skillful, alive, fast,** and **powerful**. You should further understand that **Qin Na must take the opponent by surprise**. In grabbing Qin Na you have to grasp your opponent's body, and so if your opponent is aware of your intention it will be extremely difficult for you to successfully apply the technique. In such a case you may be obliged to use a cavity strike Qin Na instead of a grabbing technique.

It is usually much easier to strike the opponent than to control him. Subduing an opponent through a Qin Na controlling technique is a way to show mercy to someone you do not want to injure. To successfully apply a grabbing Qin Na, you often need to fake or strike the opponent first to set him up for your controlling technique. For example, you can use a punch to cause your opponent to block, and when he blocks, you quickly grab his hand and use Qin Na to control him. Alternatively, you might kick his shin first to draw his attention to his leg, and immediately grab his hand and control him.

As mentioned, there are five categories of Qin Na: 1. Fen Jin or Zhua Jin (dividing the muscle/tendon or grabbing the muscle/tendon). 2. Cuo Gu (misplacing the bone). 3. Bi Qi (sealing the breath). 4. Dian Mai or Duan Mai (vein/artery press or sealing the vein/artery). 5. Dian Mai or Dian Xue (pressing primary Qi channel or cavity press). This book will discuss all of these categories in detail except the last two, which will be discussed only on an introductory level, because they require an in-depth understanding of Qi circulation, acupuncture, and specialized training techniques.

One additional point needs to be mentioned here. Very often Qin Na techniques make use of principles from several categories at once. For example, many techniques simultaneously use the principles of dividing the muscle/tendon and misplacing the bone.

1. Fen Jin or Zhua Jin 分筋 ，抓筋

(dividing the muscle/tendon or grabbing the muscle/tendon):

Fen in Chinese means to divide, Zhua means to grab and Jin means tendon, sinew, or muscle. Fen Jin or Zhua Jin Qin Na refer to techniques which tear apart the opponent's muscles or tendons. Muscles contain nerves and many Qi branch channels, so when you tear a muscle or tendon, not only do you cause sensations of pain to travel to the brain, you also directly or indirectly affect the Qi and interfere with the normal functioning of the organs. If the pain is great enough, it can disturb the Qi and seriously damage the organs, and in extreme cases even cause death. For this reason, when you are in extreme pain your brain may "give the order" for you to pass out. Once you are unconscious, the Qi circulation will significantly decrease, which will limit damage to the organs and perhaps save your life.

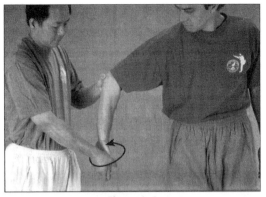

Figure 1-1

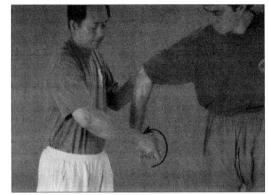

Figure 1-2

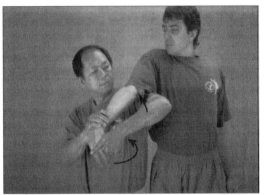

Figure 1-3

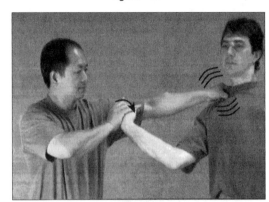

Figure 1-4

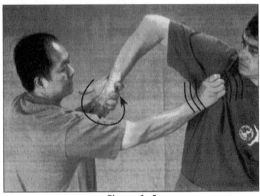

Figure 1-5

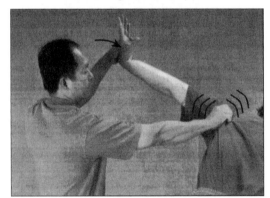

Figure 1-6

Fen Jin Qin Na uses two main ways to divide the muscle/tendon. One way is to **twist** the opponent's joint and then **bend** (Figures 1-1 and 1-2). Twisting the joint also twists the muscles/tendons. If you bend the joint at the same time, you can tear the tendons off the bone. The other method is to split and tear the muscle/tendon apart without twisting. The most common place to do this is the fingers (Figure 1-3).

Zhua Jin (grabbing the muscle/tendon) relies upon the strength of the fingers to grab, press, and then pull the opponent's large muscles or tendons. This causes pain by overextending the muscles and tendons. Common targets for Zhua Jin Qin Na are the tendon on the shoulder (Figure 1-4), under the armpit (Figures 1-5 and 1-6), on the neck (Figure 1-7),

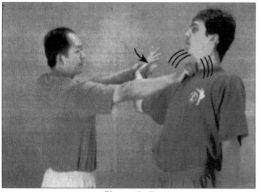

Figure 1–7

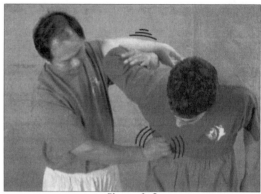

Figure 1–8

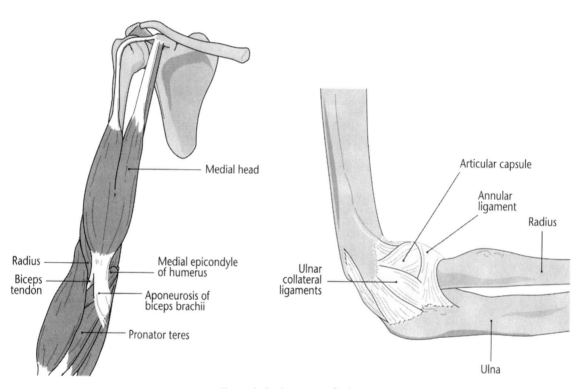

Figure 1–9. Structure of Joint

and on the sides of the waist (Figure 1-8). Zhua Jin Qin Na is used particularly by the Eagle Claw and Tiger Claw styles. Although Zhua Jin is usually classified with Fen Jin Qin Na, many Chinese martial artists separate the two categories because the principle used to divide the muscle/tendon is different.

2. Cao Gu (misplacing the bone): 错骨

Cao means wrong, disorder, or to place wrongly, and Gu means bone. Cao Gu therefore are Qin Na techniques which put bones in the wrong positions. These techniques are usually applied to the joints. If you examine the structure of a joint, you will see that the

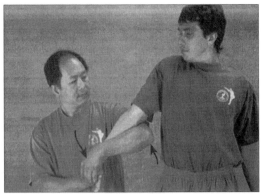

Figure 1–10

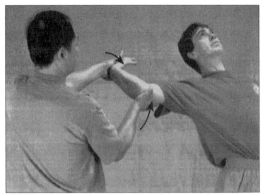

Figure 1–11

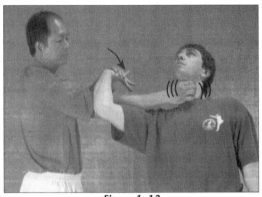

Figure 1–12

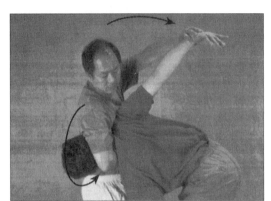

Figure 1–13

bones are connected to each other by ligaments, and that the muscles around and over the joints are connected to the bones by tendons (Figure 1-9). When a joint is bent backward (Figure 1-10) or **twisted** and **bent** in the wrong direction (Figure 1-11), it can cause extreme pain, the ligament can be torn off the bone, and the bones can be pulled apart. Strictly speaking, it is very difficult to use dividing the muscle/tendon and misplacing the bone techniques separately. When one is used, generally the other one is also more or less simultaneously applied.

3. Bi Qi (sealing the breath): 閉氣

Bi in Chinese means to close, seal, or shut, and Qi (more specifically Kong Qi) means air[4]. Bi Qi is the technique of preventing the opponent from inhaling, thereby causing him to pass out. There are three categories of Bi Qi, differing in their approach to sealing.

The first category is the direct sealing of the windpipe. You can grab your opponent's throat with your fingers (Figure 1-12), or compress his throat with your arm, and prevent him from inhaling (Figure 1-13). Alternatively, you can use your fingers to press or strike

---

4. The word "Qi" in Chinese can mean two things, depending on its context. The first meaning is air (Kong Qi) and the second is the energy which circulates in the human body. Unless otherwise noted, "Qi" in this book denotes this second meaning.

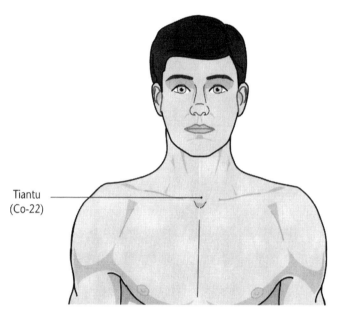

Tiantu
(Co-22)

Figure 1–14. Tiantu Cavity (Co-22)

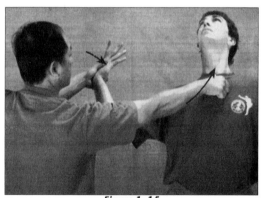

Figure 1–15

the Tiantu cavity (Co-22) on the base of his throat (Figures 1-14 and 1-15) to stop him from inhaling. Attacking this area causes the muscles around the windpipe to contract and close the windpipe.

The second category of Bi Qi is striking the muscles which surround the lungs. Because of the protection which the ribs afford, it is very difficult to strike the muscles around the lungs directly. However, some of these muscles extend beyond the ribs. When they are attacked, they contract in pain and compress the lungs, preventing inhalation. Two muscle groups in the stomach are commonly used in this way (Figure 1-16).

Finally, the last category of sealing the breath is cavity press or nerve ending strike. The principle of this category is very similar to that of the muscle strikes, the only difference being that cavities are struck rather than muscle groups. This category is normally much more difficult both in principle and technique. However, when it is done correctly it is more effective than striking the muscles.

If you take a look at the structure of the chest area, you will see that the lungs are well protected by the ribs, which prevent outside forces from damaging the lungs and other organs. You will notice also that each rib is not a single piece of bone wrapping around your body, but rather two pieces of bone, connected by strong ligaments and cartilage (Figure 1-17). When an outside force strikes the chest, the ribs act like a spring or an elastic ball to bounce the attacking force away or bounce yourself backward in order to protect the lungs and heart. This construction makes it very hard to cause the lungs to com-

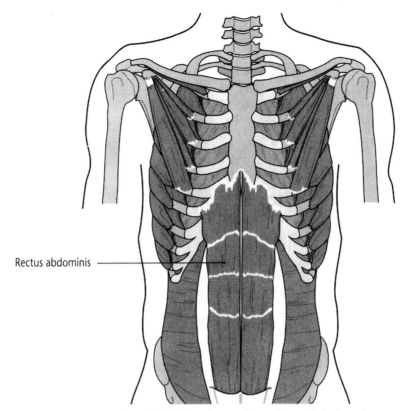

Rectus abdominis

Figure 1–16. Muscles can be used to seal the breath

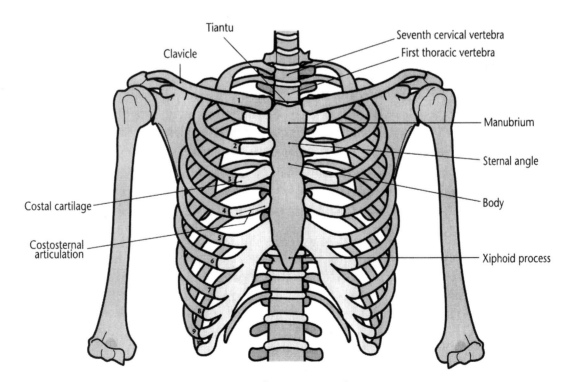

Figure 1–17. Ribs structure on chest area

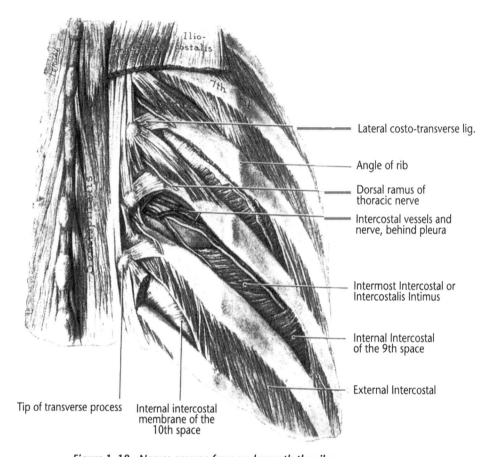

Figure 1–18. Nerves emerge from underneath the ribs

press by striking the chest. You should also understand that the muscles which are out-side the ribs will not compress the lungs when they contract, because the ribs will protect the lungs. Therefore, in order to cause contraction of the lungs you must strike particular acupuncture cavities or the ends of the nerves which emerge from the lung area under-neath the ribs (Figure 1-18). Striking these cavities accurately and at the right depth will affect the Qi in the muscles around the lungs, causing them to contract. Alternatively, you can strike the nerve endings. This causes pain to penetrate the ribs and shock the inter-nal muscles surrounding the lungs into contraction, thus sealing the breath.

4. *Dian Mai or Duan Mai* 點脈 , 斷脈

(vein/artery press or sealing the vein/artery):

Dian Mai is also known as Dim Mak, which is simply the same words spoken in a differ-ent dialect. Dian in Chinese means to point or press with a finger. Mai means Qi channels (Qi Mai), or blood vessels (Xue Mai). Therefore, Dian Mai means to strike or press either the Qi channels or the veins/arteries. When it means to strike or press the vein/artery, it is also called Duan Mai (sealing the vein/artery). Duan means to break, seal, or stop. Sometimes it is also called Tian Xue (blood press), such as when the artery in the temple is struck and ruptured. When Dian Mai means to strike or press the cavities on the Qi channels, it is also called Dian Xue (cavity press). Here, we will discuss Duan Mai and leave the discussion of Dian Xue for later.

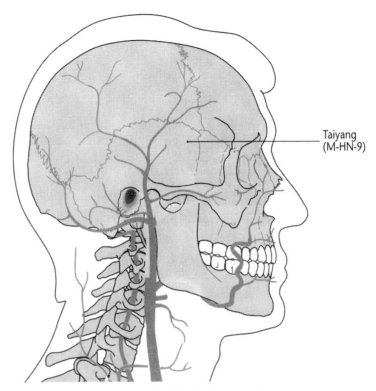

Figure 1-19. Taiyang cavity (M-HN-9) on temple

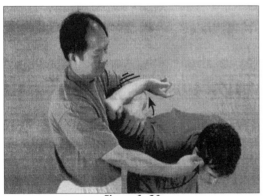

Figure 1-20

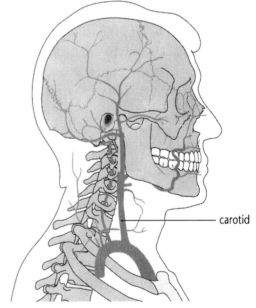

Figure 1-21. Artery (carotid) on the side of the neck

In principle, Duan Mai can be done either by striking or pressing. A striking Duan Mai Qin Na can rupture the blood vessel and stop the blood circulation, which usually causes death. For example, when the temple is struck, the muscles in that area will tighten up and rupture the artery (Figures 1-19 and 1-20). A pressing Duan Mai Qin Na can also stop or seal the blood circulation. For example, sealing the neck artery will stop the blood circulation to your head and thus cut down the oxygen supply to the brain. This will cause

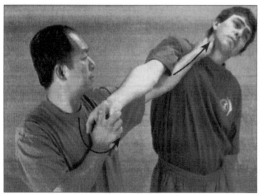

Figure 1–22

unconsciousness or even death. There are two major arteries (carotid), one on either side of your neck, which supply oxygen to your brain (Figure 1-21). When either or both of these are struck or pressed, the flow of blood to the brain can be stopped (Figure 1-22). Sometimes, the muscles on the side of the neck remain tensed. **If you do not know how to revive the victim, he will die from the lack of oxygen. Therefore, you must be careful in using sealing the vein/artery techniques. If you are not absolutely sure how to revive the person, do not use these techniques.**

5. *Dian Mai or Dian Xue* 點脈 ，點 穴
(pressing Qi channel or pressing cavity):

As mentioned, the other type of Dian Mai strikes or presses cavities on Qi channels, and is also called Dian Xue (pressing cavity). Dian means to press with a finger and Xue refers to the acupuncture cavities. The human body has more than 800 Qi cavities, mostly on the paths of the eight vessels and 12 channels. Two of the eight vessels are called the Governing and Conception Vessels (Du Mai and Ren Mai). The Qi in these two vessels circulates in a 24 hour cycle. The other 12 Qi channels are related to the 12 internal organs. The flow of Qi in these 12 channels is also related to the time of the day, with emphasis switching from one channel to the next gradually every 2 hours. Furthermore, these eight vessels and 12 channels also have seasonal and annual cycles. When the Qi circulation in these vessels and channels is stagnant or stopped, the person will sicken or die. Acupuncture is a way to readjust the Qi circulation and cure illness.

Cavity press is a method to disturb or affect the opponent's Qi circulation. There are about 108 cavities which can be struck or pressed to affect the Qi flow. Among these 108 cavities, 36 can cause death and the other 72 can cause numbness or unconsciousness. In order to make a strike effective, you must know the time of the major Qi flow (Zi Wu Liu Zhu) in that channel, the appropriate striking technique, and the depth of the cavity. We will not go into greater detail in this book, both because it is a very complicated subject, and because it can be very dangerous for a person to learn without supervision. In traditional Chinese martial society, a master will usually not pass these secrets on until he feels he can really trust a student. However, some techniques can be taught without too much danger. These cavities will not cause death, and most are attacked through the method called Zhua Xue (grabbing the cavity). If you are interested in some information about Qi flow and its timing, please refer to *"Chi Kung – Health and Martial Arts"* by YMAA.

Before we finish this section, you should understand that in Chinese martial arts you must have Jin to make your techniques effective. Jin is a way of expressing power which makes the power stronger and more penetrating. When Jin is expressed, the muscles and tendons are supported by the Qi in the body, so that the muscles and tendons reach their highest efficiency. Jin can be categorized as hard, soft-hard, or soft. When you apply a Qin Na, regardless of which category it falls into, if you do not know how to use your Jin in the technique your Qin Na will be ineffective. For example, if you do not use Jin in Fen Jin Qin Na, your opponent will have an opportunity to use his muscles to resist your muscles. If you do not use a jerking Jin in Cao Gu Qin Na, you will not be able to break or misplace the opponent's joint. In the same way, in a sealing the breath or cavity press technique, if no Jin is used, the power will not penetrate to the right depth and the technique will be ineffective. For a greater understanding of Jin, refer to the author's book: *Advanced Yang Style Tai Chi Chuan, Vol. 1; Tai Chi Theory and Tai Chi Jing.*

1-3. Different Levels of Qin Na Techniques

As with most Chinese martial arts, Qin Na is comprised of many different levels, according to different criteria or standards. In this section, we would like to define these standards according to several different systems of categorization.

First, the levels of Qin Na techniques can be divided according to how much a person understands the technique and the technical difficulty of the technique executed. The same techniques — based on the same theory and principle — can generate very different results according to an individual's expertise. Normally, this can be judged according to a few common criteria. First, a beginner's power is usually dull and stagnant, and therefore the technique is executed slowly and poorly. When an expert is performing the same technique, his power is soft and gentle, and therefore his technique is fast and effective. Second, a beginner usually cannot catch the correct angle of locking through the **feel** of the contact, while an expert can usually grasp the correct angle instinctively. Usually, this instinct will take many months of diligent practice for each technique, until they become natural and smooth. This is also the reason why a beginner needs to use more muscular, slow power.

Third, when a technique is applied by a beginner, the victim can **feel** the angle as it occurs, but when done by a Qin Na expert, he will feel nothing until he is locked in place. The reason for this is that an expert will use a flowing, circular motion. When this circular motion is used, usually you will not realize you are being locked and therefore your reaction will not be as instinctive and automatic as when someone tries to lock you at an obvious angle. Finally, when a beginner is executing a technique, usually he does not know how to coordinate with his breathing and mind, and therefore the technique is not executed as effectively as would be an expert's. This is like when you use an ax to chop a piece of wood. If you know how to place your mind on the bottom of the wood that you would like to chop, coordinating with your exhalation, you will soon find that you can break the wood much more easily than you would without such mental concentration.

Next, the levels of Qin Na techniques can be very different according to different martial styles. For example, "Small Wrap Hand" wrist Qin Na is one of the most common techniques based on the theory of "Dividing the muscle/tendon." However, because of different understanding and training methods in various martial styles, it can be used to accomplish distinctly different results, and its effectiveness can also vary. Although ostensibly the same technique, some martial styles will execute it with good speed and an accurate locking angle, while others go slowly and remain on the surface. This means that even the same technique can vary in its effectiveness, depending on the styles, the teacher and the student.

Next, the levels of Qin Na techniques can be distinguished according to different Qin Na categories discussed in the previous sections. Generally speaking, the theory and the techniques of the "Dividing Muscle/Tendon" and "Misplacing the Bone" Qin Na techniques are the easiest to learn and apply. "Grabbing the Tendon" Qin Na is harder since it needs more strength, accuracy, and the concentration of the mind to make it work. In some advanced level "Grabbing Tendon" Qin Na, the Qi and the coordination of the breathing are required. "Sealing the Vein/Artery" are the third most difficult to learn techniques. Although some of the "Sealing the Vein/Artery" Qin Na techniques applied to the neck are pretty easy to learn, most of the others are much more difficult, and require special training. Finally, "Pressing cavity" Qin Na is the hardest, since it requires in-depth knowledge about the locations of cavities, the application of specific hand forms and techniques, the time window of vulnerability associated with each cavity, and the depth of penetration required of your power to properly affect the cavity. According to Chinese medicine, Qi circulates in the body's Qi channels, and is affected and significantly influenced by the time of day and the seasons of the year. Furthermore, in order to effectively use even a small number of "pressing cavity" techniques, Jin training is required. Normally, it will take a person more than ten years of vigorous practice to understand these theories and reach the final mastery of "pressing cavity" Qin Na.

Remember, a good Qin Na is not necessarily complicated. Soon, you will realize that the simple techniques are usually faster and easier to apply. Very often, this helps make them more effective than those techniques which look fancy but take a lot of time to apply. The key to judging a good technique is to decided both how **fast** and **effective** the technique is when it is applied. Also, you should remember that almost all of the Qin Na techniques are related to the mutual angle between you and your opponent. When you set up an angle for locking, if your opponent is experienced, he can sense it and remove the angle you have set up. Furthermore, he may mount a counter-attack Qin Na technique to lock you. Therefore, the longer the time you take when you execute a technique, the greater the chance your opponent will be able to escape or even counterattack. When two Qin Na experts are practicing Qin Na, it is continuous, without an end. The reason for this is simply because every Qin Na can be countered, and again every counter Qin Na can be countered. Therefore, if both practitioners are able to **feel** or **sense** the attacks clearly and accurately, either side will be able to change the locking angle to free himself and immediately execute another Qin Na on his opponent. Naturally, to reach this stage, you will need many years of practice and accumulation of experience.

Finally, you should understand that in order to reach an in-depth level of Qin Na, you should follow the training procedures which have been used in the past. First, you should **regulate your body** until all of the physical positions are accurate. This includes the mutual angle for locking, the positioning of your body, and the correct posture for controlling. After you have mastered all of these factors, next, you should **regulate your breathing**. Correct breathing helps to manifest your power to a higher level. You will also need to **regulate your mind**. Remember, your mind leads the Qi (or bioelectricity) to the muscles and tendons to activate them for action. The more your mind can be concentrated, the more Qi can be led, and the more power you can generate. It is said: "Yi arrives, Qi also arrives" (Yi Dao, Qi Yi Dao)[5]. Once you have regulated your body, breathing, mind, and Qi, then you can raise up your spirit of controlling. This will lead you to the final level of perfect technique execution. If you are interested in knowing more about this external and internal training, please refer to *The Root of Chinese Chi Kung*, published by YMAA.

1-4. Qin Na and Health

If a person has never practiced Qin Na before, the painful feeling he or she gets through practice may cause him or her to jump to the conclusion that Qin Na is only for martial arts. In fact, only those people who have practiced Qin Na for some time realize that through practicing Qin Na, they can gain many health benefits, both physical and mental. In this section, let us review some of the health benefits which we are able to gain from practicing Qin Na.

Mental Health:

1. **Increase mental awareness.** The first benefit which a Qin Na practitioner is able to learn is building up the sense of awareness. This begins with an awareness of the wrong angles which can be harmful to the joints, tendons, and muscles. The reason for this is that Qin Na specializes in locking the joints through angles one sets up, affecting especially the tendons and ligaments. Through training, a practitioner will be able to learn the angles which can be harmful to the body. Naturally, he or she will also build up an awareness to avoid the wrong angles which can cause injury to the joints. You should remember that most bodily injury is to the joints, caused by using the wrong angle of force or postures.

2. **Build up mental endurance and establish a strong will.** After only five minutes of practice, every Qin Na beginner will realize that practicing Qin Na is a painful process. This pain is not only from the physical twisting and locking on the joints. It is also from mental struggling. We should understand that our life is painful, and that our minds are always in conflict. According to Chinese philosophy and understanding, a human has two minds, the emotional mind (Xin) and the wisdom mind (Yi). These two minds often conflict with each other. On one hand, the wisdom mind knows what we should or shouldn't do. But on the other had, the emotional mind makes a person always end up on the path to sensory satisfaction. Everybody knows that their wisdom mind is clear and has wise judgment. Unfortunately, we often surrender to our emotional mind, and suppress our wisdom mind.

   One of the main purposes of training Chinese martial arts is to establish a discipline that trains you how to use your wisdom mind to govern your emotional mind. Only

---

5. 意到，氣亦到。

then will you have a strong will. Both physical and mental hardships are necessary to accomplish this goal. When you practice Qin Na, you know both that it will be painful and that you must build up your endurance to deal with this pain in order to learn. As matter of fact, learning Qin Na is just like any other traditional martial art; a method of self-challenge. Through this challenge, you will be able to understand yourself better and more capable of comprehending the meaning of life.

3. **Understand human Qi body.** In order to control your opponents effectively, along with understanding the structure of the human physical body, you should also understand the human Qi body. For example, in order to make Cavity Press Qin Na effective, which uses grabbing, striking or finger pressing to affect the body's Qi circulation, you must have a good understanding of the distribution of Qi in your opponent's body, and the correct depth and timing of your attack.

According to Chinese medicine and Qigong practice, a person has two bodies, the physical body and the Qi body. Western medicine has reached a very high level in understanding the physical body. However, its understanding of the Qi body is still in its infancy. If you are able to understand both your physical body and your Qi body, you will be able to regulate your bodies to a healthier state. If you are interested in understanding more about the Qi body, please refer to the book: *The Root of Chinese Chi Kung* by YMAA.

4. **Train mental balance, stability, center, and root.** According to Chinese medicine and martial arts, in order to have good physical balance, stability, and centering, you must first have mental balance, stability, and centering. You should understand that the mind is the master that governs and controls the actions of your physical body. If your mind is confused and scattered, this will not only affect your decisions, but will also destroy the feeling of your physical balance and center. In addition, when you have firm mental balance, stability, centering, and rooting, you will also be able to build up your spirit of vitality.

One Qin Na training consists of "take down" techniques. In this category of training, you learn how to firm your center and root while at the same time finding your opponent's center and root to destroy them. By understanding the relationship between your own mental state and root, you will better be able to attack your enemy's spirit, and consequently disrupt his physical coordination.

5. **Make friends.** One of the invisible benefits of Qin Na training, like all other sports, is that through practice you can make so many friends. I am amazed at how often I rediscover this benefit. I have traveled to more than twelve countries in the last eight years, and have made thousands of friends. This has made my life more lovely and meaningful.

Physical Health:

1. **Stretching the physical body.** Two of the Qin Na categories are "Misplacing the Bone" and "Dividing the Muscle/Tendon." These two categories specialize in locking the joints through twisting and bending. Unless you are using Qin Na against an enemy, when you practice with your partner, you will usually not twist and bend the ligaments or tendons beyond the limit which can cause injury. Because of this, Qin Na training has become one the best ways to stretch the joints.

According to Chinese medicine and Qigong, the more we stimulate our physical body properly, the more the blood and Qi circulation can be improved. A healthy condition can be improved and strength and endurance can be increased. In fact, this is the basic theory behind Yoga. Through twisting and stretching, the deep places in the joints can be stimulated and strength can be maintained. Like Yoga, from countless practitioners' experience, Qin Na has been proven one of the best methods of stretching of the joints.

2. **Understanding the structure of the physical body.** In order to make Qin Na effective, you must also know the structure of the joints, and how the muscles and tendons relate to the action or movement of the body. Through practicing Qin Na, you will be able to gain a clearer picture of this structure. Only through understanding this physical structure may you reduce or prevent physical damage or injury to your body.

3. **Learning how to heal yourself.** Truly speaking, it does not matter how carefully both you and your partner pay attention, you will eventually experience some sort of minor injury during the learning process. The reasons for this are, first, you and your partner are excited in learning and are expecting some painful reaction from each other. Understanding this condition, you both may use power which is beyond the limits you can endure. Second, since both you and your partner are beginners, you do not yet have enough experience to see how much power you should apply to each other. This can result in injury. Normally, injury does not occur with experienced practitioners.

Once you have an injury, you will learn how to move it correctly, how to massage it, how to relax it, and how to apply herbs to expedite the healing process.

4. **Firming physical balance, stability, centering, and root.** We have discussed earlier the importance of mental and physical balance, stability, centering, and root, and how they relate to each other. Here, I would like to remind you that through practicing Qin Na, you will be able to coordinate your mental and physical centers smoothly and comfortably.

1-5. About This Book

Before continuing to read this book, you should understand a few important points:

1. Behind every joint-locking Qin Na technique, there is always one or more hidden striking techniques which can be used to injure or kill your opponent. This was necessary, especially in ancient times when guns were not available. It is often in battle, due to the slippage from sweat or the exceptional strength of the opponent, that joint locking Qin Na becomes ineffective. When this happens, you will be forced to injure or kill your opponent instead of mercifully controlling him. In this book, we will include some striking techniques for your reference.

2. In the same fighting situation, there can be many possible available Qin Na techniques and options. Some techniques may be more effective and powerful for some opponents, while others may be easier to apply for some other opponents. Some techniques emphasize speed more than strength, while others may rely easily on physical strength. The most important point is that you should treat all of the techniques as alive, and adapt them wisely and skillfully depending on the situation. That means

that when you apply your techniques, you must consider your size, power, height, and skill. In this book, you will see many of these options.

3. The same technique can be used for different situations. Because of this, in this book, you will see **the same technique used several times on different occasions**. However, you should understand an important fact: though the technique is the same, **due to different fighting situations, the way of setting up the technique can be very different**. Without knowing the trick of setting up a technique, the technique will be useless or ineffective.

4. The most unique part of this book is that Grabbing Tendon, Throwing Down, and some Cavity Press Qin Nas are also included in some of the fighting situations. This will offer you a wider freedom of techniques for your defense.

5. In every Qin Na technique, there are always one or more counter techniques. Again, in every of these counter techniques, there are also one or more counter-counter techniques. That means that if your Qin Na techniques are very skillful and you are able to catch the right timing, you will be able to counter any Qin Na. Since some of the counter attack Qin Na have been discussed in the book: *Analysis of Shaolin Chin Na – Instructor's Manual*, we will not repeat them here.

In order to have a better foundation, other than reading this book, you should also read Analysis of *Shaolin Chin Na – Instructor's Manual*, published by YMAA. This book will help you build up a firm theoretical foundation and classify all of the different techniques. If you are also interested in "pressing cavity" Qin Na, you may obtain the general concepts and applications for some simple techniques from my first book: Shaolin Chin Na.

As mentioned earlier, though this book can offer you theory and pictures, it cannot offer you the continuous movement of the action. With the help of the companion videotape, you will be able to see the action, and this will lead you to a better understanding of how a technique can be executed. Finally, even if you have books and videotapes, if you do not have the correct feeling, you will often miss the key angles and points for effective locking. Participating in Qin Na seminars offered by qualified masters is also highly recommended. From seminars, you can be led on to the right path in just a few days or even a few hours. This could save you a lot of confusion and wondering.

Next, you should always have a humble and appreciative mind. Those who are humble and appreciative will continue to absorb knowledge, while those who become satisfied will become impervious to it. It is said in Chinese society: "Satisfaction loses and humility gains."[6]

In the second chapter, Qin Na techniques against barehand attacks will be introduced. These include Qin Na control against open handed attacks, such as chops and palm strikes, and against the different kinds of fist attacks. In the third chapter, follow up Qin Na techniques - used when your punches are blocked or intercepted - will be discussed. Next, Qin Na techniques against various types of kicks will be reviewed in the fourth chapter.

---

6. 滿招損，謙受益。

In order to offer the reader some idea of how Qin Na can be used to defend against weapons, some techniques against knife attack are covered in Chapter 5. One of the most popular applications of Qin Na is against an opponent's grabbing. Therefore, in the sixth chapter, Qin Na techniques against wrist, forearm, chest, shoulder, and neck grabbing will be summarized. Finally, some offensive Qin Na, which can be used quite effectively by security personnel or police officers, will be introduced in Chapter 7.

Finally, Chinese masters always say: "Practice makes perfect." You should practice, practice, and practice. The only trick to perfecting an art once you understand the basic theories and principles is through constant practice. From practice, your techniques will become ever more skillful, and your understanding will grow ever deeper. Remember, when you practice with a partner you should avoid hurting each other intentionally. Always control your power. A good martial artist should always know how to control his power. Some Qin Na injuries can be permanent. For example, once a ligament is detached from the bones in the joint, the damage will be permanent, and the only way to repair it is through surgery.

▪ Chapter **2** ▪

QIN NA AGAINST

BAREHAND ATTACKS

2-1. Introduction

Among all possible conflicts, the barehand attack is the most basic, and probably the most common. This chapter will focus on those Qin Na techniques which can be used against various forms of barehand attack.

The next section introduces those techniques which can be used against an opponent who is ready to attack you with open hands (i.e. - not made into fists). In section 2-3, some techniques against chopping will be discussed, and in section 2-4, techniques which can be used to counter different palm strikes will be reviewed. Finally, effective Qin Na skills against various fist attacks will be covered in the last section.

2-2. Qin Na Against Open Hand

In Chinese martial arts, there are many styles, such as Baguazhang (Figure 2-1), Xingyiquan (Figure 2-2), Tiger Claw (Figure 2-3), Long Fist (Figure 2-4), or White Crane (Figure 2-5), that specialize in using the palms for attack and defense. Because of this, it is very common that, prior to an attack, the hands of these stylists are opened in a ready position. This presents the opportunity to apply some finger Qin Na techniques. Generally speaking, finger Qin Na techniques against open hands are fast and very effective. Remember though, that if your opponent's fingers are closed, it will be more difficult, if not impossible, to use these techniques.

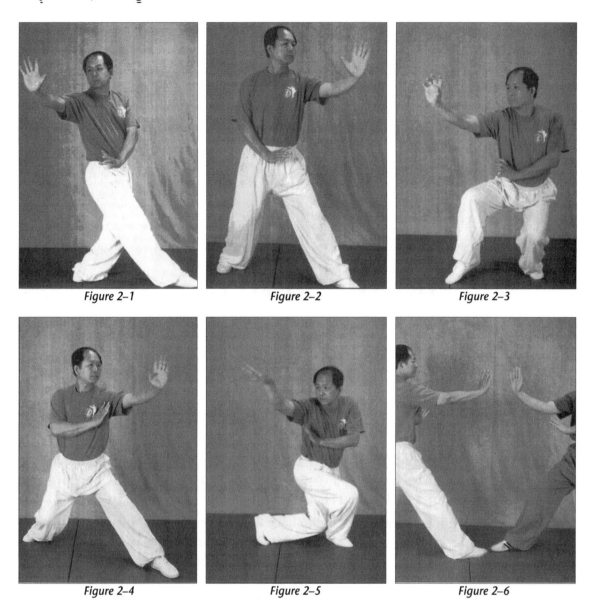

| Figure 2–1 | Figure 2–2 | Figure 2–3 |

| Figure 2–4 | Figure 2–5 | Figure 2–6 |

I. RIGHT HAND AGAINST RIGHT HAND

Technique #1: White Crane Nods Its Head

(Bai He Dian Tou) 白鶴點頭

When your opponent's right hand is extended forward with his palm opened (Figure 2-6), step your left leg beside his right leg while using your right hand to grab his fingers and press downward (Figure 2-7). The angle of pressing is very important. You should press until the back of your palm is bending downward (Figure 2-8). After you have locked your opponent at the correct angle, immediately press downward and then lead (do not pull) him down to the ground, and use your left hand to pull his hair down and control his head (Figure 2-9). In order to make your opponent's entire body lie on the ground, you may lead him straight down and forward first, and then follow with a circular motion. This will destroy his stability. If you have locked your opponent's finger joints at the right

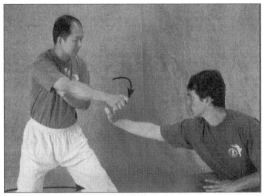
Figure 2–7

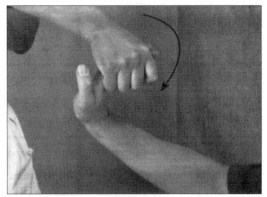
Figure 2–8

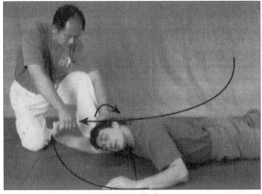
Figure 2–9

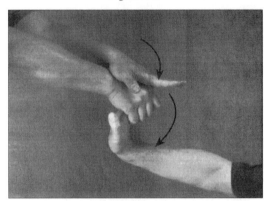
Figure 2–10

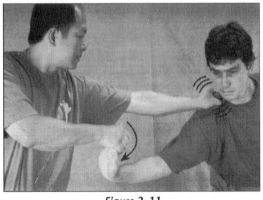
Figure 2–11

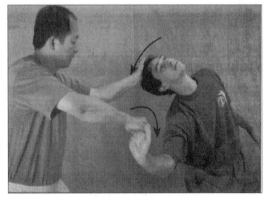
Figure 2–12

angle, you should not need to use much power to lead him down. If your hands are weak, you may use both hands to accomplish the same goal (Figure 2-10).

After you have locked your opponent's right hand, you can also use your left hand to grab and squeeze his shoulder tendon (Figure 2-11). This will prevent his right arm from moving.

In addition, right after your have locked your opponent's right hand, you may immediately use your left hand to grab his hair and pull his head backward to take him down (Figure 2-12). If your opponent's hair is short and hard to grab, use your left hand or forearm to push his throat or neck backward while sweeping his right leg forward with your left leg (Figure 2-13). This will make him fall backward.

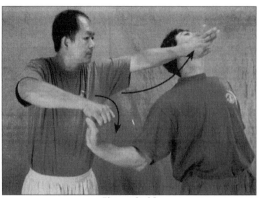

Figure 2–13

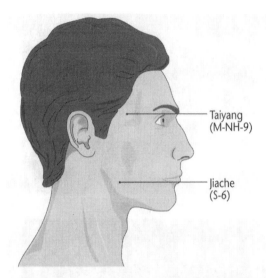

Taiyang
(M-NH-9)

Jiache
(S-6)

Figure 2–14, Taiyang (M-NH-9), Jaicha (S–6)

Finally, if you discover that you cannot control your opponent's right hand effectively, then you should immediately use your left fist to punch his right eye, Taiyang (M-NH-9)(temple), or Jiache (S-6)(jaw) to injure him (Figures 2-14 and 2-15). If your target is the jaw, your opponent may lose consciousness. However, if your target is the temple, you may rupture the artery located in the temple area and thus kill him. Never do such a thing unless it is absolutely necessary.

Theory:

Misplacing the Bone (base of fingers), Grabbing Tendon (shoulder), Taking Down, and Cavity Strike Qin Na. When you grab your opponent's fingers, you may grab all four (except the thumb), three, two, or even one finger. The whole idea is to bend the base joints of the fingers backward until the ligaments are strained or torn off. When this happens, you may cause a significant pain and lock your opponent in place.

Technique #2: White Crane Twists Its Neck

(Bai He Niu Jing) 白 鶴 扭 頸

In terms of action, this technique is very similar to technique #1. However, in theory, it is very different. If your opponent takes the same position with his right palm opened, again first use your right hand to grab his right finger(s). After you have grabbed your opponent's right hand, turn his hand to your right and then bend to lock his pinkie's tendon into position just slightly over his ring finger (Figure 2-16). Finally, press him down to the ground (Figure 2-17). Again, you may use a circular motion to make your opponent's chest touch the ground. After your opponent's elbow reaches the ground, use his elbow for leverage, and increase the twisting and bending pressure against the ground. This will produce significant pain in his pinkie's tendon. When you apply this technique, it is very important that, in order to lock your opponent at a correct angle, **his elbow must always be kept lower than his wrist**. Again, you may use both hands to execute this technique (Figure 2-18). To prevent him from biting you, use your left hand to pull his hair backward (Figure 2-19) or simply push his right jaw away (Figure 2-20).

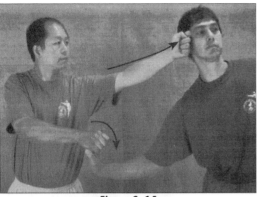

Figure 2–15

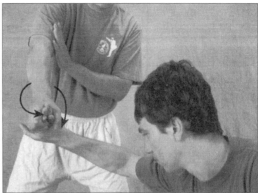

Figure 2–16

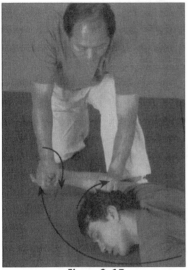

Figure 2–17

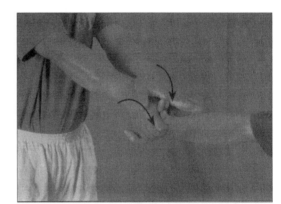

Figure 2–18

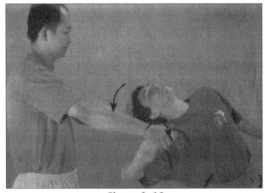

Figure 2–19

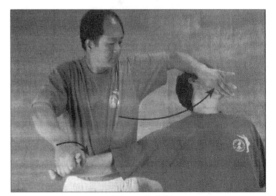

Figure 2–20

Since the control angle and the position where you stand are similar to the previous techniques, you may also apply the same techniques for tendon grabbing, taking down, and cavity striking for this technique.

Theory:

Dividing the Muscle/Tendon (pinkie). After you have grabbed your opponent's fingers and twisted to your right, place his fingers at the correct angle for locking. Right after twisting, if you immediately bend his fingers backward, you will have twisted and bent the pinkie's tendon, resulting in serious pain.

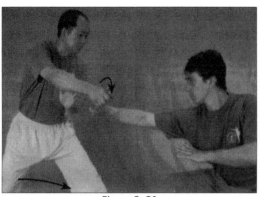

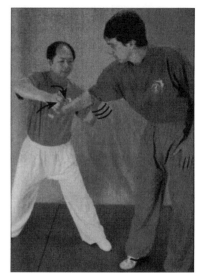

Figure 2–21

Figure 2–22

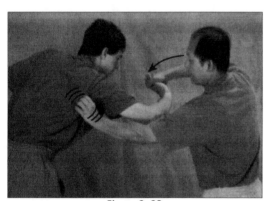

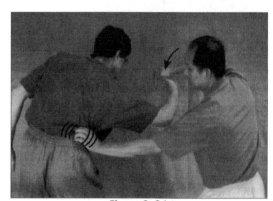

Figure 2–23

Figure 2–24

Technique #3: Lift the Elbow to Break the Wing

(*Tai Zhou Ao Chi*) 抬肘拗翅

If your opponent takes the same position as in the previous technique, with his right palm opened, again first use your right hand to grab his right finger(s). After you have locked your opponent's finger joints on his right hand, turn his hand to your right and lock his pinkie's tendon into position (Figure 2-21). Then, increase the pressure on his pinkie, while using your left hand to generate leverage by lifting the elbow upward and pressing toward his pinkie for controlling (Figure 2-22).

If the distance between you and your opponent is suitable, you may use you left hand to grab the rear tendon under his armpit (Figure 2-23) or the tendon on the sides of his waist (Figure 2-24).

To take him down, you may place your left forearm on his throat area and sweep your left leg forward to make him fall (Figure 2-25). You may also use your left hand to press his *Shaohai* (H-3) cavity or *Quchi* (Li-11) cavity (Figures 2-26 to 2-27) to make his arm numb. In addition, you may use the knuckle of your left index finger to strike the nerves on his side ribs to seal his breath (Figure 2-28). Naturally, you may also use your left leg to kick his right leg to break it or make it bend (Figure 2-29).

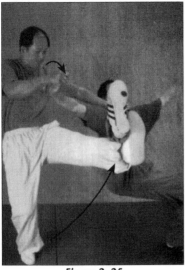

Figure 2–25

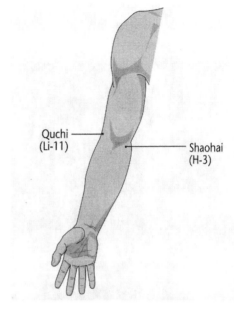

Figure 2–26, Shaohai (H-3) and Quchi (Li-11)

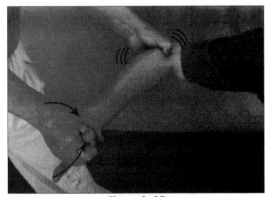

Figure 2–27

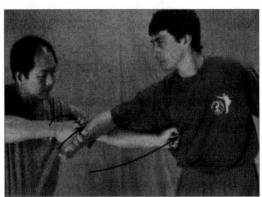

Figure 2–28

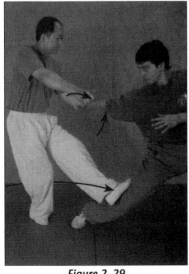

Figure 2–29

Theory:

Dividing the Muscle/Tendon (pinkie). After you have grabbed your opponent's fingers and twisted to your right, you have placed his fingers at the correct angle for locking. You should increase your bending pressure and keep his elbow lower than his wrist. When you lift his elbow up with your left hand, you will generate sufficient leverage for locking.

If you strike the nerves on the side ribs, due to the pain, the internal muscles surrounding the lungs will contract and thus seal the breath.

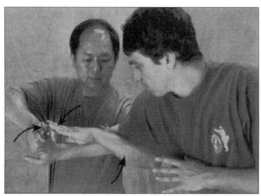

Figure 2–30

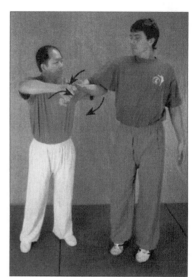

Figure 2–31

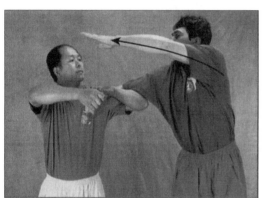

Figure 2–32

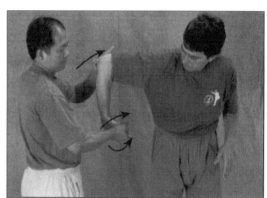

Figure 2–33

Technique #4: White Crane Covers Its Wings

(Bai He Yan Chi) 白鶴掩翅

This is an option for the pinkie tendon lock. After you have grabbed your opponent's fingers, turn them to your right, and bend them backward to lock the pinkie's tendon. Step your left leg behind his right leg and at the same time, use the inside crook of your left elbow to lock and lift up his elbow while using the left hand to help increase the turning and bending pressure of your opponent's pinkie tendon (Figure 2-30). In order to prevent your opponent from kicking you, you should increase the bending pressure until his heels are off the ground (Figure 2-31). When you use this technique, it is very important that you stand beyond the reach of your opponent's left hand (Figure 2-32).

Theory:

Dividing the Muscle/Tendon (pinkie). When you twist and bend your opponent's pinkie downward, his right elbow will automatically move downward in order to release the pressure. At this time, if you use the crook of your left elbow to stop his right elbow going down, you can produce great pain in his pinkie tendon. This pain feels like it is shooting up through your opponent's forearm.

28

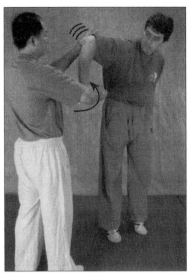

Figure 2–34

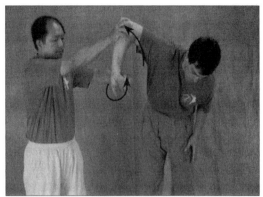

Figure 2–35

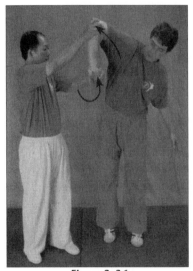

Figure 2–36

Technique #5: Hands Embrace a Guitar

(Shou Bao Pi Pa) 手抱琵琶

If your opponent takes the same position as in the previous technique, with his right palm opened, again first use your right hand to grab his right fingers. After you have locked your opponent's right hand finger joints, twist his hand counterclockwise and lock his pinkie's tendon into position (Figure 2-33). While you are doing this, you also use your left hand to push his right elbow to your right. Finally, increase the pressure on his pinkie while using the left hand to generate leverage for controlling (Figure 2-34). You should adjust your locking angle until his heels are off the ground.

Theory:

Dividing the Muscle/Tendon (pinkie and entire arm). After you grab your opponent's fingers and twist to your right, you have placed his fingers at the correct angle for locking. With the leverage of the left hand, you may generate great pain in his pinkie.

Technique #6: Large Roc Twists Its Wing

(Da Peng Ao Chi) 大鵬拗翅

In the last technique, right after you twist your opponent's hand, you may immediately use your left hand to grab his right fingers and twist them counterclockwise while using your right hand to hold his elbow in position (Figure 2-35). In order to prevent him from hitting you with his left hand, you should move your body to his right side. This will generate great pain and force his heels off the ground (Figure 2-36).

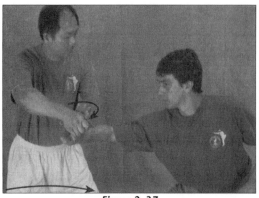
Figure 2–37

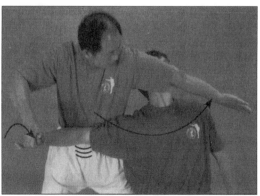
Figure 2–38

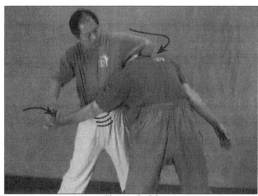
Figure 2–39

Theory:

Dividing the Muscle/Tendon (pinkie). The angle of locking on your opponent's right hand is very important. Only with an accurate angle, may you lock your opponent effectively.

Technique #7: Arm Wraps Around the Dragon's Neck

(Bi Chan Long Jing) 臂纏龍頸

In this technique, again you use your right hand to grab your opponent's right fingers, twist and bend them while also stepping your left leg to his right hand side (Figure 2-37). Next, place his right elbow against your stomach to lock his pinkie tendon, continuously circling your left arm around his neck (Figure 2-38) and finally locking him upward (Figure 2-39). If you increase the circling pressure, you may seal the artery, interrupting the oxygen supply to your opponent's brain and making him pass out. However, you should never do this unless it is absolutely necessary, since this technique is fatal.

Theory:

Dividing the Muscle/Tendon (pinkie), Misplacing the Bone (neck), or Sealing the Artery/Vein (neck). When you place your opponent's elbow on your stomach, you provide good leverage for increasing pressing power against his pinkie tendon. There are two large blood vessels on the sides of the neck, the carotid artery and the jugular vein, which supply blood to the brain. Increasing the pressure on either side of the neck over these blood vessels can starve the brain, causing unconsciousness and death.

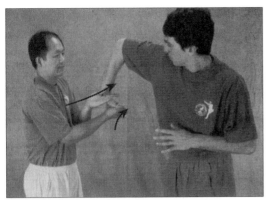

Figure 2–40

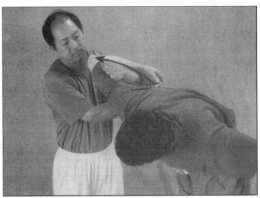

Figure 2–41

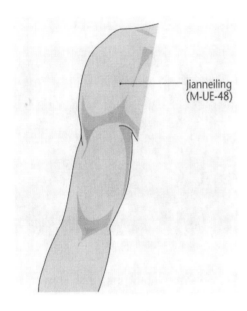

Figure 2–42, Jianneiling (M-UE-48)

Jianneiling
(M-UE-48)

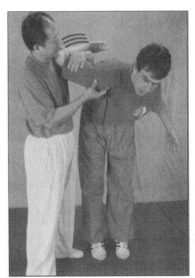

Figure 2–43

Technique #8: Pressing Shoulder with Single Finger and Extending the Neck for Water

(Yi Zhi Ding Jiang and Yin Jing Qiu Shui) 一指頂肩，引頸求水

In this technique, right after you have grabbed and twisted your opponent's hand, immediately push his arm upward and toward his right side (Figure 2-40), while simultaneously coiling your left hand around his elbow area to lock his arm (Figure 2-41). Right after you have locked his arm, lift it up to increase the pain in his shoulder, while using your index finger to press the *Jianneiling* cavity (M-UE-48)(Figures 2-42 and 2-43). This will cause significant pain in the shoulder area. You should increase the pressing pressure on your index finger until your opponent's heels leave the floor. Alternatively, you may use

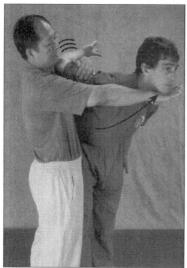

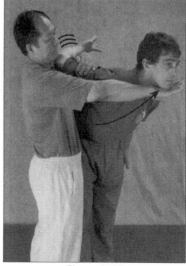

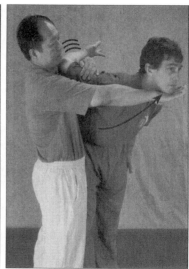

| Figure 2–44 | Figure 2–45 | Figure 2–46 |

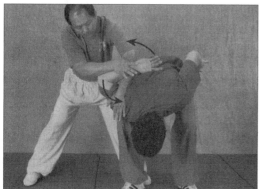

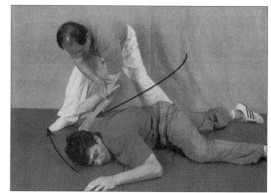

| Figure 2–47 | Figure 2–48 |

your right hand to push his chin upward (Figure 2-44). You may also push his chin to his left and upward (Figure 2-45) or grab his hair and pull it toward you (Figure 2-46). This will also increase the pain.

When your opponent's right arm is locked behind him, you may disable him to prevent further attack. To take him down, you simply press your left hand downward while lifting your left elbow (Figure 2-47). This will generate great pain in his shoulder. While you are doing this, you should also step your right leg backward, circling him down to the ground and locking him there (Figure 2-48).

In addition, since your right hand is free, you may use it to attack anywhere on the front side of his body, such as grabbing the neck tendon (Figure 2-49), front tendon under the armpit (Figure 2-50), throat, groin, or attacking the solar plexus (Figure 2-51). You may even use your right knee to kick his face, while pulling his head down with your right hand (Figure 2-52).

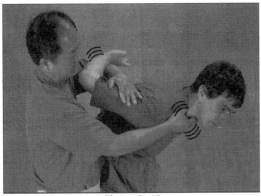

Figure 2–49

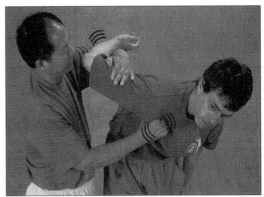

Figure 2–50

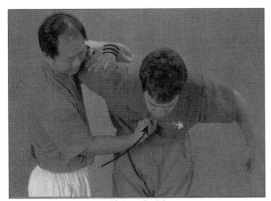

Figure 2–51

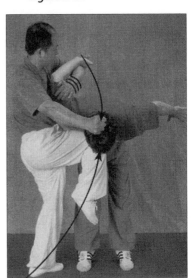

Figure 2–52

Theory:

Misplacing the Bone (shoulder), and Cavity Press (*Jianneiling* cavity). When you use your left arm to lock your opponent's right arm and lift it upward, you have generated a strain on his right shoulder's tendons and ligaments. This action also exposes his *Jianneiling* cavity for your cavity press attack. Without an accurate locking position for the shoulder, the cavity press will not be effective.

Technique #9: White Crane Bores the Bush

(Bai He Chuan Cong) 白鶴穿叢

In this technique, after you have turned your opponent's wrist and locked his pinkie's tendon, step your right leg beside his right leg and place your left hand on his right elbow (Figure 2-53). With the help of your left hand, you are now able to lock your opponent's entire right arm behind his back by controlling his right hand pinkie (Figure 2-54). In order to control his pinkie effectively, you should increase the pressure toward the pinkie side

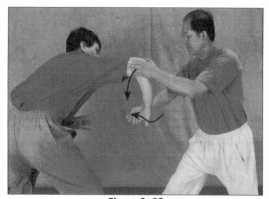

Figure 2–53

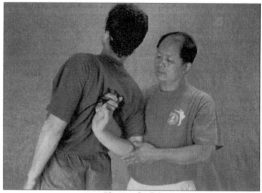

Figure 2–54

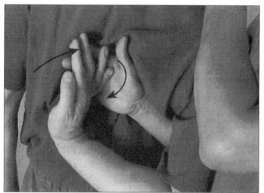

Figure 2–55

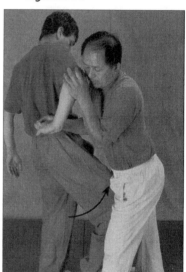

Figure 2–56

(Figure 2-55). It is very important to know that when you step in to lock his right arm behind him, you **should not step in with your left leg** since it will also expose your groin to attack (Figure 2-56). In order to control your opponent more efficiently, you may also use your left hand to pull either his second, middle, or ring fingers backward to increase the pain (Figure 2-57). Alternatively, you may also use your left hand to grab his hair and pull his head down to control him (Figure 2-58) or use your left arm to circle his throat to seal his breath (Figure 2-59).

Theory:

Dividing the Muscle/Tendon (pinkie) and Misplacing the Bone (shoulder). When you step your right leg beside your opponent's right leg, you use your left hand to lock his elbow to provide good leverage for the pinkie tendon lock. Once you have locked him in position with the leverage of your chest and the right hand, you can release your left hand for many other options. Once you have locked your opponent's hand behind his back, if you lift his arm upward, you may also induce tearing in the ligaments of his shoulder.

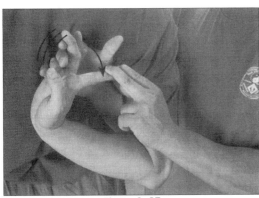

Figure 2–57

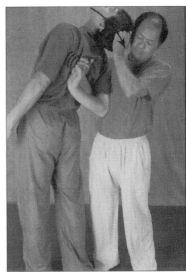

Figure 2–58

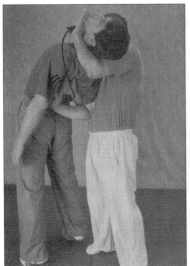

Figure 2–59

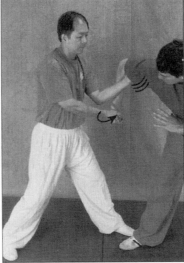

Figure 2–60

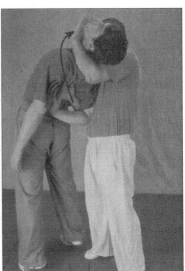

Figure 2–61

Technique #10: Large Python Turns Its Body

(Da Mang Fan Shen) 大蟒翻身

There is another option for the last technique: after you have locked your opponent's pinkie and right elbow, step your left leg beside his right leg while also coiling your left hand around his right arm (Figure 2-60), followed with the right leg stepping, while turning your body and locking his pinkie and elbow in place (Figure 2-61). In order to set up the correct angle, you should also use your left hand to control your opponent's elbow while you are turning. Right after you have completed your turning, you will be able to press your opponent's wrist and elbow down and lock him on the ground (Figure 2-62).

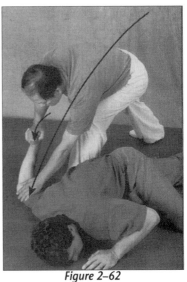

Figure 2–62

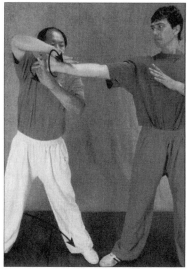

Figure 2–63

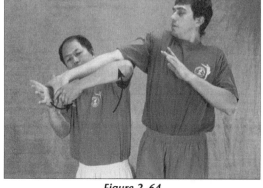

Figure 2–64

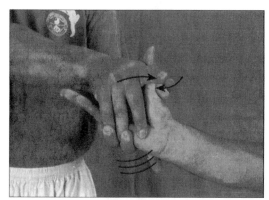

Figure 2–65

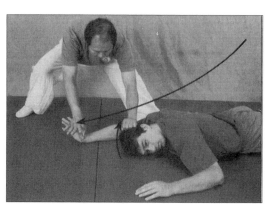

Figure 2–66

Theory:

Dividing the Muscle/Tendon (while turning) and Misplacing the Bone (the base joints of the fingers). First, you use the method of locking the pinkie tendon to immobilize your opponent's action, then continue with your stepping and body's turning. Finally, press his elbow down and increase the twisting pressure on his finger joints. When you apply this technique, you are using the entire body's turning power to twist and lock your opponent's fingers and elbow.

Technique #11: Twist the Snake's Neck with Fingers or Thumb Press

(Zhi Ban She Jing or Mo Zhi Ya) 指扳蛇頸， 姆指壓

First you circle your right hand around his right wrist and use your left hand to grab your opponent's right ring finger and pinkie, while also stepping your left leg to the right side of your opponent (Figure 2-63). Immediately turn your left hand clockwise until his palm faces upward, and at the same time split his ring finger and pinkie away from the other fingers (Figure 2-64). While you are doing this, you should also use your left elbow to lock his right arm upward into position. Next, use your thumb and index finger to lock and generate pressure on the ligaments in your opponent's thumb joint (Figure 2-65). Finally, lead him down to the ground (Figure 2-66).

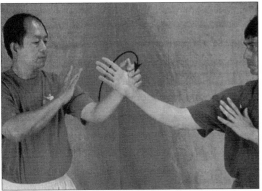

Figure 2–67

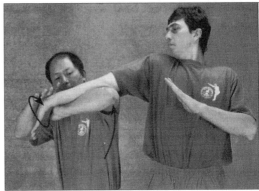

Figure 2–68

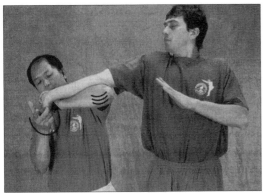

Figure 2–69

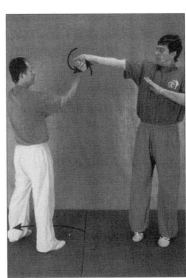

Figure 2–70

When you use your index finger and thumb to control your opponent's thumb, you place your index finger on its second joint, and your thumb on its base joint. Then generate pressure from the leverage of these two fingers. If you do not have enough power with your right hand, you may add your left hand to double the pressure. You should control your opponent until his entire right arm touches the ground. Alternatively, if your right hand is strong enough to lock his thumb alone, you may also use your left hand to grab his hair and pull his head toward you.

Theory:
Misplacing the Bone (thumb), although the leverage of the thumb and the index finger may generate great pressure on the base joint of the thumb and tear the ligament off. To make sure this technique is effective, you should use both hands as much as possible. This will allow you to generate more pressure for locking.

Technique #12: The Hand Locks the Dragon's Tail or Small Finger Hook

(Shou Kou Long Wei or Xiao Zhi Kou) 手扣龍尾， 小指扣

In this technique, first you use your left hand to cover your opponent's right hand and grab his thumb (Figure 2-67). Next, turn his hand until his palm faces upward, while also using your left elbow to lock his arm near the elbow (Figure 2-68). While you are doing this, you should also step to your opponent's right side in order to avoid his left hand's strike. Without hesitation, use your right hand to grab his pinkie (Figure 2-69) and lock him upward until his heels are off the ground (Figure 2-70).

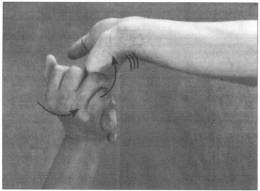

Figure 2–71

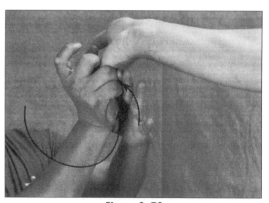

Figure 2–72

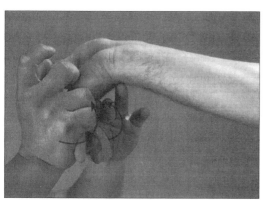

Figure 2–73

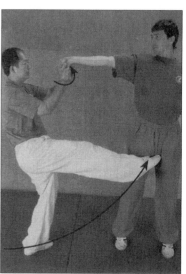

Figure 2–74

When you control your opponent's pinkie, place your ring finger on the pinkie's base joint and bend your wrist, until your index finger is pointing upward (Figure 2-71). If you find that you do not have enough power to lock your opponent upward, you may also use your left index finger to press your right ring finger to double the controlling strength (Figure 2-72). Alternatively, you may also use your left hand to bend any of his other fingers down to secure the lock (Figure 2-73).

When you are locking your opponent, if your opponent's pinkie somehow slips away, immediately use your right leg to kick his groin (Figure 2-74).

Theory:

Misplacing the Bone (pinkie). From the leverage of your hooking the wrist, you will be able to lock the base joint of your opponent's pinkie and produce great pain. If you continue to increase the pressure, the joint can pop out.

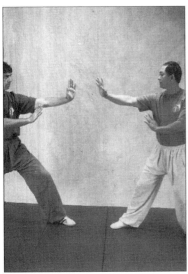
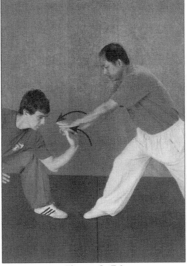
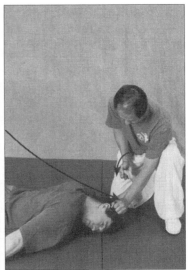

| Figure 2–75 | Figure 2–76 | Figure 2–77 |

II. RIGHT HAND AGAINST LEFT HAND

In this sub-section, we will discuss some Qin Na techniques which can be used when your opponent extends his left hand out with palm opened, while you use your right hand to control him.

Technique #1: White Crane Nods Its Head

(Bai He Dian Tou) 白鶴點頭

When your opponent's left hand is extended forward with his palm opened (Figure 2-75), use your right hand to grab his fingers and press downward (Figure 2-76). In order to grab his fingers easily and with the proper angle, you should circle your right hand to your left and then directly forward to his fingers. In addition, the angle of pressing is very important. To help the control, you may again use your left hand to press his fingers backward. You should press until the back of your palm is bending downward. After you have locked your opponent at the correct angle, immediately press downward and lead (do not pull) your opponent down to the ground (Figure 2-77). If you have locked your opponent's finger joints at the right angle, you should not need too much power to lead him down. If your hands are much smaller than his, simply grab only his ring finger and pinkie to do the job.

Theory:

Misplacing the Bone (base of the fingers). When you grab your opponent's fingers, you may grab all four (except the thumb), three, two, or even one finger. The whole idea is to bend the base joints of the fingers backward until the ligaments are strained or torn off. When this happens, you may cause significant pain and lock your opponent in place.

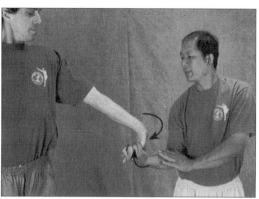

Figure 2–78

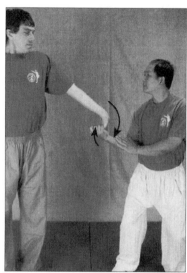

Figure 2–79

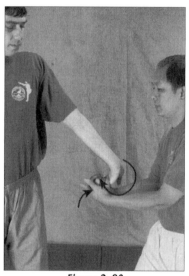

Figure 2–80

Technique #2: Rotating the Sky Post

(Niu Zhuan Tian Zhu) 扭轉天柱

Once you have grabbed your opponent's left hand with your right hand, immediately rotate his left hand clockwise until his palm faces upward (Figure 2-78). Next, bend your wrist to increase the pressure on your opponent's fingers and lock him upward (Figure 2-79). To make the control more effective and increase the pain in your opponent's fingers, you may also use your left hand to push your opponent's left fingers upward (Figure 2-80). You should continue to increase your pressure until his heels are off the ground.

Theory:

Misplacing the Bone (base of the fingers). When you grab your opponent's fingers, you may grab all four fingers (excepting the thumb), three, two, or even one finger. The whole idea is to bend the base joints of the fingers backward until the ligaments are strained or torn off. When this happens, you cause excruciating pain and lock your opponent in place.

Technique #3: White Crane Covers Its Wings

(Bai He Yan Chi) 白鶴掩翅

For this technique, first grab your opponent's left fingers, turn them to your right, and bend them backward to lock the tendons of the index finger. At the same time, step your left leg beside his left leg (Figure 2-81). Next, move your left arm under his right elbow and reach his index finger (Figure 2-82). Finally, press his index finger downward to generate

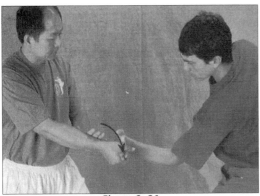

Figure 2–81

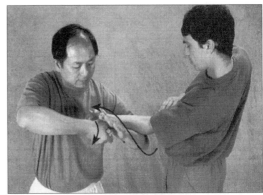

Figure 2–82

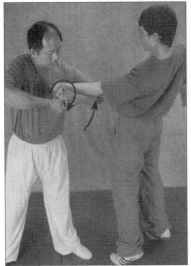

Figure 2–83

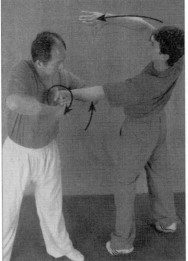

Figure 2–84

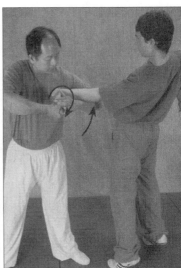

Figure 2–85

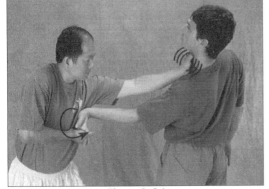

Figure 2–86

pain and lock him upward (Figure 2-83). When you use this technique, it is very important to stand beyond the reach of your opponent's right hand (Figure 2-84).

You may sweep your left leg backward against your opponent's left leg to make him fall (Figure 2-85). Alternatively, you may use your left hand to grab his throat (Figure 2-86).

Theory:

Dividing the Muscle/Tendon (index finger) and Misplacing the Bone (elbow and index finger). The index finger is usually stronger than the pinkie. Therefore, in order to generate pain, the angle of control must be accurate.

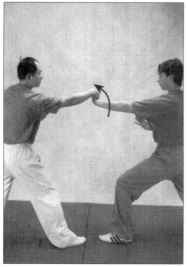

Figure 2–87

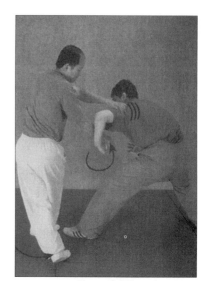

Figure 2–88

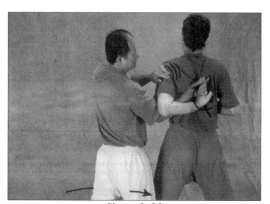

Figure 2–89

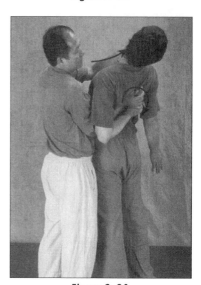

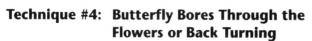

Technique #4: Butterfly Bores Through the Flowers or Back Turning

Figure 2–90

(Hu Die Chuan Hua or Fan Bei Zhuan) 蝴蝶穿花，反背轉

In this technique, first use your right hand to cover your opponent's left fingers and grab them (Figure 2-87). Next, rotate your grabbing hand downward and then behind his back, while stepping your left leg behind your right leg (Figure 2-88). While you are doing this, also use your left hand to hold his left upper-arm to prevent him from stepping backward and freeing himself. Finally, step your right leg behind his left leg and lock him up high (Figure 2-89). In order to increase the locking leverage, you may use your left hand to push his chin up and to his right (Figure 2-90). You should **increase your right hand's twisting pressure** on his wrist until his heels leave the ground. You may also use your left hand to grab his hair and pull his head down or to his left (Figure 2-91).

Theory:

Misplacing the Bone (shoulder and the base joint of the left hand). The key to this control is in your right hand's rotation. The more you increase your rotational pressure, the more the pain will increase in your opponent's fingers. In addition, the position of the control should be as high as possible, which also significantly

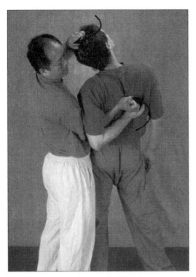

Figure 2–91

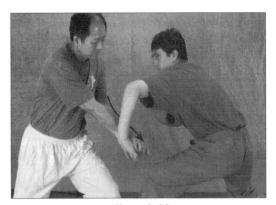

Figure 2–92

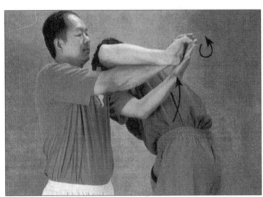

Figure 2–93

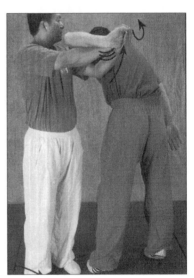

Figure 2–94

increases the pain in his shoulder. When you use your left hand to grab your opponent's hair or to push his head upward, you will destroy his centering sense and put him in a posture from which it is harder to resist you.

Technique #5: White Ape Offers the Fruit

(Bai Yuan Xian Guo) 白猿獻果

Though it looks similar, the control of this technique is different from that of the last one. Once again, when your opponent faces you with his left palm opened, use your right hand to cover and grab his left fingers while stepping your left leg beside his left leg (Figure 2-92). Then, you twist your fingers downward and toward his back, while at the same time stepping your right leg beside your left leg, bringing your feet together (Figure 2-93). While you are doing this, place your left hand against your right hand. Finally, use both hands to lift your opponent's left hand upward and increase the tension on his shoulder joint (Figure 2-94). This will force his heels off the ground. In order to prevent your opponent from turning, you should also press your left shoulder close to his left shoulder.

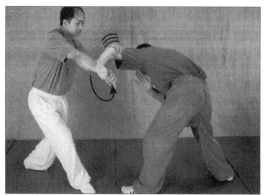

Figure 2–95

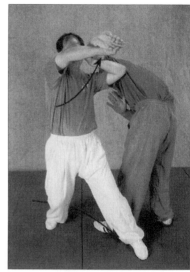

Figure 2–96

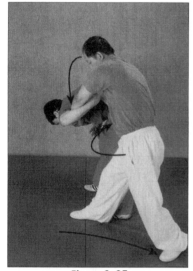

Figure 2–97

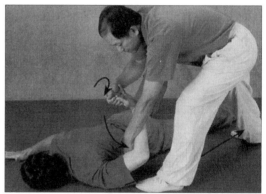

Figure 2–98

Theory:

Misplacing the Bone (shoulder) and Dividing the Muscle/Tendon (wrist). The key to controlling is in your right hand's rotation. The more you increase your rotational pressure, the more the pain will increase in your opponent's fingers. In addition, the distance between your opponent's hand and back should be accurate. **His arm should not be too straight or too bent**. Proper distance makes the technique most effective. Furthermore, the position of the control should be high, which significantly increases the pain in his shoulder. However, if you continue to increase the lifting power, you may pop out your opponent's shoulder joint

Technique #6: Large Python Turns Its Body

(Da Mang Fan Shen) 大蟒翻身

In this technique, first you use your right hand to grab your opponent's left fingers and circle them downward (Figure 2-95). Continue to twist them counterclockwise while stepping your left leg beside your opponent's left leg, and push your left forearm upward against your opponent's elbow (Figure 2-96). Continuing your rotation, use your left hand to push your opponent's left elbow while lifting your right hand (Figure 2-97). In order to prevent your opponent from rolling over and releasing the controlling pressure, right after you have pressed him down, step your right leg backward and use your left hand to pull his elbow toward you, while still twisting his fingers with your right hand to increase the pressure on his hand and lock him in place (Figure 2-98).

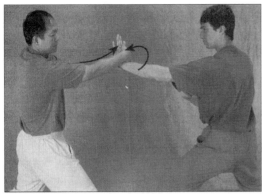

Figure 2–99

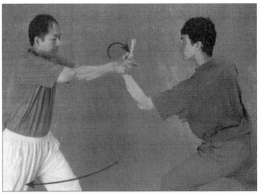

Figure 2–100

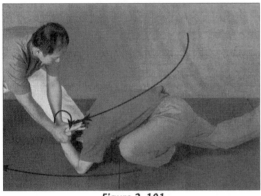

Figure 2–101

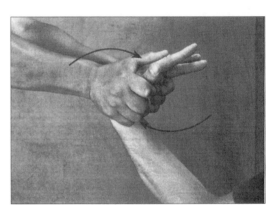

Figure 2–102

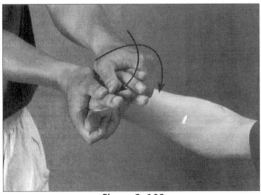

Figure 2–103

Theory:
Dividing the Muscle/Tendon (entire arm, especially the hand). When you turn your body, you should use the entire body's turning power. Right after you press your opponent down to the ground, it is very easy for him to roll forward and free himself from your control. To prevent him from doing so, use your left hand to pull his elbow inward and at the same time twist his hand outward to increase the pain and lock him in place.

Technique #7: White Ape Worships the Buddha or Reverse Wrist Press

(Bai Yuan Bai Fo or Fan Ya Wan) 白猿拜佛，反壓腕

In this technique, you again use your right hand to cover the wrist while your left hand clamps upward to hold your opponent's wrist (Figure 2-99). Rotate your opponent's wrist clockwise until his palm faces upward while stepping your right leg backward (Figure 2-100). Finally, press him down until his left elbow touches the ground (Figure 2-101). The leverage of pressing is generated from the thumb and pinkie of each hand, working together (Figure 2-102). Alternatively, when you control his wrist, you may also twist and bend your opponent's hand clockwise to increase the pressure on his pinkie (Figure 2-103).

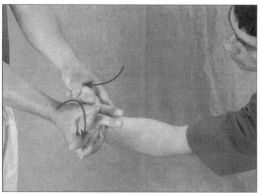

Figure 2–104

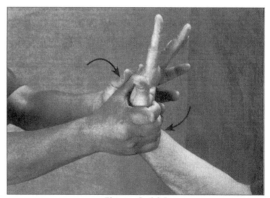

Figure 2–105

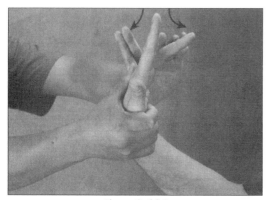

Figure 2–106

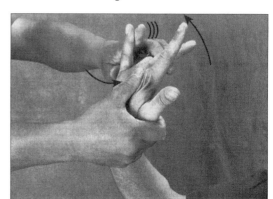

Figure 2–107

In this technique, if your opponent tenses his wrist, it will be very difficult for you to control him. You must then use your left hand to attack his left eye first, to move his attention away from his wrist, then immediately apply the technique.

Theory:
Dividing the Muscle/Tendon (wrist). The key to the control is in using the entire structure of both hands to generate the pressing pressure instead of only using the thumbs.

Technique #8: Fingers Lock the Dragon's Tail or Turning Finger Dividing

(Zhi Suo Long Wei or Zhuan Fen Zhi) 指鎖龍尾 ，轉分指

You will sometimes encounter an opponent who is double jointed, which makes the previous technique ineffective. In this case, right after you have twisted and bent his wrist, immediately use your left thumb to press his left pinkie backward to control him (Figure 2-104).

Alternatively, right after you have twisted and bent his wrist (Figure 2-105), use your left hand to split open your opponent's ring finger and pinkie (Figure 2-106). Then, immediately twist his ring finger and pinkie while using your right hand to pull the base of his thumb backward (Figure 2-107). This will lock him in place.

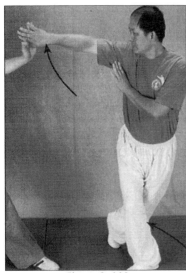
Figure 2–108

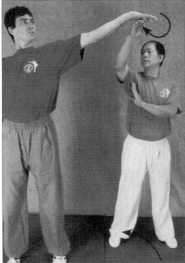
Figure 2–109

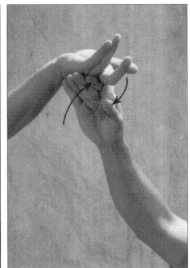
Figure 2–110

Theory:

Dividing the Muscle/Tendon (wrist and pinkie), Misplacing the Bone (pinkie). When you twist and press your opponent's ring finger and pinkie, you use your thumb and index finger to generate leverage to lock his pinkie, while using your other three fingers to hook and pull his ring finger.

Technique #9: Hand Twists the Snake's Neck or Upward Finger Turn

(Shou Niu She Jing or Shang Fen Zhi) 手扭蛇頸，上分指

In this technique, first turn your right palm to the right, so that it faces your opponent's left palm, while stepping your left leg behind your right leg (Figure 2-108). This will set up an easy angle to grab his index finger. Next, use your right hand to grab your opponent's left index finger and twist it clockwise until the palm faces upward, while stepping your right leg again to reposition yourself on his left hand side (Figure 2-109). Finally, use the leverage of your thumb, index and middle fingers to bend your opponent's fingers down and lift his body upward, until his heels are off the ground (Figure 2-110).

Theory:

Misplacing the Bone (base of the index finger). When your right hand approaches your opponent's left hand, move your hand upward under his left hand. This will help you set up a good angle for your grip. In addition, it will also make it harder for your opponent to see your hand coming.

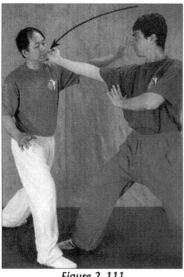
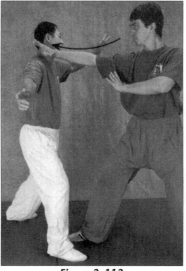
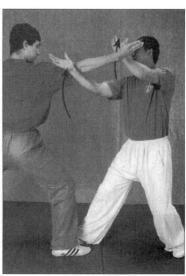

| *Figure 2–111* | *Figure 2–112* | *Figure 2–113* |

2-3. Qin Na Against Chopping

Many martial styles specialize in using the edge of the palm to chop their target. Generally, these types of techniques target the neck area. When some specific areas of the neck are struck, a person can be knocked down and rendered unconscious. In this section, we will introduce some Qin Na techniques which can be used to counter such chops to the neck.

Here you should understand that, when your opponent is chopping you, his hand is opened. Because of this, many of the previously introduced Qin Na techniques against opened hands can easily be applied. In this section, we will not repeat all of these techniques. Instead, we will review some Qin Na techniques which exemplify the intercepting and locking principles that characterize this type of situation.

In order to make the techniques clear, we would like to divide this section into two parts. The first part introduces those techniques which can be used against chopping attacks from the side (Figure 2-111). The second part discusses techniques which can be used against diagonal chopping attacks (Figure 2-112).

I. AGAINST SIDEWAYS CHOPPING

Technique #1: Twist the Wing with Both Hands or Forward Upward Turning

(Shuang Shou Ban Chi or Qian Shang Fan) 雙手扳翅， 前上翻

If your opponent chops the left side of your neck with his right hand, first repel the strike with your left forearm, while placing your right arm under his right elbow (Figure 2-113). Immediately use the back of your right thumb to pull his elbow toward you, while

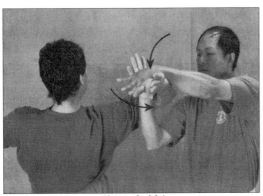

Figure 2–114

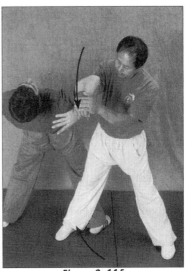

Figure 2–115

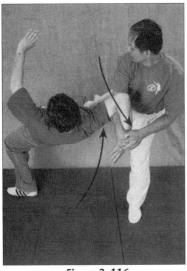

Figure 2–116

pushing your left hand forward (Figure 2-114). Finally, step your right leg behind his right leg, bend his forearm downward and lock your opponent's arm in place (Figure 2-115). You may also use your right leg to sweep your opponent's right leg and make him fall (Figure 2-116). It is very important that you stand on the right side of your opponent's body to avoid his left hand's strike.

Theory:

Misplacing the Bone (elbow). When you apply this technique, your opponent's arm may be stiff; this can make it harder for you to bend his arm. The key to making his arm bend is to use your inner wrist area (thumb side) to hook downward while pushing your left arm upward. This will provide you with good leverage to bend his arm. In this technique, if you jerk your power suddenly, you can pop out your opponent's elbow.

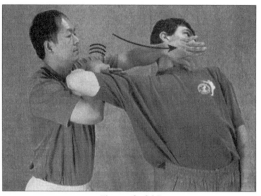

Figure 2–117

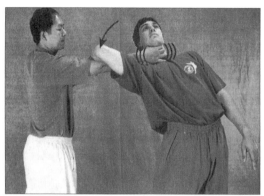

Figure 2–118

Technique #2: Lock the Elbow, Push the Neck and Lock the Elbow, Seal the Throat

(Suo Zhou Tui Jing and Suo Zhou Feng Hou) 鎖 肘 推 頸 ， 鎖 肘 封 喉

In the last technique, right after you have locked your opponent's right arm, use your right hand to hold his right wrist and press it downward, while using your left hand to push his chin to his left (Figure 2-117). This will produce significant pain and lock him upward until his heels are off the ground.

Alternatively, you may let your left hand take over the lock and free you right hand to grab your opponent's throat (Figure 2-118).

Theory:
Misplacing the Bone (elbow), Dividing the Muscle/Tendon (shoulder and neck) and Seal the Breath (throat).

Technique #3: White Tiger Turns Its Head or Upward Elbow Wrap

(Bai Hu Fan Shou or Shang Chan Zhou) 白 虎 返 首 ， 上 纏 肘

In this technique, instead of repelling the chopping with the left forearm, use your left forearm near the wrist area to cover the chop, while stepping your right leg back to avoid it (Figure 2-119). When you cover the chop, also use your right hand to clamp upward to control your opponent's wrist. Next, twist your opponent's wrist counterclockwise with your left hand, while circling your right arm around his right arm (Figure 2-120). Continue circling your right arm until his right arm is locked in place (Figure 2-121). Your body should be behind your opponent's.

Theory:
Dividing the Muscle/Tendon (wrist) and Misplacing the Bone (elbow). When you rotate your arms to lock your opponent, you should use your entire body to direct the motion. Your rotational power can then be strong. In order to generate pain, the leverage generated from your left hand's twisting and right hand's lifting is very important (Figure 2-122).

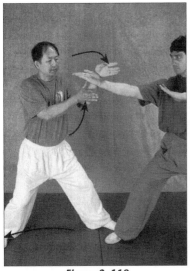

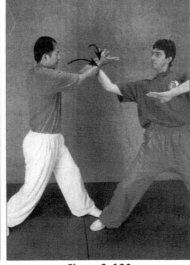

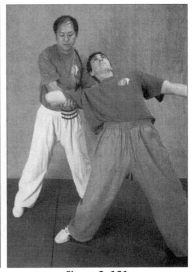

Figure 2–119

Figure 2–120

Figure 2–121

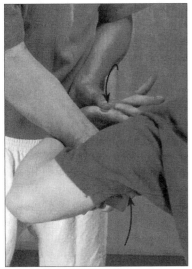

Figure 2–122

Technique #4: Fingers Lock the Dragon's Tail or Turning Finger Dividing

(Zhi Suo Long Wei or Zhuan Fen Zhi)
指鎖龍尾，轉分指

In this technique, use your left forearm to cover the chop, while stepping your right leg back to avoid it (Figure 2-123). As you cover the chop, also use your right hand to clamp upward to grab your opponent's wrist and hand. Next, immediately rotate both your hands counterclockwise until your opponent's right palm faces upward (Figure 2-124). Bend your opponent's fingers toward him, and at the same time use your right thumb and index finger to separate his ring finger and pinkie (Figure 2-125). Then, use your thumb to press the base joint of his pinkie while pulling back his ring finger to generate pain (Figure 2-126). Your left hand should continue to grab your opponent's thumb area, pulling it backward to generate good leverage for your right hand control. You should control him by leading him down to the ground (Figure 2-127).

Theory:

Dividing the Muscle/Tendon (wrist) and Misplacing the Bone (pinkie base joint). The pain in your opponent's pinkie is generated from the twisting power of your index finger and thumb, while the other three fingers lock your opponent's ring finger. With good coordination, you can generate extreme pain in your opponent.

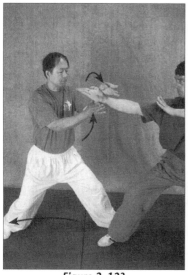

Figure 2–123

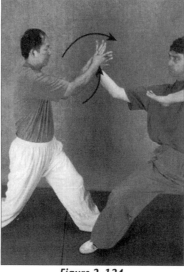

Figure 2–124

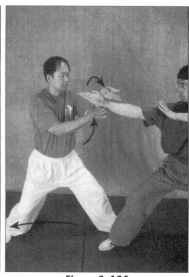

Figure 2–125

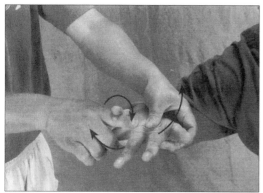

Figure 2–126

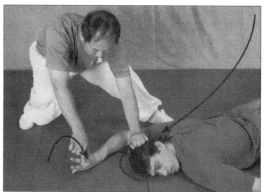

Figure 2–127

Technique #5: The Old Man Carries the Fish on His Back

(Lao Han Bei Yu) 老漢背魚

In the previous technique, after you have covered and clamped the chop (Figure 2-128), immediately turn your body to your right (Figure 2-129) and bow forward to generate pressure on your opponent's elbow and shoulder joints (Figure 2-130). If you increase your controlling pressure or jerk your locking arms, you may rip his shoulder out of the socket.

In this technique, if you continue your turning while moving your opponent's arm to your right shoulder (Figure 2-131), you may use your right leg to sweep backward and to your opponent's right leg to take him down (Figure 2-132). In addition, while you are locking your opponent behind your back, you may free your right hand and use your right elbow to strike his back (Figure 2-133).

Theory:

Misplacing the Bone (shoulder and elbow). The angle at which you control your opponent's arm is very important. If you opponent's arm is either too straight or too bent, the control will not be effective. With an accurate angle, you may generate great pain in your opponent's shoulder (Figure 2-134).

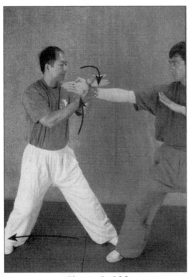

Figure 2–128

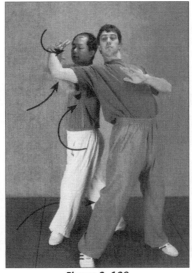

Figure 2–129

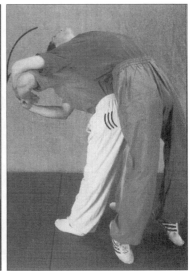

Figure 2–130

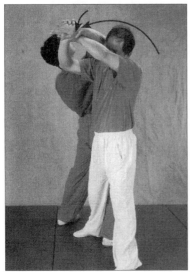

Figure 2–131

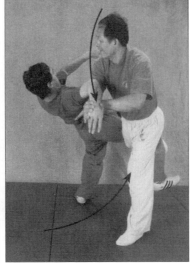

Figure 2–132

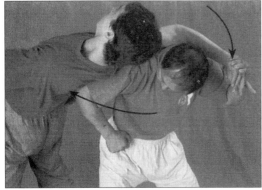

Figure 2–133

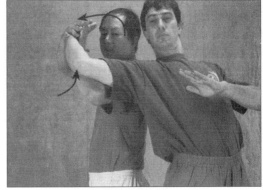

Figure 2–134

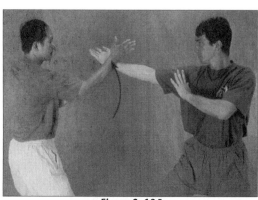

Figure 2-135

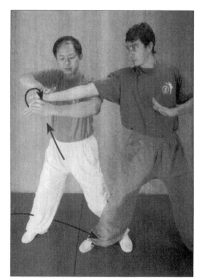

Figure 2-136

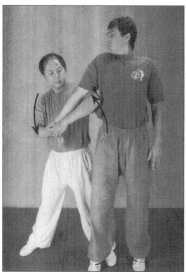

Figure 2-137

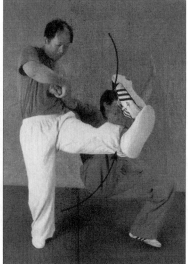

Figure 2-138

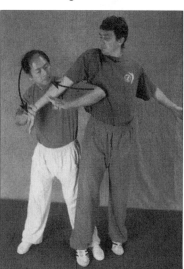

Figure 2-139

Technique #6: Hands Prop a Large Beam or Prop Up Elbow

(Shou Ban Da Liang or Shang Jia Zhou) 手扳大樑，上架肘

When your opponent chops you with his right hand, you may also use your right forearm to intercept by covering (Figure 2-135). While you are doing this, you should step your left leg backward. Immediately after your right hand has covered the chop, step your left leg behind his right leg, place your left elbow against his elbow, circle your right hand to the outside of his arm and grab his wrist while your left hand is grabbing his right fingers (Figure 2-136). Finally, with the leverage of the right hand and the left elbow, lock your opponent's right arm (Figure 2-137). You should continue exerting the locking pressure until your opponent's heels are off the ground.

To take your opponent down, simply sweep your left leg forward to your opponent's right leg while pushing your left hand backward against his chest (Figure 2-138). You may also use your left elbow to strike the nerves on the side of his rib cage to seal his breath (Figure 2-139).

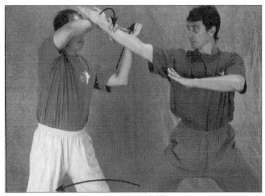

Figure 2–140

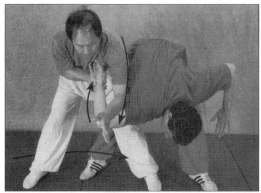

Figure 2–141

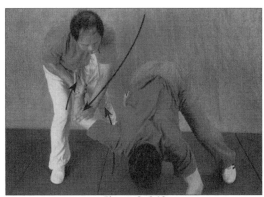

Figure 2–142

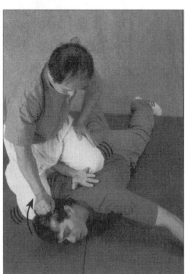

Figure 2–143

Theory:

Misplacing the Bone (elbow). Your right hand's interception of the chop is very important. With the correct angle of interception, you are able to lead your opponent's chopping energy into your locking position without difficulty.

Technique #7: Luo Han Bows or Small Elbow Wrap

(Luo Han Xing Li or Xiao Chan Zhou) 羅漢行禮 ， 小纏肘

In this technique, first use your right arm to repel the chop, and grab his wrist while stepping your right leg backward (Figure 2-140). While you are doing this, also press your left forearm upward against your opponent's right elbow. Next, step your left leg to the front of his right leg while circling your left hand down, and lift up your right hand (Figure 2-141). Finally, pull your opponent's right arm toward the front of your body to destroy his stability, while bowing and sweeping your left leg backward to make him fall (Figure 2-142). When your opponent is on the ground, lock his arm behind his back. Using both of your legs, you will be able to lock him there firmly (Figure 2-143).

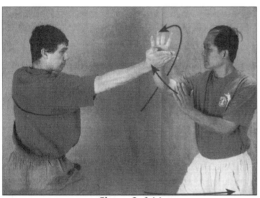
Figure 2–144

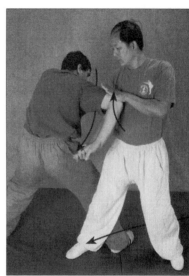
Figure 2–145

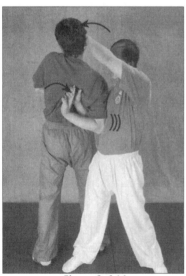
Figure 2–146

Theory:

Misplacing the Bone (elbow and shoulder). Your right hand's interception of your opponent's chop and the left hand's upward pressing on his elbow are very important. Without proper intercepting, it will be extremely difficult to grab your opponent's forearm. In order to make your opponent fall, after you have locked him, you should **pull him to your front to destroy his balance**, while sweeping your left leg backward. Once your opponent is on the ground, if necessary, you may rotate his arm toward his head and pop his shoulder out of joint.

Technique #8: White Crane Bores the Bush

(Bai He Chuan Cong) 白鶴穿叢

When your opponent is chopping you, his hand will be opened. Because of this, you will be able to use most of the Qin Na techniques against open hands, which were introduced earlier. Here, we will only review a few of them for your references.

When your opponent chops you with his right hand, first step your left leg back, while using your right hand to grab your opponent's right hand fingers (Figure 2-144). As you do this, you should clamp your left hand upward to grab his right wrist. Immediately step your right leg behind his right leg and circle his hand down, while at the same time pushing his elbow upward (Figure 2-145). Finally, lock his arm behind his back and push his chin away with your left hand (Figure 2-146).

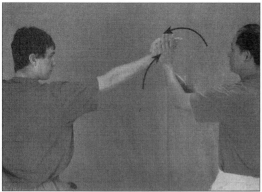

Figure 2–147

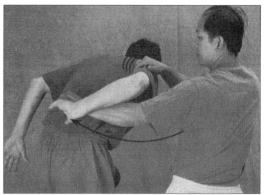

Figure 2–148

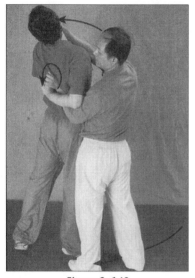

Figure 2–149

Theory:

Misplacing the Bone (base of the fingers). The most important key to successful control is correct interception. Through practice, and using your left hand to assist your right, you should be able to intercept the chopping easily.

Technique #9: Butterfly Bores Through the Flowers or Back Turning

(Hu Die Chuan Hua or Fan Bei Zhuan) 蝴蝶穿花，反背轉

When your opponent chops you with his right hand, first step your right leg backward while using your left hand to cover and grab your opponent's right fingers (Figure 2-147). As you do this, also use your right hand to clamp upward, helping the left hand's grabbing. Immediately step your right leg behind your left leg, circling your left hand down and to his back (Figure 2-148). While you are doing this, also use your right hand to hold his right shoulder - preventing him from stepping backward and escaping. Finally, step your left leg behind your opponent, and lock his arm behind his back (Figure 2-149). To prevent him from attacking you with his left hand, you should use your right hand to push his chin upward.

Theory:

Misplacing the Bone (shoulder and base joints of the fingers). The distance between you and your opponent is very important for the interception. If the proper distance is kept, the technique can be so fast and smooth that you are able to control your opponent with very little effort.

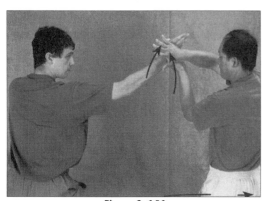

Figure 2–150

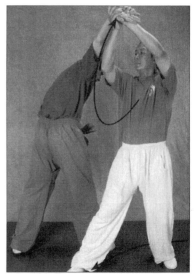

Figure 2–151

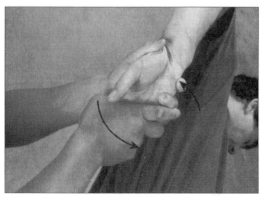

Figure 2–152

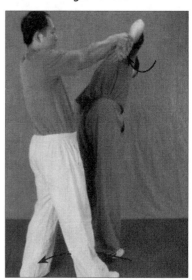

Figure 2–153

Technique #10: Send the Devil to Heaven

(Song Mo Shang Tian) 送魔上天

When your opponent chops the left side of your neck with his right hand, first step your right leg back to avoid it, while also using both your hands to block and grab your opponent's right wrist and hand (Figure 2-150). Immediately step your right leg to his right and use your entire body to rotate and twist his arm (Figure 2-151). Finally, use your left hand to twist his wrist and pinkie, while grabbing his fingers with your right hand and bending them downward (Figure 2-152). You should increase your twisting pressure until your opponent's heels are off the ground (Figure 2-153).

Theory:

Dividing the Muscle/Tendon (wrist) and Misplacing the Bone (shoulder). The trick to making this technique effective is that you execute it while your opponent's mind is still on chopping. Another important point is that, when you have locked your opponent in the final position, you should emphasize the pinkie's twisting, which is both efficient and effective.

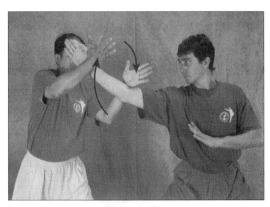

Figure 2–154

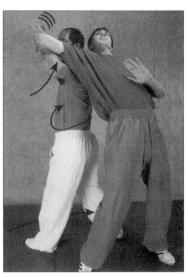

Figure 2–155

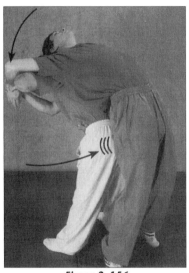

Figure 2–156

II. AGAINST DIAGONAL CHOPPING

Generally, when your opponent applies a diagonal chopping technique, it is because one of your arms is wide opened. This allows the chop to reach you easily. Therefore, if your opponent is chopping your right neck with his right hand, usually your right arm will be opened and consequently, it will be very hard to intercept with your right arm. Because of this, we will only introduce those defensive techniques which use the left hand to intercept.

Technique #1: The Old Man Carries the Fish on His Back

(Lao Han Bei Yu) 老漢背魚

When your opponent uses his right hand to chop your right neck, step your right leg backward while using your left forearm to intercept the chop at his elbow, and use your right hand to clamp upward on his wrist (Figure 2-154). Right after intercepting, use both hands to grab your opponent's wrist, while pressing your left elbow upward against his elbow and turning your body to your right (Figure 2-155). Finally, bow your body forward to lock your opponent's right arm behind your back (Figure 2-156).

Theory:

Misplacing the Bone (shoulder). In order to lock your opponent's shoulder effectively, the angle of locking must be accurate. If his arm is either too straight or too bent when you turn your body and pull, the locking will not be effective.

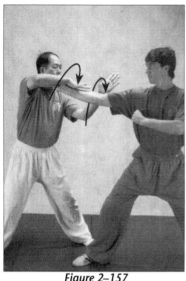
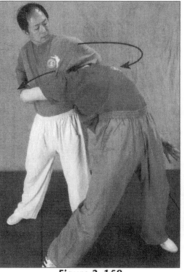
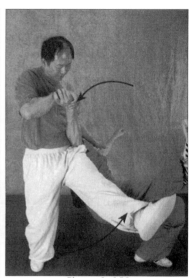

Figure 2–157	*Figure 2–158*	*Figure 2–159*

Technique #2: Arm Wraps Around the Dragon's Neck

(Bi Chan Long Jing) 臂 纏 龍 頸

In the last technique, right after you intercept with both of your hands (Figure 2-157), immediately grab his right wrist with your right hand, while at the same time circling your left arm around his neck to lock it (Figure 2-158). When you are doing this, you should lock his right arm against your chest. In this technique, if you increase the squeezing pressure, you can seal the oxygen supply to your opponent's brain. However, you should not do so unless it is absolutely necessary, since this may cause death. In this technique, if you sweep your opponent's right leg with your left leg, you will make him fall (Figure 2-159).

Theory:
Misplacing the Bone (elbow) and Sealing the Artery (neck). In order to lock your opponent's arm efficiently in front of your chest, his elbow must be bent. To do this, right after your left hand intercepts, use both your hands to bend his arm to press against your chest and immediately follow with the neck lock.

Technique #3: Twist the Wrist and Lock the Neck

(Niu Wan Suo Jing) 扭 腕 鎖 頸

In this technique, use your left hand to cover while using your right hand to clamp your opponent's right hand upward (Figure 2-160). Next, circle his hand to his right (your left), and use your left hand to grab his right fingers, twisting and pressing them downward (Figure 2-161). Finally, while your left hand locks his right wrist and twists it downward, use your right hand to push upward on the back of his neck (Figure 2-162). While you are doing this, you should also step your right leg behind his right leg. This will put him into an awkward position to resist your control (Figure 2-163). You can continue to press with your right arm and press down with your left arm while sweeping your right leg backward to take your opponent down (Figure 2-164).

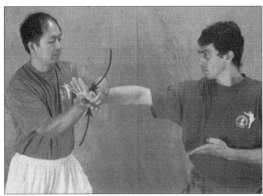

Figure 2–160

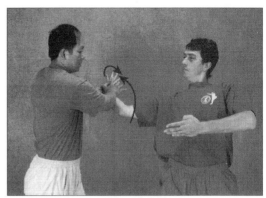

Figure 2–161

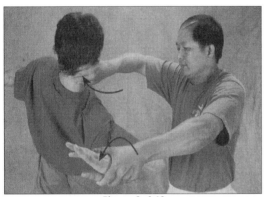

Figure 2–162

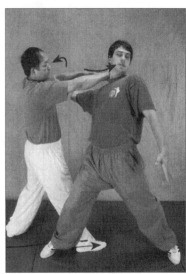

Figure 2–163

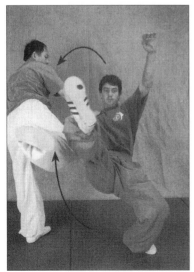

Figure 2–164

Theory:

Dividing the Muscle/Tendon (wrist) and Misplacing the Bone (neck). Stepping your right leg behind his right leg to avoid your opponent's left hand attack is very important. In addition, you should twist his left wrist until his body leans backward. This will stop him from generating any strong resistance or striking power with his left hand.

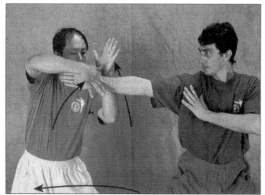

Figure 2–165

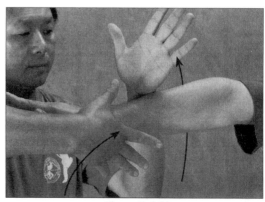

Figure 2–166

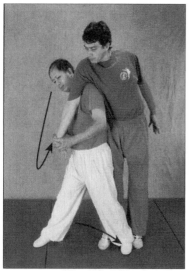

Figure 2–167

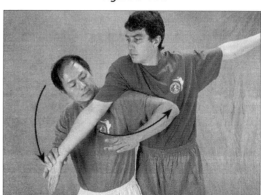

Figure 2–168

Technique #4: One Post to Support the Heavens

(Yi Zhu Ding Tian) 一柱頂天

When your opponent chops you with his right hand, step your right leg backward while using your left forearm near the wrist area to intercept the chop (Figure 2-165). As you are doing this, also clamp your right hand upward to grab his right wrist (Figure 2-166). Next, step your left leg to the front of his right leg while using both hands to grab your opponent's wrist and keep his entire arm straight. Finally, lift his arm upward to increase the pressure on his shoulder (Figure 2-167). You should continue lifting until his heels are off the ground. In addition, you should stand at an angle to his right side, so that it is harder for your opponent's left hand to attack you.

If necessary, you may use your left elbow to strike your opponent's solar plexus (Figure 2-168).

Theory:

Misplacing the Bone (elbow and shoulder). In this technique, you control the elbow to lock your opponent's arm in position and lift the arm upward to tear off the ligaments in the shoulder. Once you have your opponent in this locked position, if you jerk your body forward, you may pop his shoulder out. In addition, in order to increase the pain and lock him better, you may place the back of his upper arm on your shoulder. This will generate great pain on the tendons located in his upper arm.

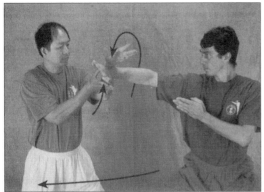

Figure 2–169

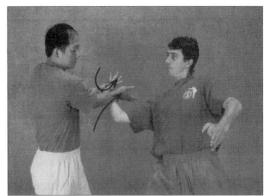

Figure 2–170

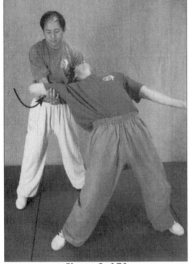

Figure 2–171

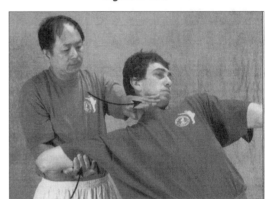

Figure 2–172

Technique #5: White Tiger Turns Its Head or Upward Elbow Wrap

(Bai Hu Fan Shou or Shang Chan Zhou) 白虎返首 ，上纏肘

In this technique, while you intercept with your left hand, you also use your right hand to clamp your opponent's wrist (Figure 2-169). Immediately circle both hands counterclockwise, and step your left leg behind his right leg (Figure 2-170). Finally, use your left hand to grab and twist your opponent's right wrist, while at the same time using your right hand to lift your opponent's elbow (Figure 2-171). With the combined leverage of the left and right hands you will be able to control him effectively as you squeeze both hands in toward one another.

In order to improve the effectiveness of your control, you may use your right arm and the right side of your stomach area to lock his right arm while using your left hand to push his chin away to his left (Figure 2-172).

Theory:

Dividing the Muscle/Tendon (wrist) and Misplacing the Bone (elbow). In order to make the control more effective, your left hand must twist your opponent's hand strongly. With the leverage from the right hand controlling the elbow, the pain generated will be more significant. When you position your right hand, it should be **on the upper-arm and as close as possible to the elbow**. In addition, your right palm should be facing upward. When you circle both of your hands to control, you should use the entire body to generate power.

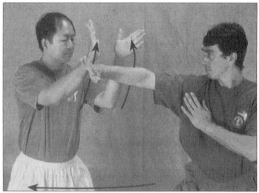

Figure 2–173

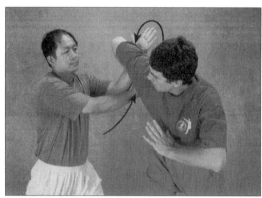

Figure 2–174

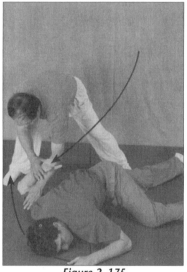

Figure 2–175

Technique #6: Spiritual Dragon Waves Its Tail or Reverse Elbow Wrap

(Shen Long Bai Wei or Fan Chan Zhou)

神龍擺尾，反纏肘

In this technique, you step your right leg backward and intercept your opponent's chop with both of your forearms (Figure 2-173). Next, use your right hand to grab his right wrist and push his arm upward to keep it bent, while at the same time coiling your left hand around his right arm (Figure 2-174). Next, release your right hand while you continue using your left arm to lock his right arm, and step your right leg backward, making a circle as you press him down until his body reaches the ground (Figure 2-175).

Theory:

Misplacing the Bone (shoulder and elbow). When applying this technique, you should keep your opponent's arm bent all the time. If he is able to straighten his arm, he will be able to get out. The trick to keeping his arm bent is to **use your right hand and left upper-arm to help**. Once your opponent is on the ground, if you continue your forward pressure, you may easily pop his shoulder joint out of its socket.

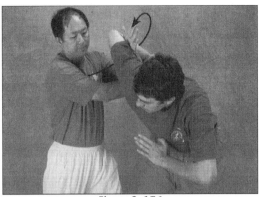

Figure 2–176

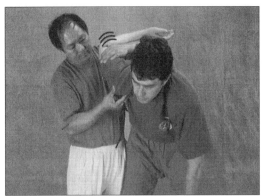

Figure 2–177

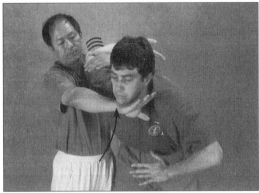

Figure 2–178

Technique #7: Pressing Shoulder with a Single Finger and Extending the Neck for Water

(Yi Zhi Ding Jiang and Yin Jing Qiu Shui) 一指頂肩 ， 引頸求水

In the last technique, when you lock your opponent's arm behind him, all of the tendons and ligaments in his shoulder become very tense (Figure 2-176). At this moment, if you press your index finger into his *Jianneiling* cavity (M-UE-48), you will be able to create tremendous pain in his shoulder area (Figure 2-177). Alternatively, you may use your right hand to push his chin upward (Figure 2-178). This will also increase his pain.

Theory:

Misplacing the Bone (shoulder), and Cavity Press (*Jianneiling* cavity). When you use your left arm to lock your opponent's right arm and lift it upward, you generate a strain in his right shoulder's tendons and ligaments. This action also exposes his *Jianneiling* cavity for your cavity press attack. Without an accurate lock of the shoulder joint, the cavity press will not be effective.

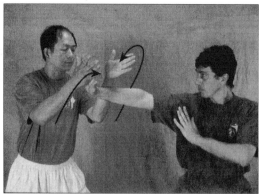

Figure 2–179

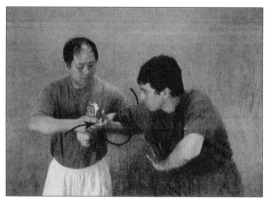

Figure 2–180

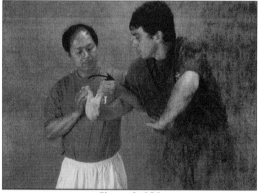

Figure 2–181

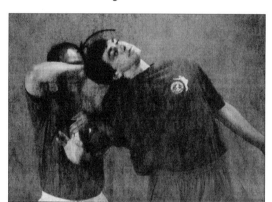

Figure 2–182

Technique #8: The Hand Bends the Pine Branch

(Shou Ban Song Zhi) 手扳松枝

Right after you intercept your opponent's chop with your left forearm, immediately use your right hand to grab all four fingers on his right hand (Figure 2-179). Next, bend his fingers backward while moving your left hand under his right arm (Figure 2-180). Finally, use your left hand to grab and bend his index and middle fingers, or his pinkie backward (Figure 2-181). You should continue your pressure until his heels are off the ground. In order to prevent him from attacking you with his left hand, you should use your right hand to grab his hair and pull it to your right (Figure 2-182).

Theory:

Misplacing the Bone (index finger). In this technique, first you use your right hand to control your opponent's right fingers, then your left hand takes over and locks his index finger. The advantage of this technique is that your opponent is able to walk with you while he is under your control. In a practical situation, if your opponent tries to use his left hand to unlock your left hand control, simply use your right hand to punch his temple or nose. Alternatively, you may increase your pulling on his hair, and this will put him into an awkward position to unlock his index finger.

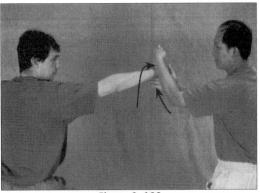

Figure 2-183

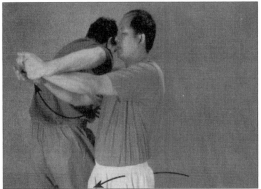

Figure 2-184

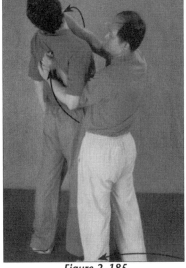

Figure 2-185

Technique #9: Butterfly Bores Through the Flowers or Back Turning

(Hu Die Chuan Hua or Fan Bei Zhuan)

蝴蝶穿花，反背轉

When your opponent chops the right side of your neck with his right hand, again use your left hand to intercept, while also using your right hand to clamp upward and finally grab his right fingers (Figure 2-183). Immediately step your right leg behind his right leg, while circling your left hand down and then behind his back (Figure 2-184). Finally, step your left leg behind his right leg and raise your left hand to lock his arm (Figure 2-185). Again, you should beware of his left hand strike. In order to avoid him from hitting you with his left hand, use your right hand to push his chin upward. This will destroy his center and balance, and prevent him from generating a powerful attack.

Theory:

Misplacing the Bones (shoulder) and Dividing the Muscle/Tendon (fingers). To make the control effective, you should **rotate his fingers as much as possible until his heels are off the ground**. In order to prevent your opponent from attacking you with his left hand, you should re-position yourself to his right side, and keep away from his left hand. If you can also use your right hand to push his chin to his left and upward, you can stop him from further attack. Note that your right knee is in a good position and angle to kick his groin.

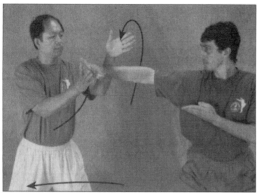

Figure 2–186

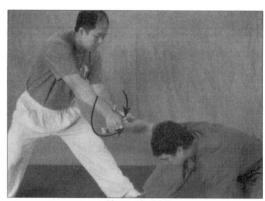

Figure 2–187

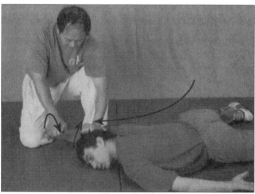

Figure 2–188

Technique #10: White Crane Twists Its Neck

(Bai He Niu Jing) 白鶴扭頸

Once again you use your left hand to intercept your opponent's right hand while clamping upward with your right hand (Figure 2-186). Immediately use your right hand to grab his fingers, twisting and bending to lock his ring finger and pinkie. While you are doing this, step your right leg backward. Finally, press his fingers down to the ground (Figure 2-187). You should continue your pressing until your opponent's elbow touches the ground. In order to improve your control, you may also use your left hand to press downward on your right thumb to increase the power. After you have pressed your opponent down to the ground, use your left hand to grab his hair and pull it backward (Figure 2-188). This will prevent him from biting you.

Theory:
Dividing the Muscle/Tendon (base joint of the pinkie). To make this control effective, the angle of locking is very important. If you keep your opponent's arm either too straight or too bent, the technique will be ineffective. With an accurate angle, your opponent's pinkie tendon can be locked without too much effort. If you find that you are losing your control, you may use your right leg to kick his groin or throat. However, this is very likely to cause the death of your opponent, and you should not do so unless your life is in danger.

2-4. Qin Na Against Palm Strike

There are two common types of Palm Strike. The first strikes forward to the chest or slightly upward to the chin or face. The other presses downward to the abdomen area to seal the breath. In this section, we will focus on Qin Na techniques against these two possible attacks.

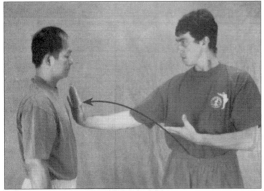

Figure 2-189

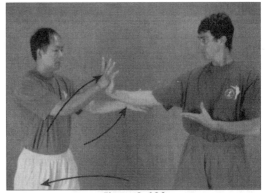

Figure 2-190

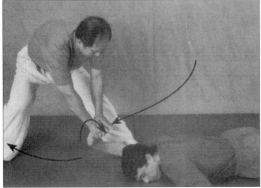

Figure 2-191

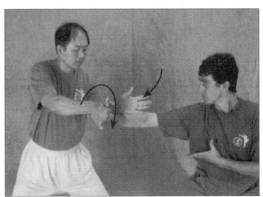

Figure 2-192

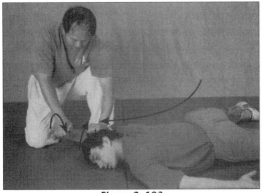

Figure 2-193

Since the hand must be opened for palm strikes, many of the Qin Na techniques used against an open hand can also be applied here. However, you should still pay attention to how to intercept and set up for the accurate locking angle.

I. PALM STRIKING FORWORD TO THE CHEST

Technique #1: White Crane Nods Its Head or White Crane Twists Its Neck

(Bai He Dian Tou or Bai He Niu Jing)
白鶴點頭，白鶴扭頸

When your opponent strikes your chest with his right palm (Figure 2-189), intercept his arm with your left hand, and at the same time use your right hand to grab his right fingers (Figure 2-190). When you are doing this, also step your right leg backward. Finally, press his fingers backward until his elbow touches the ground (Figure 2-191). Alternatively, you may twist his hand to your right and then bend (Figure 2-192). This will control his pinkie's tendon, rather than the base of his fingers. Additionally, you may use your left hand to grab his hair to prevent him from biting your fingers (Figure 2-193). Another option to the first technique is, when you use your right hand to grab, instead of grabbing all of the fingers, only grab any two of his fingers. The pain generated this way

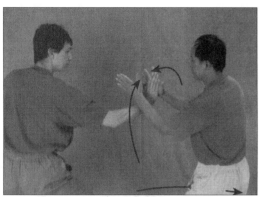

Figure 2–194

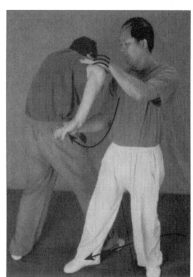

Figure 2–195

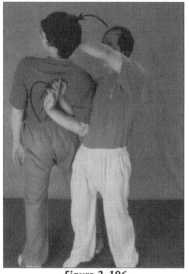

Figure 2–196

Theory:

Misplacing the Bone (base of the finger joints in the first technique) and Dividing the Muscle/Tendon (pinkie tendon in the second technique). Although this technique was introduced previously, you should still note how to intercept and set up the correct angle for locking.

Technique #2: White Crane Bores the Bush

(Bai He Chuan Cong) 白鶴穿叢

In the last technique, after you have grabbed your opponent's hand with your right fingers (Figure 2-194), twist and bend his right wrist, and then circle down and toward his back while using your left hand to hold up his elbow and step your right leg behind his right leg (Figure 2-195). Finally, sandwich his right arm between your right hand and right chest to lock him there (Figure 2-196). To make this technique more effective, after you have locked your opponent's arm behind him, you should increase the pressure on his pinkie.

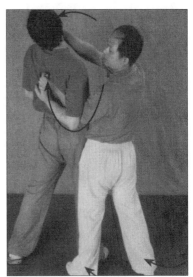

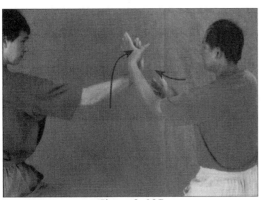

Figure 2–197

Figure 2–198

Theory:

Misplacing the Bone (shoulder) and Dividing the Muscle/Tendon (pinkie). Right after you have twisted and bent your opponent's hand, you should continue to maintain pressure to prevent your opponent's resistance or escape. When you move his arm behind him, you should keep his arm as high as his nipple area; this will lock his entire arm effectively.

Technique #3: Butterfly Bores Through the Flowers or Back Turning

(Hu Die Chuan Hua or Fan Bei Zhuan) 蝴蝶穿花，反背轉

When your opponent strikes you with his right palm, use your left hand to cover his right hand and grab his fingers. In order to make the grabbing more effective, you may again use your right hand to help, by sandwiching your opponent's hand between your hands (Figure 2-197). While you are doing this, you should step your right leg back to set up a good angle. Right after your left hand grabs, you should immediately circle your opponent's hand behind his back. Through bending your opponent's fingers backward, you can control him effectively (Figure 2-198). You should continue your pressure until his heels are off the ground. In order to make the control more effective, you should use your right hand to push his chin upward. Naturally, you should beware of any attack from the other hand.

Theory:

Misplacing the Bone (shoulder and base joints of the fingers). When you move his hand behind him, you should keep the movement at the same level as his nipple. This will lock his entire arm instead of just his fingers.

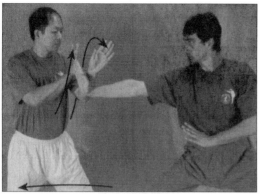

Figure 2–199

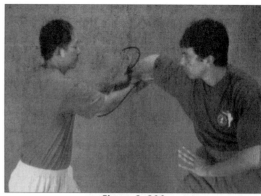

Figure 2–200

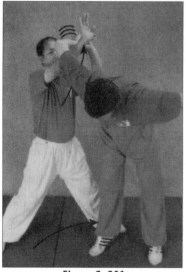

Figure 2–201

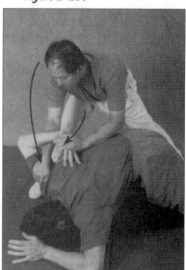

Figure 2–202

Technique #4: Lion Worships the Buddha or Large Wrap Elbow

(Shi Zi Bai Fo or Da Chan Zhou) 獅子拜佛，大纏肘

In this technique, first use your left hand to cover your opponent's right hand while also stepping your right leg backward (Figure 2-199). Next, circle your left hand around his right arm and grab his right wrist, while also circling your right arm around his right arm until it reaches the elbow (Figure 2-200). When you do this, you should step your left leg behind his right leg while lifting his right arm for locking (Figure 2-201). Finally press him to the ground (Figure 2-202).

Theory:

Misplacing the Bone (shoulder) and Dividing the Muscle/Tendon (wrist). When you circle your right arm to lock your opponent's arm behind him, you should use the entire body's power instead of just the arm. In addition, in order to lock him efficiently, you should place your hand on his upper-arm near the elbow area instead of on his shoulder. Because of the strength of the shoulder, if you place your hand there, he may reverse the situation by simply circling his arm forward.

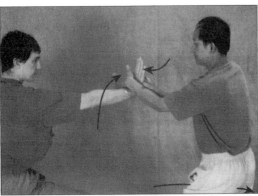

Figure 2-203

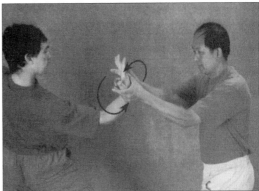

Figure 2-204

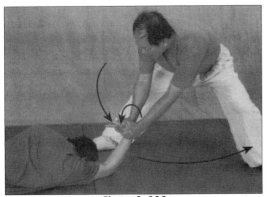

Figure 2-205

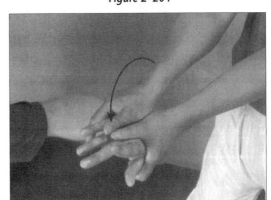

Figure 2-206

Technique #5: White Ape Worships the Buddha or Reverse Wrist Press

(Bai Yuan Bai Fo or Fan Ya Wan) 白猿拜佛 , 反壓腕

In this technique, you again step your right leg backward and use your left hand to cover your opponent's right hand, while clamping upward and grabbing his right hand (Figure 2-203). Immediately turn your opponent's wrist counterclockwise until his palm faces upward (Figure 2-204) and then press it down while stepping your left leg backward (Figure 2-205). You should press him down until his elbow touches the ground. When you press him down, you may twist his hand to the side slightly, and thereby generate more pressure on his pinkie tendon (Figure 2-206). This can result in more pain.

Theory:

Dividing the Muscle/Tendon (wrist and pinkie). To make the control efficient, you must generate good leverage between your thumbs and pinkies. Once you have locked the hand, press downward with the entirety of both your hands, instead of just the thumbs.

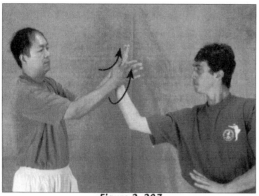

Figure 2–207

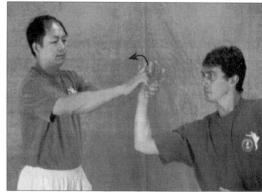

Figure 2–208

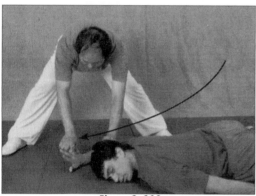

Figure 2–209

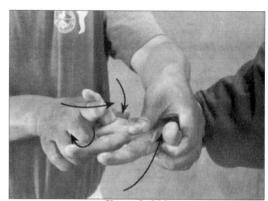

Figure 2–210

Technique #6: Fingers Lock the Dragon Tail or Turning Finger Dividing

(Zhi Suo Long Wei or Zhuan Fen Zhi) 指鎖龍尾，轉分指

This technique is an option to the last technique. In this technique, right after you have grabbed your opponent's right wrist and turned it counterclockwise until the palm faces upward (Figure 2-207), immediately use your right thumb and index finger to split his pinkie from his other four fingers (Figure 2-208). Finally, twist your index finger and thumb to lock and press your opponent's pinkie in place (Figures 2-209 and 2-210). You should press him down until his elbow touches the ground.

Theory

Misplacing the Bone (pinkie). From the beginning until your opponent's pinkie is locked, you should not let your left hand lose control of his right wrist. When you use your index finger and thumb to lock his pinkie, the leverage generated from your index finger and thumb is very important. Without good leverage, the control will be ineffective.

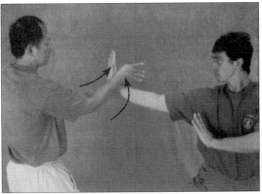

Figure 2–211

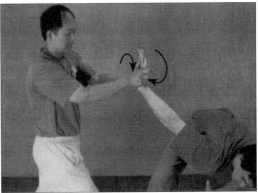

Figure 2–212

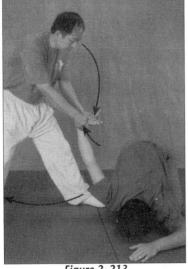

Figure 2–213

Technique #7: Wild Chicken Spreads Its Wings

(Ye Ji Zhan Chi) 野雞展翅

In this technique, use your right hand to cover your opponent's right hand, while also clamping upward with your left hand to grab your opponent's right wrist (Figure 2-211). Immediately after the grab, turn your opponent's wrist clockwise until his palm faces upward (Figure 2-212). Finally, step your right leg backward and press him down (Figure 2-213). You should press him down until his elbow touches the ground.

Theory:
Dividing the Muscle/Tendon (wrist). When you grab, you are using the entirety of both your hands, and when you turn your opponent's hand clockwise, you should use your entire body instead of just the arms. When you press your opponent down, the **power is generated from the leverage of your pinkie and the thumb area**. Keep trying until you find the most effective angle and leverage.

Technique #8: One Post to Support the Heavens

(Yi Zhu Ding Tian) 一柱頂天

In this technique, again use your right hand to cover your opponent's right hand, while also using the left hand to clamp his right wrist (Figure 2-214). Immediately circle your right hand to grab your opponent's right wrist, while also turning your body clockwise to place his right arm on your shoulder with the palm facing upward (Figure 2-215). Finally, use both hands to push your opponent's arm upward to generate pain in his shoulder (Figure 2-216). You should continue exerting your pushing strength until your opponent's heels are off the ground.

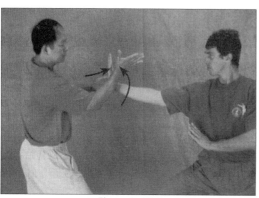

Figure 2–214

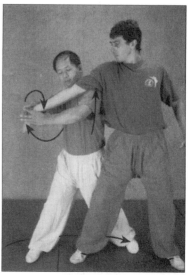

Figure 2–215

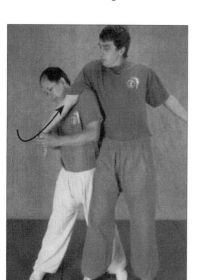

Figure 2–216

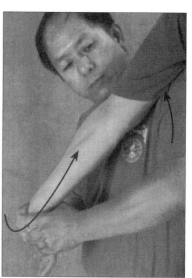

Figure 2–217

Theory:

Misplacing the Bone (shoulder). If the angle of your opponent's arm is set correctly, with the leverage of your shoulder and hands, you should be able to lock him very easily. In order to make the technique more effective, you may place the back side of his upper-arm on your shoulder while executing the technique (Figure 2-217). This will generate great pain in the tendons of his upper-arm. Naturally, you must beware of a possible attack from his left hand. That is why you must control him until his heels are off the ground. This will prevent him from generating any power to attack.

Technique #9: Twist Wrist and Press Elbow and
The Old Man Is Promoted to General

(Niu Wan Ya Zhou and Lao Han Bai Jiang) 扭腕壓肘 ， 老漢拜將

Again, first step your right leg backward and cover your opponent's right palm with your right hand and coil around his wrist to grab it, while placing your left forearm on his

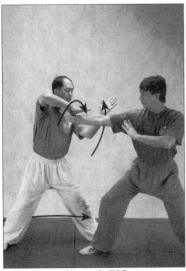
Figure 2–218

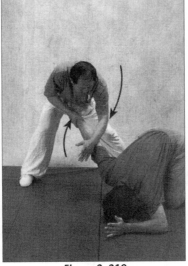
Figure 2–219

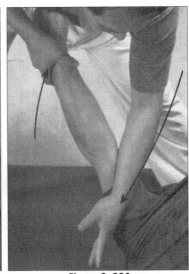
Figure 2–220

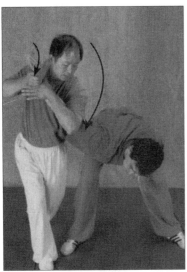
Figure 2–221

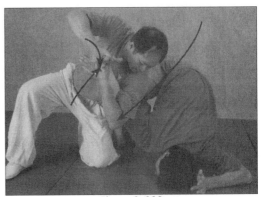
Figure 2–222

elbow (Figure 2-218). Next, bow forward and use the leverage of your right hand and left forearm to press him down until he is on the ground (Figure 2-219). Alternatively, you may use your left forearm to press the tendon on the back of your opponent's upper-arm (Figure 2-220). This also generates pain and therefore controls your opponent.

Using the same theory, you may also place your opponent's elbow under your left armpit area (Figure 2-221), and use the leverage of your hands and left shoulder to press him down to the ground (Figure 2-222).

Theory:
Misplacing the Bone (elbow), Dividing the Muscle/Tendon (wrist), and Pressing the Tendons (upper-arm). From your right hand's twisting, you set up the correct angle for the elbow's pressing. With the leverage of your left forearm (or shoulder) and right hand, you can generate great pain in the elbow.

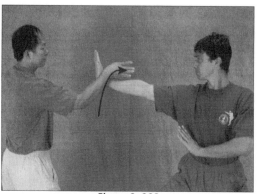

Figure 2–223

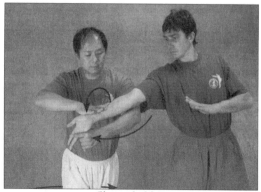

Figure 2–224

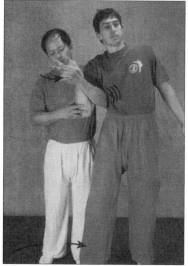

Figure 2–225

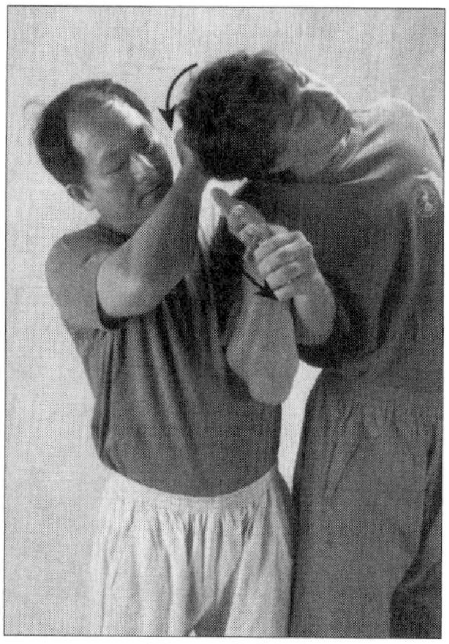

Figure 2–226

Technique #10: Hand Bends the Dragon's Tail

(Shou Ban Long Wei) 手扳龍尾

When your opponent attacks you with his right palm, first use your right hand to cover his hand (Figure 2-223). Next, circle your right hand around his forearm to grab his wrist while also using your left hand to grab his index and small fingers (Figure 2-224). When you do this, you should step your left leg forward and to his right hand side while placing your left arm under your opponent's right arm. Finally, use your left hand to pull back your opponent's index finger and pinkie against your chest to control him (Figure 2-225). When you use this technique, pay attention to where you stand. In order to prevent your opponent from attacking you with his left hand, after you have locked his index finger and pinkie with your left hand, use your right hand to grab his hair and pull and twist his head to his left (Figure 2-226). Alternatively, you may use your right hand to push his chin upward.

Theory:

Misplacing the Bone (index finger and pinkie). When you lock your opponent, his forearm should be sandwiched between your chest and hand.

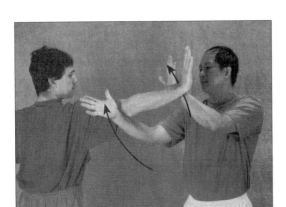

Figure 2–227

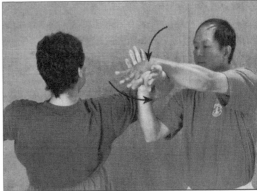

Figure 2–228

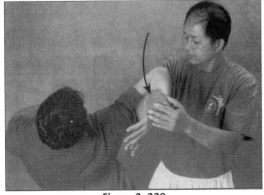

Figure 2–229

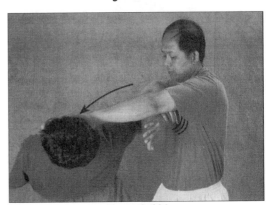

Figure 2–230

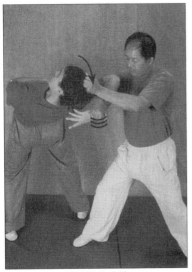

Figure 2–231

Technique #11: Twist the Wing with Both Hands or Forward Upward Turning

(Shuang Shou Ban Chi or Qian Shang Fan)
雙手扳翅，前上翻

When your opponent attacks you with his right palm, turn your body to your left and use your left forearm to block upward, while placing your right arm under his elbow (Figure 2-227). Immediately after blocking, push your left forearm forward while using your right wrist area to pull his elbow toward you (Figure 2-228). Finally, step your right leg behind his right leg and use both of your arms to lock your opponent's right arm (Figure 2-229). In order to prevent your opponent from attacking you with his left hand, you may use your right arm to lock the elbow, while using your left hand to push his chin toward his left (Figure 2-230). You may also grab his hair

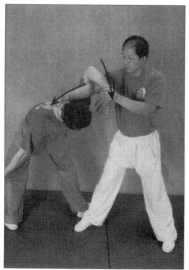

Figure 2–232

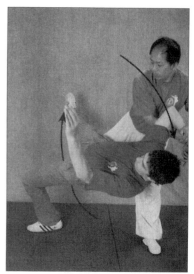

Figure 2–233

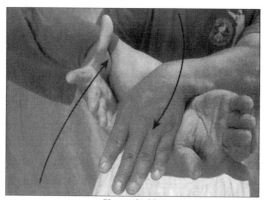

Figure 2–234

and pull it down (Figure 2-231). Naturally, you may use your right hand to grab his throat (Figure 2-232) or sweep your right leg backward to make your opponent fall (Figure 2-233).

Theory:

Misplacing the Bone (elbow and neck). In order to make his arm bend for your locking, while your are pushing your left forearm forward and downward, you should also use the area on the base of your thumb to pull inward on his elbow (Figure 2-234). The leverage and the angle of locking are very important. With good leverage and correct locking, if you jerk your power, you may pop your opponent's elbow out of the socket quite easily.

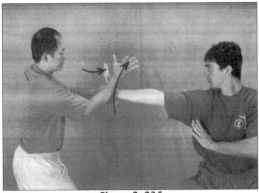

Figure 2–235

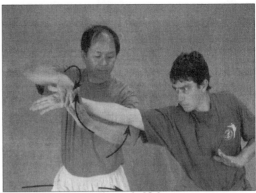

Figure 2–236

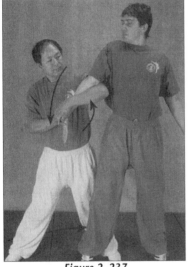

Figure 2–237

Technique #12: Hands Prop a Large Beam or Prop Up Elbow

(Shou Ban Da Liang or Shang Jia Zhou)
手扳大樑，上架肘

When your opponent attacks you with his right palm, again use your right hand to cover his hand while stepping your left leg backward (Figure 2-235). Then, immediately coil your right hand around his wrist, direct it to your right, and grab it (Figure 2-236). While you are doing so, you should also step in with your left leg, and use your left elbow to push upward on his right elbow. Finally, use the leverage of your hands and left elbow to lock him upward until his heels are off the ground (Figure 2-237). You should position yourself where your opponent cannot strike you with his left hand.

Theory:
Misplacing the Bone (elbow). With the good leverage generated from your left elbow and right hand, you should be able to lock him easily. In this technique, if you generate a jerking Jin, you may easily break your opponent's elbow.

II. PALM PRESSING DOWNWARD TO THE ABDOMEN
In Chinese martial arts, it is very common to use the palm to press downward against the stomach and abdominal areas (Figure 2-238). When these two areas are pressed, the muscles connected to the upper chest will contract, and therefore the breath can be sealed. Here, we will introduce some Qin Na Techniques which can be used against palm pressing to these areas.

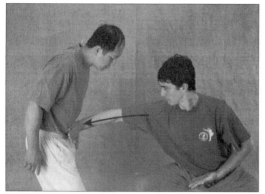

Figure 2–238

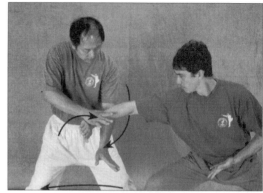

Figure 2–239

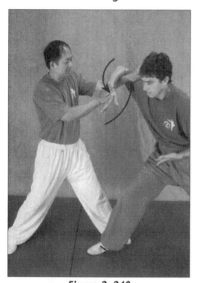

Figure 2–240

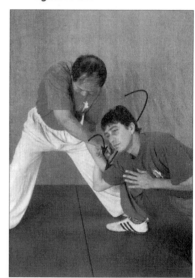

Figure 2–241

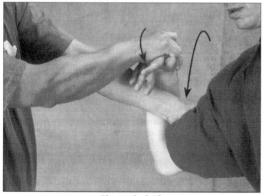

Figure 2–242

Technique #1: Low Outward Wrist Press

(Xia Wai Ya Wan) 下外壓腕

When your opponent uses his right palm to press downward against your stomach area, first step your right leg backward, and use your left forearm to intercept his press by repelling it to your right (Figure 2-239). While you are doing this, also use your right hand to grab his wrist. Next, circle your left forearm upward and then downward to coil around your opponent's forearm (Figure 2-240). Finally, use your left hand to control his forearm until it is vertical to the ground, while using your right hand to press his hand downward to generate pain in his wrist (Figure 2-241).

Theory:

Dividing the Muscle/Tendon (wrist). In this technique, you do not generate any pain in your opponent's elbow. Your left hand serves only to lock the arm in the correct position for your right hand control (Figure 2-242). The major pain comes from the wrist. The leverage of **control is generated from the base of your right palm and thumb and the middle finger grabbing the wrist**.

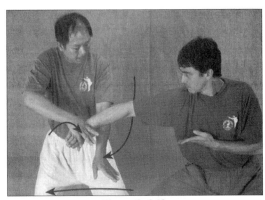

Figure 2–243

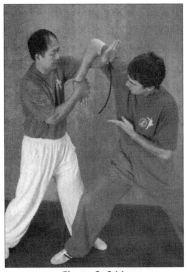

Figure 2–244

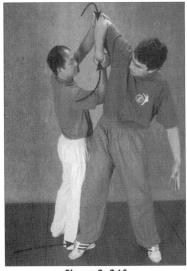

Figure 2–245

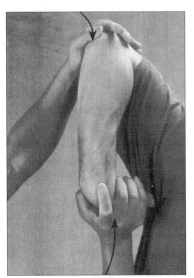

Figure 2–246

Technique #2: Single Hand to Support the Heavens or Press the Wrist Up

(Zhi Shou Cheng Tian or Shang Ya Wan) 隻手撐天，上壓腕

When your opponent uses his right palm to press downward against your stomach area, first step your right leg backward and use your left forearm to intercept his press by repelling it to your right (Figure 2-243). While you are doing this, also use your right hand to grab his wrist. Next, use your left hand to push his elbow upward while pressing his hand to control his wrist (Figure 2-244). You should position yourself where your opponent cannot easily strike you with his left hand. Finally, place your left hand on his elbow, and using the leverage of your left hand and right hand, lock your opponent upward (Figure 2-245). You must increase the upward pressing strength until his heels are off the ground. This can also prevent him from hitting you with his left hand.

Theory:

Dividing the Muscle/Tendon (wrist). In this technique, the major pain originates from the wrist. In order to increase the efficiency of the control, you may **squeeze both of your hands against each other** (Figure 2-246). You should position your-

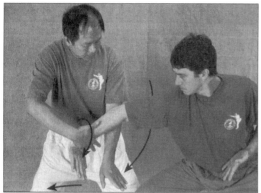

Figure 2–247

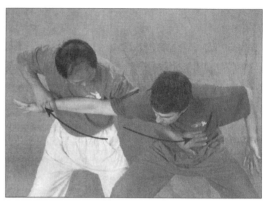

Figure 2–248

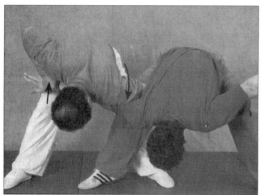

Figure 2–249

self on the right side of your opponent to prevent him from attacking you with his left hand.

Technique #3: Two Children Worship the Buddha

(Shuang Tong Bai Fo) 雙童拜佛

When your opponent uses his right palm to press downward against your stomach area, first step your right leg backward and use your left forearm to intercept his press by repelling it to your right (Figure 2-247). While you are doing so, also use your right hand to grab his wrist. Next, slide your left arm under his armpit, and use your left upper-arm to press against the tendon on the back of his upper-arm (Figure 2-248). Finally, bow forward to increase the pressure on his upper-arm to generate pain (Figure 2-249).

Theory:

Pressing the Tendon (upper-arm) and Misplacing the Bone (elbow). In order to control your opponent more efficiently, you may press **your left shoulder forward and pull your right hand backward**. This generates strong controlling leverage. This technique can only control your opponent temporarily, instead of long term. This will offer you an opportunity for a quick right hand attack to his face. It is very difficult to dislocate your opponent's elbow with this technique.

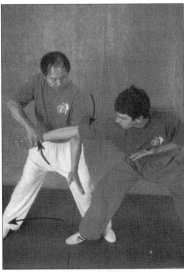

Figure 2–250

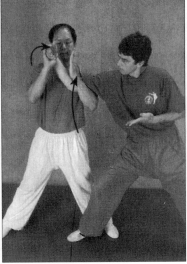

Figure 2–251

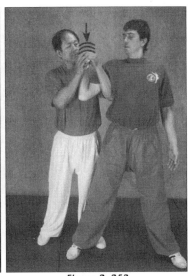

Figure 2–252

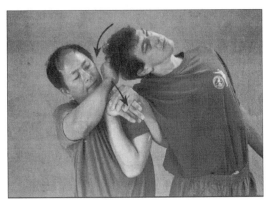

Figure 2–253

Technique #4: Feudal Lord Invites to Dinner

(Ba Wang Qing Ke) 霸王請客

When your opponent uses his right palm to press downward against your stomach area, first step your right leg backward and use your left forearm to intercept his press by repelling it to your right (Figure 2-250). While you are doing so, also use your right hand to grab his wrist. Next, bend your left elbow and use your left arm to lock your opponent's right arm, while your right hand lifts up your opponent's hand (Figure 2-251). Finally, use both of your hands to press your opponent's hand downward to generate pain in his wrist (Figure 2-252). You should increase your pressure until his heels are off the ground. If you are afraid of your opponent's left hand attack, you may simply use your left hand to control his wrist and use your right hand to grab his hair (Figure 2-253).

Theory:
Dividing the Muscle/Tendon (wrist). Right after your intercept, you should use your left arm to press his elbow while pulling his right hand backward with your right hand. This will lock his arm right at the beginning of this technique. The natural reaction of your opponent against your action is to bend his arm in order to protect his elbow from being locked. You then simply follow his bending to lock him upward. The final control leverage is generated from your hands, pressing the base joints of your fingers and left elbow to sandwich your opponent's forearm. Occasionally, you will encounter someone who is double jointed in his wrist. This technique then becomes ineffective. Once you realize this, immediately use your left hand to lock the wrist, while using your right hand to bend his pinkie backward to control him.

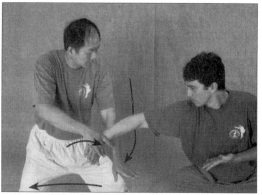

Figure 2-254

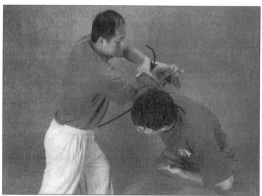

Figure 2-255

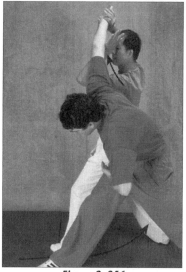

Figure 2-256

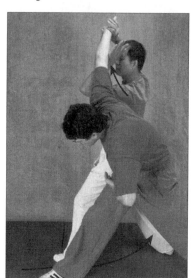

Figure 2-257

Technique #5: Large Python Turns Its Body

(Da Mang Fan Shen) 大蟒翻身

When your opponent uses his right palm to press downward against your stomach area, first step your right leg backward and use your left forearm to intercept his press by repelling it to your right (Figure 2-254). While you are doing so, also use your right hand to grab his wrist. Next, swing his arm to his left while placing your left forearm under his right elbow (Figure 2-255). Then, rotate your body under his right arm while pressing your left forearm against his elbow (Figure 2-256). Finally, bow forward while pressing his elbow down with your left forearm (Figure 2-257). You should press until his elbow touches the ground.

Theory:

Misplacing the Bone (elbow and shoulder). When you rotate and press your opponent downward, you should use your entire body's power. In this technique, if your opponent is very skillful and fast, he will be able to roll forward and therefore release himself from your control. To prevent this, you may step your right leg back to circle his body while pressing downward. This will enable you to lock him down to the ground.

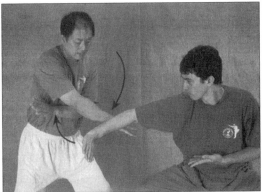

Figure 2-258

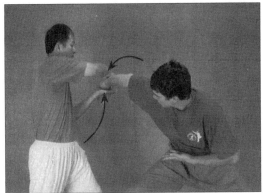

Figure 2-259

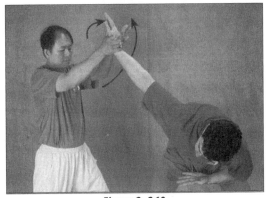

Figure 2-260

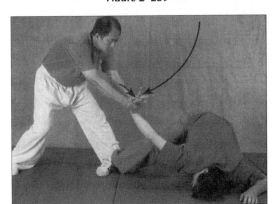

Figure 2-261

Technique #6: Wild Chicken Spreads Its Wings

(Ye Ji Zhan Chi) 野雞展翅

In this technique, use your right hand to repel your opponent's right arm while placing your left hand under your right arm (Figure 2-258). Next, grab your opponent's right hand with your left hand, while moving your right hand to his right wrist and grabbing it (Figure 2-259). Right after the grab, immediately turn your opponent's wrist clockwise while still bending his wrist (Figure 2-260). Finally, use your entire body's power to press him down (Figure 2-261). You should press him down until his left elbow touches the ground.

Theory:

Dividing the Muscle/Tendon (wrist). When you grab his wrist, you are using the entirety of both your hands to grab instead of only using fingers, and when you turn your opponent's hand clockwise, you should use your entire body instead of just using arms. When you press your opponent down, the power is generated from the leverage of your pinkie and thumb area, and the power is generated from your body. Keep trying until the most effective angle and leverage are found.

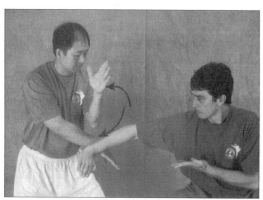

Figure 2–262

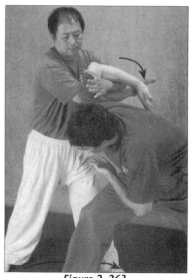

Figure 2–263

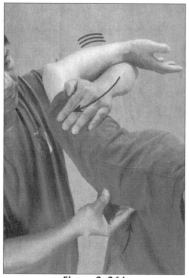

Figure 2–264

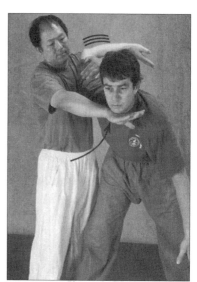

Figure 2–265

Technique #7: Pressing Shoulder with Single Finger and Extending the Neck for Water

(Yi Zhi Ding Jiang and Yin Jing Qiu Shui) 一指頂肩 ， 引頸求水

In this technique, first use your right forearm to repel your opponent's attack to your right, while placing your left arm above his elbow (Figure 2-262). Next, press his right elbow down and coil your left hand around his right arm until reaching his elbow (Figure 2-263). This will place his right arm behind him. Finally, use your left arm to lift his right arm upward and behind him. At this stage, all of the tendons and ligaments in your opponent's shoulder are very tensed. You should press your index finger on his *Jianneiling* cavity (M-UE-48) to generate great pain in his shoulder area (Figure 2-264). You should increase the pressing pressure on your index finger until your opponent's heels are off the floor. Alternatively, you may use your right hand to lift his chin upward (Figure 2-265) or grab and pull his hair (Figure 2-266). This will also produce great pain.

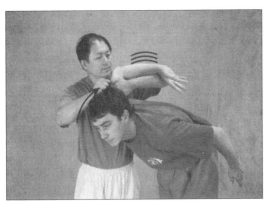

Figure 2-266

Theory:

Misplacing the Bone (shoulder) and Cavity Press (*Jianneiling* cavity). When you use your left arm to lock your opponent's right arm and lift it upward, you generate a strain on his right shoulder's tendons and ligaments. This action also exposes his *Jianneiling* cavity for your cavity press attack. Without an accurate locking position for the shoulder, the cavity press will not be effective.

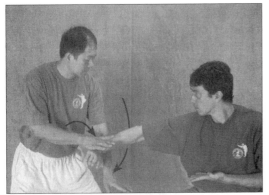

Figure 2-267

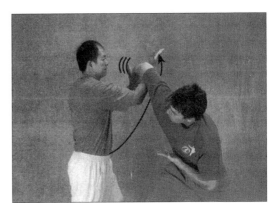

Figure 2-268

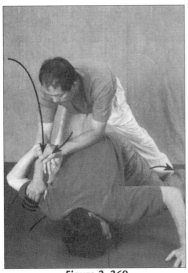

Figure 2-269

Technique #8: Lion Worships the Buddha or Large Wrap Elbow

(Shi Zi Bai Fo or Da Chan Zhou) 獅子拜佛，大纏肘

When your opponent strikes your abdomen area with his right palm, use your left forearm to repel the attack to your right, while using your right hand to grab his right wrist (Figure 2-267). Next, coil your right hand around his forearm and push his arm to his right while also using your left hand to grab his right wrist (Figure 2-268). Finally, step your left leg behind him while circling your right arm and press him down to the ground (Figure 2-269).

Theory:

Misplacing the Bone (shoulder) and Dividing the Muscle/Tendon (wrist). When you circle your right arm to lock your opponent's arm behind him, you should use the entire body's power instead of just the arm. In addition, in order to lock him effectively, you should place your hand on his upper-arm, near the elbow area, instead of on his shoulder. If you place your hand on his shoulder, because of its strength, he may reverse the situation by simply circling his arm forward.

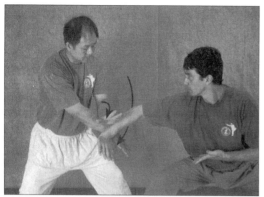

Figure 2–270

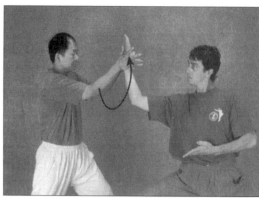

Figure 2–271

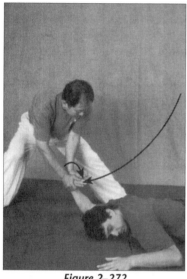

Figure 2–272

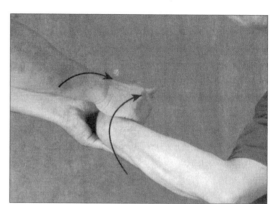

Figure 2–273

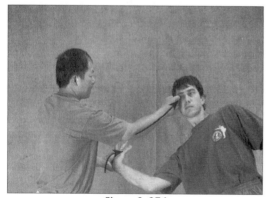

Figure 2–274

Technique #9: White Ape Worships the Buddha or Reverse Wrist Press

(Bai Yuan Bai Fo or Fan Ya Wan)
白猿拜佛，反壓腕

In this technique, first use your right forearm to repel your opponent's attack to your right, while also placing your left hand above his right forearm (Figure 2-270). Next, use both of your hands to turn your opponent's wrist counterclockwise until the palm faces upward (Figure 2-271). Finally, use both hands to press and bend his wrist to generate pain (Figure 2-272). You may also twist his hand to his right in order to generate pain in the pinkie area (Figure 2-273). You should continue to press until his elbow touches the ground. If necessary, you may use your left hand to strike his nose or eyes (Figure 2-274).

Theory:

Dividing the Muscle/Tendon (wrist). To make the control effective, you must generate good leverage between your thumbs and pinkies. Once you have locked the hand, press downward with the entirety of both of your hands instead of just the thumbs.

2-5. Qin Na Against Fist Strike

Before we discuss the Qin Na techniques against fist strikes, you should first recognize two important facts. First, the main difference between Qin Na against open hands and fist strikes is that, in fist attacks, your opponent's fingers are closed, and it is difficult, if not impossible, to apply finger Qin Na against him. Therefore, Qin Na against fist attacks must focus on the wrist, elbow, or shoulder.

Second, when your opponent attacks you with his fist, he has several options. He may punch your head, chest, or abdominal areas. He may also punch you straight with the front side of his fist, attack you with the side of his fist to your face or temple, or strike you with an uppercut to your chin or abdomen. In this section, we will discuss Qin Na techniques against fist attacks by dividing them into three main subsections: punches to the head, the chest, and the abdomen. The category of punches to the head will again be divided into three categories: straight punches, sideways back fist strikes, and uppercuts. Chest punches likewise will be categorized according to four possible methods of intercepting. Finally, Qin Na techniques against abdominal punches will be divided into two groups, the straight punch and the uppercut.

I. AGAINST HEAD PUNCH

A. STRAIGHT PUNCH

Technique #1: Twist the Wing with Both Hands or Forward Upward Turning

(Shuang Shou Ban Chi, Qian Shang Fan) 雙手扳翅，前上翻

If your opponent punches at your head with his right fist, first you repel the strike with your left forearm while placing your right forearm under his elbow area (Figure 2-275). Immediately after repelling, use your forearm near the thumb area to pull his elbow toward you, while pushing your left hand forward (Figure 2-276). Finally, lock your opponent's right arm in place (Figure 2-277). You may also use your right leg to sweep your opponent's right leg and make him fall (Figure 2-278). It is very important that you should stand on the right side of your opponent's body to avoid his left hand's strike.

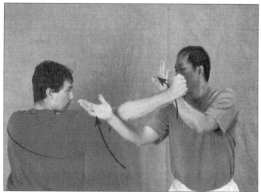

Figure 2–275

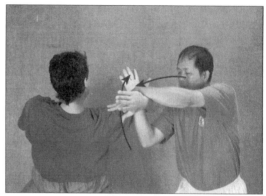

Figure 2–276

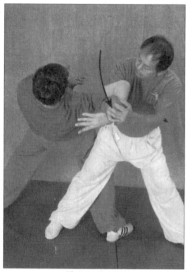

Figure 2–277

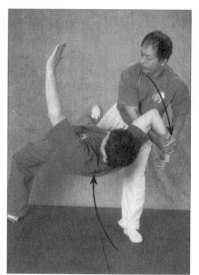

Figure 2–278

Theory:

Misplacing the Bone (elbow). When you apply this technique, your opponent's arm may be stiff; this makes it harder for you to bend his arm. The key to make his arm bend is to use the wrist area on your thumb side to hook his elbow downward, while pushing your left arm upward. This will provide you with good leverage to bend his arm. In this technique, if you jerk your power suddenly, you may pop out your opponent's elbow.

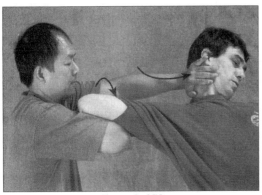

Figure 2–279

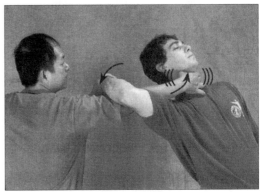

Figure 2–280

Technique #2: Lock the Elbow and Push the Neck or Lock the Elbow and Seal the Throat

(Suo Zhou Tui Jing or Suo Zhou Feng Hou) 鎖肘推頸 ， 鎖肘封喉

In the last technique, right after you have locked your opponent's right arm, you may use your right hand to continue to lock the arm while using your left hand or forearm to press against your opponent's neck (Figure 2-279).

Alternatively, you may let your left hand take over the locking, and free you right hand to grab your opponent's throat (Figure 2-280).

Theory:

Misplacing the Bone (elbow), Dividing the Muscle/Tendon (shoulder and neck), or Sealing the Breath (throat).

Technique #3: Luo Han Bows or Small Elbow Wrap

(Luo Han Xing Li or Xiao Chan Zhou) 羅漢行禮 ， 小纏肘

In this technique, first you repel the punch to your right with your right forearm and grab the wrist while placing your left hand on your opponent's elbow (Figure 2-281). Next, step your left leg to the front of your opponent's right leg while circling your left forearm upward and then downward, at the same time pulling your right hand downward and then inward (Figure 2-282). Finally, pull your opponent's right arm toward the front of your body to destroy his stability, while bowing and sweeping your left leg backward to make him fall (Figure 2-283). When your opponent is on the ground, lock his arm behind his back. With the help both of your legs, you will be able to lock him there firmly (Figure 2-284).

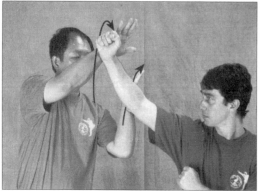

Figure 2–281

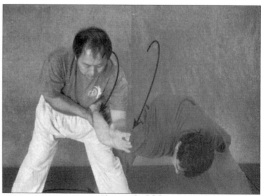

Figure 2–282

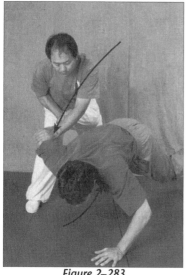

Figure 2–283

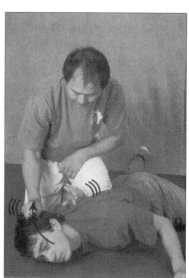

Figure 2–284

Theory:

Misplacing the Bone (elbow and shoulder). In order to make your opponent fall, after you have locked him, you should **pull him to your front to destroy his balance, while sweeping your left leg backward**. Once your opponent is on the ground, if necessary, you may rotate his arm toward his head and pop his shoulder out of joint.

Technique #4: Pressing Shoulder with Single Finger and Extending the Neck for Water

(Yi Zhi Ding Jiang and Yin Jing Qiu Shui) 一指頂肩，引頸求水

In this technique, again use your right forearm to repel your opponent's punch to your right while placing your left forearm on his elbow area (Figure 2-285). Next, hook down with your right hand, grab his wrist, and then push his arm upward while coiling your left arm around his arm and finally placing your hand behind his elbow (Figure 2-286). With the level of your left elbow and hand, now you may lock your opponent's arm behind him. You should lift his arm upward to generate tension in his shoulder. In this situation, if you press your index finger on his *Jianneiling* cavity (M-UE-48), you will be able to generate great pain

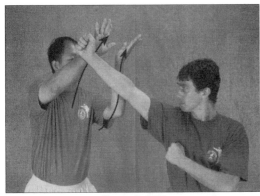

Figure 2–285

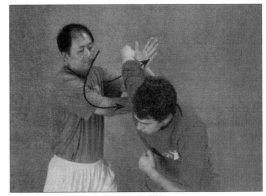

Figure 2–286

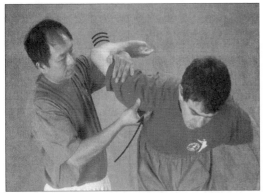

Figure 2–287

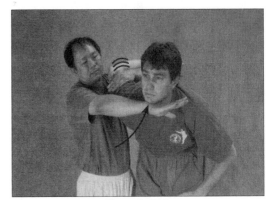

Figure 2–288

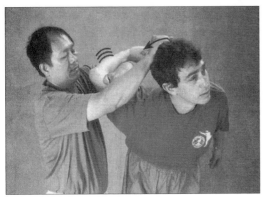

Figure 2–289

in his shoulder area (Figure 2-287). You should increase the pressure on your index finger until your opponent's heels leave the floor. Alternatively, you may use your right hand to push his chin upward (Figure 2-288). This will increase the pain greatly. Naturally, you may use your right hand to grab his hair and pull to generate good leverage for your control (Figure 2-289).

Theory:
Misplacing the Bone (shoulder), and Cavity Press (*Jianneiling* cavity). When you use your left arm to lock your opponent's right arm and lift it upward, you put a strain on his right shoulder's tendons and ligaments. This action also exposes his *Jianneiling* cavity for your cavity press attack. Without the accurate locking position of the shoulder, the cavity press will not be effective.

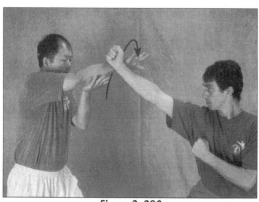

Figure 2–290

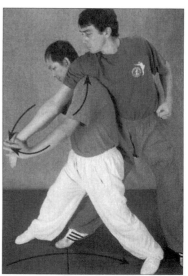

Figure 2–291

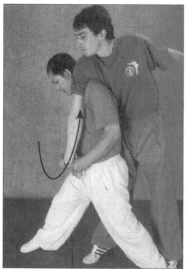

Figure 2–292

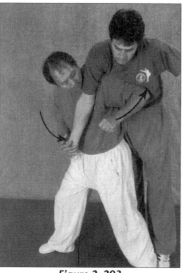

Figure 2–293

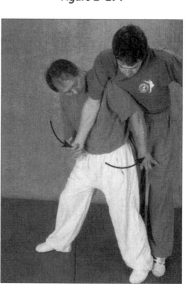

Figure 2–294

Technique #5: One Post to Support the Heavens
(Yi Zhu Ding Tian) 一柱頂天

When your opponent punches at your head with his right fist, first use your right forearm to repel his punch to your right (Figure 2-290). Next, hook your right hand down and grab his wrist with both or your hands and turn his palm to face upward, while stepping your left leg to the front of his right leg and placing the back of his upper-arm over your left shoulder (Figure 2-291). Finally, lift his arm upward to generate pain in his shoulder (Figure 2-292). You should keep lifting until his heels are off the ground. The position where you stand should be as far as possible beyond the reach of his left hand.

If your opponent intends to attack you with his left hand, immediately use your left elbow to strike his solar plexus, while still holding his arm in position with your right hand (Figure 2-293). You may also use your left hand to strike his groin (Figure 2-294).

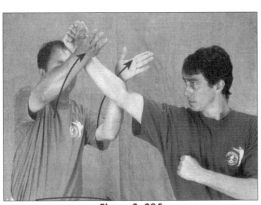

Figure 2–295

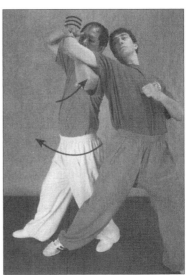

Figure 2–296

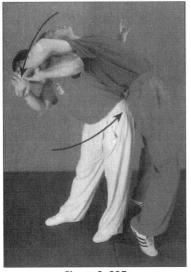

Figure 2–297

Theory:

Misplacing the Bone (shoulder). When you turn your opponent's arm to make his palm face upward, you have twisted the tendons and ligaments in his shoulder into a tensed condition. If you lift his arm upward, the lifting will cause the ligaments to tear off. Further lifting will dislocate the shoulder joint. In order to produce more pain, you may place your opponent's upper-arm tendon on your shoulder while you are executing this technique.

Technique #6: The Old Man Carries the Fish on His Back

(Lao Han Bei Yu) 老漢背魚

When your opponent uses his right fist to punch your head, step your right leg backward while using your left forearm to intercept his punch on his right elbow and your right forearm on his wrist area (Figure 2-295). Right after the interception, pull your left hand downward and turn your body to your right (Figure 2-296). Finally, bow your body forward and position your opponent's right arm behind your back (Figure 2-297).

Theory:

Misplacing the Bone (shoulder). In order to lock your opponent's shoulder effectively, the angle of locking must be accurate. When you turn your body and pull, if your opponent's arm is either too straight or too bent, the locking will not be effective.

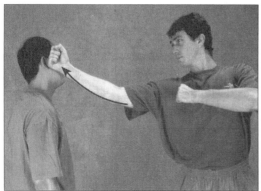

Figure 2–298

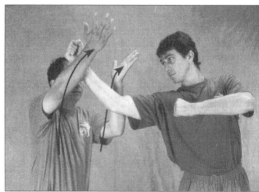

Figure 2–299

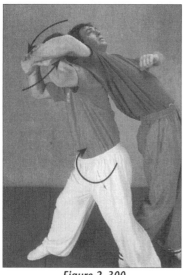

Figure 2–300

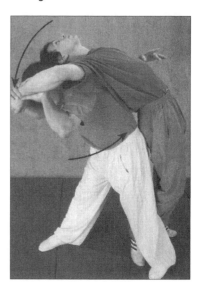

Figure 2–301

B. SIDEWAYS BACK FIST STRIKE

Technique #1: The Old Man Carries the Fish on His Back

(Lao Han Bei Yu) 老漢背魚

When your opponent uses his right back fist to strike your right temple (Figure 2-298), use your left hand to intercept his elbow and right hand at his wrist while stepping back with your right leg (Figure 2-299). Right after the interception, push your left forearm downward, turning your body to your right (Figure 2-300). Finally, bow forward and pull his arm downward with both of your hands to lock his right arm behind your back (Figure 2-301).

Theory:
Misplacing the Bone (shoulder). In order to lock your opponent's shoulder effectively, the angle of locking must be accurate. When you turn your body and pull, if your opponent's arm is either too straight or too bent, the lock will not be effective.

Technique #2: White Tiger Turns Its Head or Upward Elbow Wrap

(Bai Hu Fan Shou or Shang Chan Zhou) 白虎返首，上纏肘

In this technique, while you intercept with your left hand, also use your right hand to clamp your opponent's wrist (Figure 2-302). Immediately circle both of your hands coun-

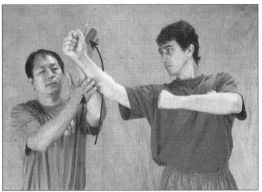

Figure 2–302

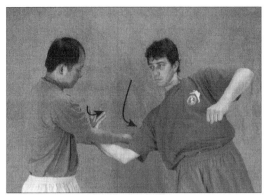

Figure 2–303

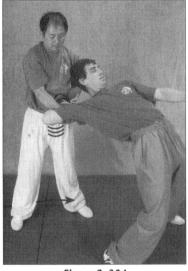

Figure 2–304

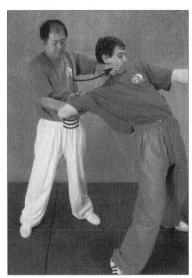

Figure 2–305

terclockwise and use your left hand to grab your opponent's hand, then continue to coil your right hand until reaching his elbow area (Figure 2-303). Finally, lift his elbow upward with your right hand while twisting his wrist with your left hand to lock him up (Figure 2-304). When you execute this technique, you should also reposition yourself behind your opponent so that he cannot attack you with his left hand. With the leverage from the left and right hands, if you squeeze both sides in, you will be able to control him effectively.

In order to increase the effectiveness of the control, you may lock his right arm with your right hand and stomach, while using your left hand to push his right neck to the left (Figure 2-305).

Theory:

Dividing the Muscle/Tendon (wrist) and Misplacing the Bone (elbow). In order to make the control effective, you should forcefully twist your opponent's hand. With the leverage of your left hand and right hands, the pain generated can be very significant. When you position your right hand, it should be on the upper-arm, as close as possible to the elbow. In addition, your right palm should be facing upward. When you circle both of your hands to control, you should use the entire body to generate power.

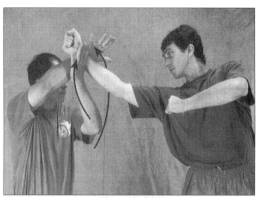

Figure 2–306

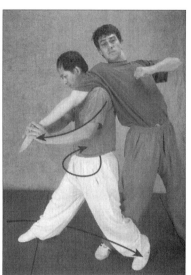

Figure 2–307

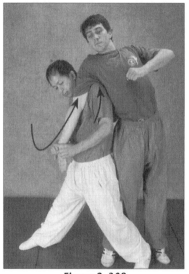

Figure 2–308

Technique #3: One Post to Support the Heavens
(Yi Zhu Ding Tian) 一柱頂天

When your opponent attacks your right temple with his right back fist, first use your right forearm to repel his punch while also clamping your right hand upward on his wrist (Figure 2-306). Next, grab his wrist with both of your hands and turn until his palm is facing upward, while turning your body to your right and placing his upper-arm over your left shoulder (Figure 2-307). Finally, pull his arm down until it is almost vertical to the ground and then lift it upward (Figure 2-308). You should keep lifting until his heels are off the ground, and you should stand as far as possible beyond the reach of his left hand.

Theory:
Misplacing the Bone (shoulder). When you turn your opponent's arm to make his palm face upward, you twist the tendons and ligaments in his shoulder to a tensed condition. If you lift his arm upward, it will cause the ligaments to tear off. Further lifting will dislocate the shoulder joint. When you execute this technique, you may place his upper-arm tendon on your shoulder to increase the pain.

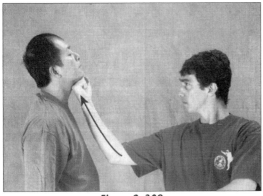

Figure 2–309

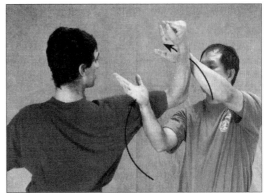

Figure 2–310

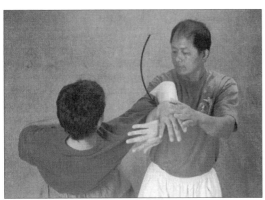

Figure 2–311

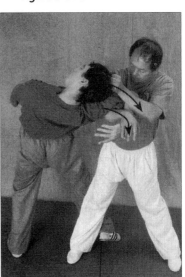

Figure 2–312

C. UPPERCUT PUNCHES TO THE CHIN

Technique #1: Twist the Wing with Both Hands or Forward Upward Turning

(Shuang Shou Ban Chi or Qian Shang Fan) 雙手扳翅，前上翻

If your opponent throws an uppercut punch at your chin with his right fist (Figure 2-309), first you repel his strike to your left with your left forearm, while also placing your right forearm on his elbow area (Figure 2-310). Next, using the leverage of the left hand and your right wrist, bend his right arm and lock it in place (Figure 2-311). In order to control him more effectively, you may let your right hand take over the arm control while using your left hand to pull his hair backward or to push his neck to his left (Figure 2-312). You may also sweep your right leg backward to your opponent's right leg and make him fall. In this technique, it is very important that you stand on the right hand side of your opponent's body to avoid his left hand's strike.

Theory:

Misplacing the Bone (elbow). When you apply this technique, your opponent's arm may be stiff, and this makes it harder for you to bend his arm. The key to making his arm bend is to use the wrist area on your thumb side to hook downward, while pushing your left arm upward. This will provide you with good leverage to bend his arm. In this technique, if you jerk your power suddenly, you may pop out your opponent's elbow joint.

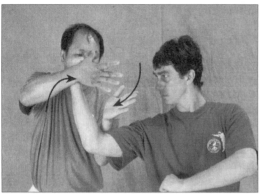

Figure 2-313

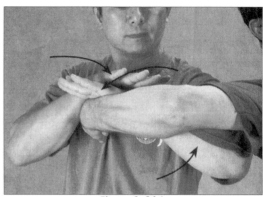

Figure 2-314

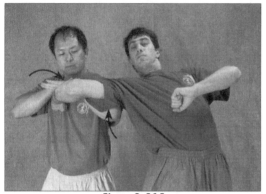

Figure 2-315

Technique #2: Daoist Greets with Hands
(Dao Zi Zuo Ji) 道子作揖

When your opponent throws an uppercut punch at your chin with his right fist, first turn your body to your right and use your left forearm to intercept his elbow, while using the right arm to cover his wrist (Figure 2-313). Then, immediately push your left elbow forward while rotating your right arm backward (Figure 2-314). Finally, lock him into position (Figure 2-315). If necessary, you may dislocate his elbow.

Theory:
Misplacing the Bone (elbow). When you execute this technique, you should beware of his left hand punch. The angle of lock between his upper-arm and forearm is very important. Too straight or too bent will make the technique ineffective.

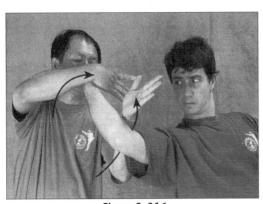

Figure 2–316

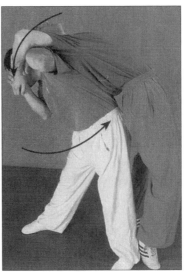

Figure 2–317

Technique #3: The Old Man Carries the Fish on His Back

(Lao Han Bei Yu) 老漢背魚

This is an alternative technique from the last one. When your opponent uses his right fist to uppercut punch your chin, use your right forearm to cover his wrist while using your left forearm to push his right elbow to your right (Figure 2-316). Right after the interception, immediately turn your body to your right and lock your opponent's right arm behind your back (Figure 2-317).

Theory:

Misplacing the Bone (shoulder). In order to lock your opponent's shoulder effectively, the angle must be accurate. When you turn your body and pull, if your opponent's arm is either too straight or too bent, the locking will not be effective.

Technique #4: Luo Han Bows or Small Elbow Wrap

(Luo Han Xing Li or Xiao Chan Zhou) 羅漢行禮，小纏肘

When your opponent throws an uppercut punch at your chin with his right fist, step your right leg back while using your right forearm to repel his attack. As you do so, also place your left hand under his right elbow (Figure 2-318). Next, step your left leg in front of his right leg while circling both of your arms and bowing forward (Figure 2-319). Then, pull him toward the front of your body to destroy his stability and at the same time sweep your left leg backward to make him fall (Figure 2-320). Once he is on the ground, lock his arm behind his back (Figure 2-321). With the help of both your legs, you will be able to lock him there firmly. You may also use both of your hands to twist his head and lock his neck.

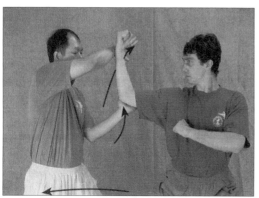

Figure 2–318

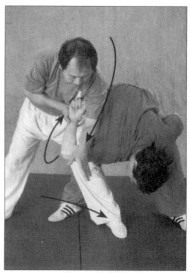

Figure 2–319

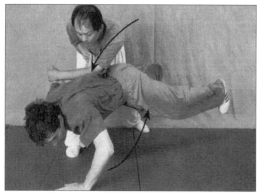

Figure 2–320

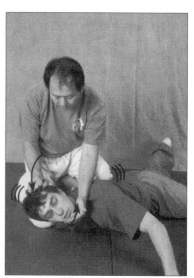

Figure 2–321

Theory:

Misplacing the Bone (elbow). Your right arm's interception of the punch and the left hand's position on his elbow are very important. With the correct rotation of both arms, you can control your opponent's right arm easily. In order to make your opponent fall, after you have locked him you should pull him to your front to destroy his balance, while sweeping your left leg backward. Once your opponent is on the ground, you may push his arm toward his head and pop his shoulder out of joint.

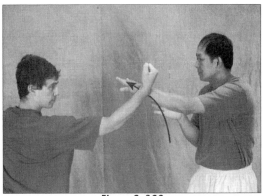

Figure 2–322

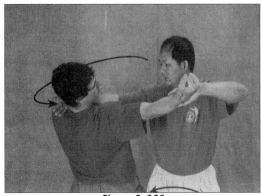

Figure 2–323

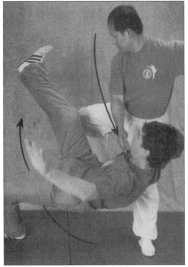

Figure 2–324

Technique #5: The Lame Man Shows His Courtesy

(Bo Zi You Li) 跛子有禮

When your opponent uses his right hand to punch upward to your chin, use your left forearm to repel his punch to your left (Figure 2-322). After your repel, immediately step your right leg behind his right leg and use your right arm to circle his neck (Figure 2-323). Finally, sweep your right leg backward while pressing your right arm forward to make your opponent fall (Figure 2-324).

Theory:

Taking Down. One of the most effective techniques against uppercut punches is the take down. The reason for this is simply that, when your opponent is executing an uppercut punch, the distance between you and him must be close. This will allow you to reach his center and destroy his balance easily. To prevent your opponent from grabbing you with his right hand while falling, right after your interception, try to grab his right arm or shoulder or even push it forward.

II. Against Chest Punch

Because of its improper punching angle, the hook punch to the chest is seldom used. The more common attack to the chest is the straight punch, aimed at the solar plexus or the nipple area. Because straight chest punches are so common in Chinese martial arts, many Qin Na techniques have been developed against them. In this section, we will introduce some of the most common Qin Na techniques which can be used against the straight chest punch. In order to categorize the techniques and make them clear, we will assume that your opponent punches you with his right fist, and the techniques will be discussed

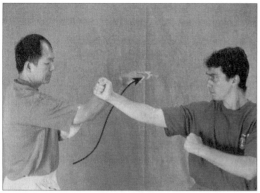

Figure 2–325

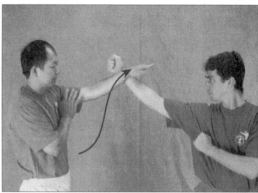

Figure 2–326

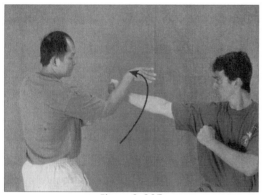

Figure 2–327

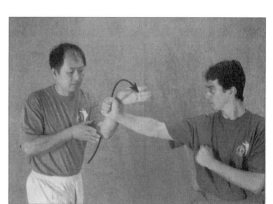

Figure 2–328

by dividing them into four categories: repelling to the right with the right hand (Figure 2-325), repelling to the left with the left hand (Figure 2-326), covering to the left with the right hand (Figure 2-327), and covering to the right with the left hand (Figure 2-328).

A. REPELLING TO THE RIGHT WITH THE RIGHT HAND

Technique #1: Forward Wrist Press, Upward Wrist Press, and Low Inward Wrist Press

(Qian Ya Wan, Shang Ya Wan, and Xia Nei Ya Wan) 前壓腕，上壓腕，下內壓腕

When your opponent punches at your chest with his right fist, use your right forearm to repel the punch to your right while also placing your left hand on his elbow (Figure 2-329). Immediately grab his wrist with your right hand and use the base of your right palm to press his hand, while squeezing your left hand against his elbow (Figure 2-330). With the leverage of both of your hands, you will be able to lock your opponent forward (Figure 2-331), upward (Figure 2-332), or downward, all toward his chest (Figure 2-333).

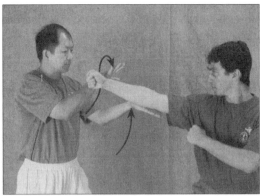

Figure 2–329

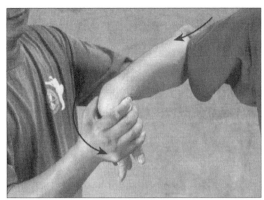

Figure 2–330

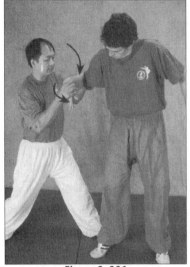

Figure 2–331

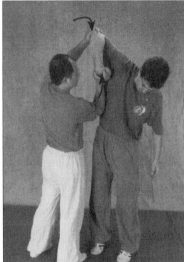

Figure 2–332

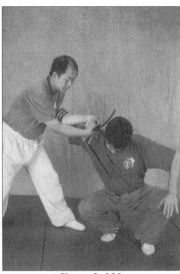

Figure 2–333

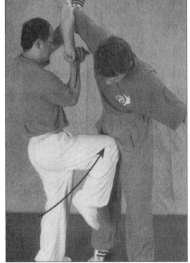

Figure 2–334

Theory:

Dividing the Muscle/Tendon (wrist). In this technique, if your opponent is double jointed in his wrist, your control may not be effective. Once you discover this, immediately use your right knee to kick his groin (Figure 2-334).

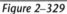

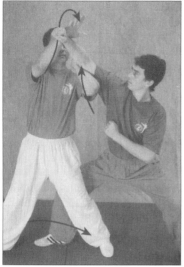

Figure 2–335

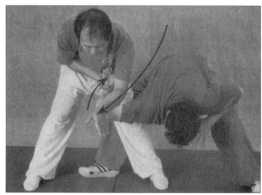

Figure 2–336

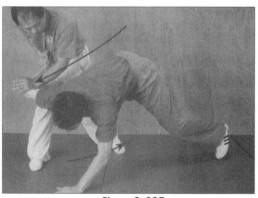

Figure 2–337

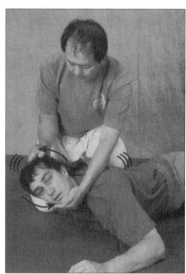

Figure 2–338

Technique #2: Luo Han Bows or Small Elbow Wrap

(Luo Han Xing Li or Xiao Chan Zhou) 羅漢行禮, 小纏肘

In this technique, right after you have repelled the punch, step your left leg to the front of your opponent's right leg, while using your right hand to grab his right wrist and press your left forearm upward against your opponent's right elbow (Figure 2-335). Next, bow your body forward while rotating both of your hands and pulling your opponent's right arm toward the front of your body to destroy his stability (Figure 2-336). Finally, sweep your left leg backward to make your opponent fall (Figure 2-337). When your opponent is on the ground, lock his arm behind his back and use both of your hands to twist his neck (Figure 2-338). With the help of both of your legs, you will be able to lock him there firmly.

Theory:

Misplacing the Bone (elbow). Your right hand's interception of the punch and the left hand's upward pressing on your opponent's elbow are very important. With

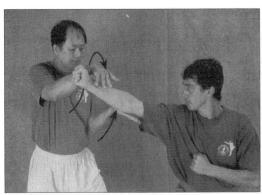

Figure 2-339

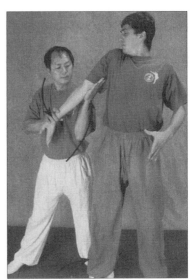

Figure 2-340

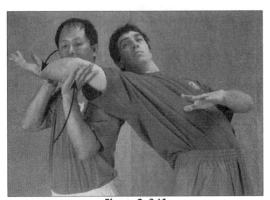

Figure 2-341

correct intercepting, you will be able to lock his arm in place easily. In order to make your opponent fall, after you have locked him, you should pull him to your front to destroy his balance, while sweeping your left leg backward. Once your opponent is on the ground, if necessary, you may push his arm toward his head and pop his shoulder out of joint.

Technique #3: Heaven King Supports the Pagoda or Upward Elbow Press

(Tian Wang Tuo Ta or Shang Ya Zhou) 天王托塔，上壓肘

Once you have repelled your opponent's right fist attack, immediately grab his wrist while placing your left hand on his elbow (Figure 2-339). Next, step in with your left leg and press his wrist down with your right hand, while lifting his elbow upward with your left hand (Figure 2-340). You should increase your controlling power until his heels are off the ground. You should keep yourself on the right hand side of your opponent. This will prevent him from attacking you with his left hand.

Theory:

Misplacing the Bone (elbow). The leverage generated from both of your hands is the key to the control. From the beginning, you should keep your opponent's elbow as straight as possible. If he keeps it bent, it will be difficult to lock him with this technique. However, if he bends his elbow before you have locked him in place, you should immediately push his elbow forward while pulling his wrist toward you (Figure 2-341). In this case, you will still be able to lock him.

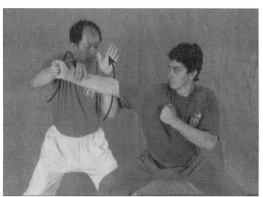

Figure 2–342

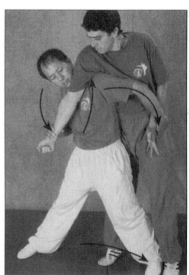

Figure 2–343

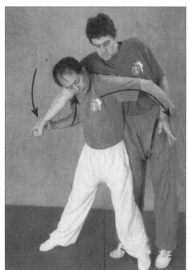

Figure 2–344

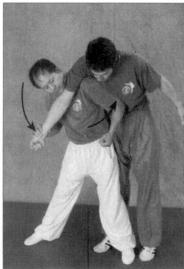

Figure 2–345

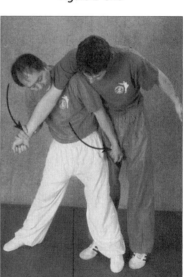

Figure 2–346

Technique #4: Carry a Pole on the Shoulder

(Jian Tiao Bian Dan) 肩挑扁擔

In this technique, again use your right forearm to repel your opponent's punch, and then immediately hook it down while using your left hand to push his elbow to keep his arm straight (Figure 2-342). Next, step your left leg to the front of his right leg, and place your opponent's upper-arm over your left shoulder and lock him (Figure 2-343). In order to prevent him from attacking you with his left hand, you should circle your left arm to wrap his left arm or simply grab it. Through the leverage of your right hand and left shoulder, you can lock him up until his heels are off the ground.

You may also place his arm on your right shoulder (Figure 2-344). Though this will allow you to generate more locking strength, you also take a risk because your opponent will be able to punch you more easily with his left hand. Therefore, you should use your left arm to seal his left arm's movement.

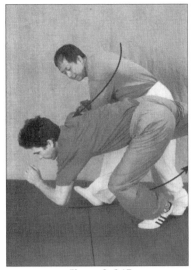

Figure 2–347

If necessary, your left elbow can strike his solar plexus (Figure 2-345). Alternatively, you can also use your left hand to attack his groin to injure him (Figure 2-346). If you push your left arm forward while sweeping your left leg backward, you will be able to take him down (Figure 2-347).

Theory:

Misplacing the Bone (elbow). In order to generate good leverage, you should pull his right hand backward while thrusting your left shoulder forward as in the first option discussed. For the second option, simply pull down his right hand and place his elbow on your right shoulder.

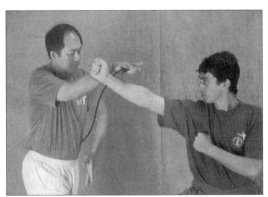

Figure 2–348

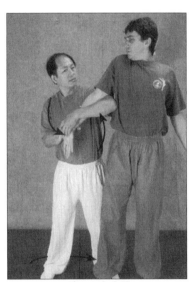

Figure 2–349

Technique #5: Hands Prop a Large Beam or Prop Up Elbow

(Shou Ban Da Liang, Shang Jia Zhou) 手扳大樑，上架肘

When your opponent punches you with his right fist, again use your right arm to intercept his punch (Figure 2-348). Then, immediately step your left leg behind his right leg while placing your left elbow under his right elbow. Finally, use the leverage generated from your hands and left elbow to lock him up until his heels are off the ground (Figure 2-349). Again, you should reposition yourself to avoid his left hand attack.

Theory:

Misplacing the Bone (elbow). When you use your left arm to lock his elbow, to make the technique effective, the position for locking has to be exactly on the elbow. Truly speaking, this technique is safer than the last one. However, you need a strong arm to generate the strong leverage for locking. In this technique, if you suddenly jerk your left arm upward while pushing both of your hands downward, you may break his elbow.

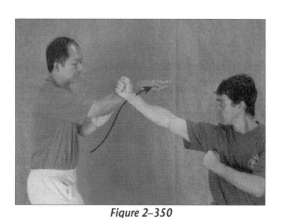

Figure 2–350

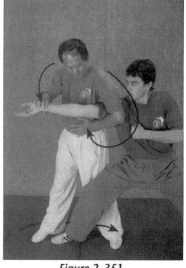

Figure 2–351

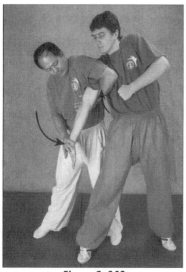

Figure 2–352

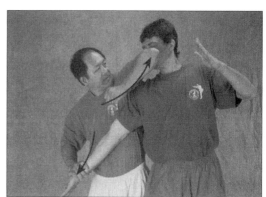

Figure 2–353

Technique #6: Hands Holding a Large Beam

(Shou Wo Da Liang) 手握大樑

After the right repelling interception with your right hand (Figure 2-350), step your left leg behind his right leg while circling your left arm around his right arm (Figure 2-351). Finally, lift your left forearm upward against his upper-arm tendon, while pushing his wrist downward (Figure 2-352). This will generate great pain in his upper-arm.

If you find you cannot control your opponent easily, simply use your left elbow to strike his face (Figure 2-353).

Theory:

Misplacing the Bone (elbow and shoulder) and Pressing Tendon (upper-arm). In this technique, you should beware of your opponent's left hand attack. In addition, if you are shorter than your opponent, it will be harder for your to lock his upper-arm tendon.

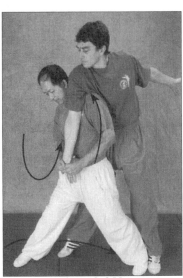

Figure 2–355

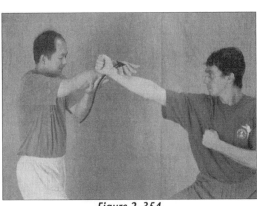

Figure 2–354

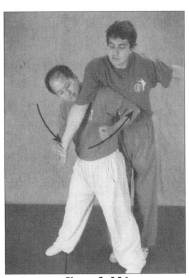

Figure 2–356

Technique #7: One Post to Support the Heavens

(Yi Zhu Ding Tian) 一柱頂天

Right after intercepting with your right forearm, hook your hand down (Figure 2-354). Next, step your left leg to the front of his right leg while placing your left shoulder under his upper-arm, and then lift the arm straight upward (Figure 2-355). When you execute this technique, you should use both hands to grab your opponent's wrist and keep his entire arm straight and vertical to the ground. You should continue your lifting until his heels are off the ground. In addition, you should stand where it is harder for your opponent's left hand to attack.

If necessary, you may use your left elbow to strike the solar plexus to injure your opponent (Figure 2-356).

Theory:

Misplacing the Bone (elbow and shoulder). In this technique, you control the elbow to lock your opponent's arm in position, and lift the arm upward to tear off the ligament of the shoulder. In this locking position, if you jerk your body forward with your opponent's arm, you may pop out his shoulder.

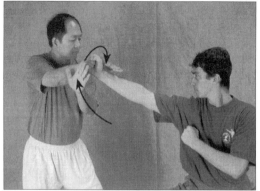

Figure 2–357

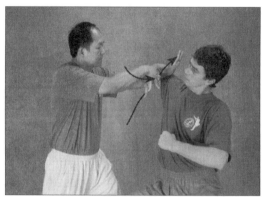

Figure 2–358

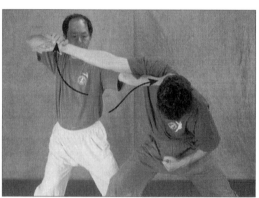

Figure 2–359

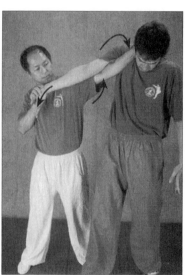

Figure 2–360

Technique #8: Roast Peking Duck

(Bei Ping Kao Ya) 北平烤鴨

In this technique, again use your right forearm to intercept your opponent's punch while placing your left hand under your right arm (Figure 2-357). Next, hook your right hand down to grab his right wrist and push toward him to bend his right arm, while inserting your left hand under his right arm and reaching the back side of his neck (Figure 2-358). Then, circle your right hand until his right palm faces upward to keep his right arm straight (Figure 2-359). Finally, straighten your left arm and push upward on his upper-arm to lock him (Figure 2-360). You should increase your locking power until his heels are off the ground.

Theory:
Misplacing the Bone (elbow and shoulder). Once you have locked your opponent's arm in place, if you push your left hand down against his right shoulder (i.e., your left wrist is bending downward), you may produce significant pain in his shoulder.

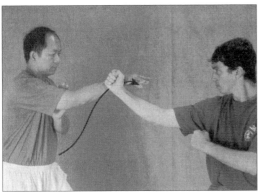

Figure 2–361

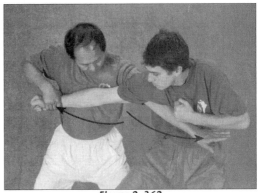

Figure 2–362

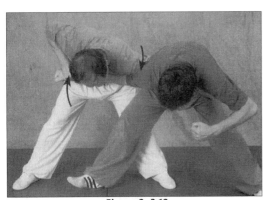

Figure 2–363

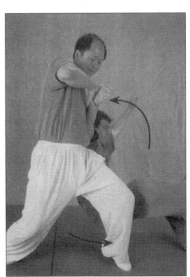

Figure 2–364

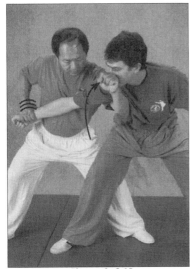

Figure 2–365

Technique #9: Two Children Worship the Buddha

(Shuang Tong Bai Fo) 雙童拜佛

In this technique, again use your right forearm to intercept your opponent's right punch (Figure 2-361). Next, pluck down and grab his right wrist while stepping your left leg behind his right leg, and insert your left arm under his right arm to reach his stomach area (Figure 2-362). Finally, pull your right hand backward and thrust your chest out while bowing the body downward (Figure 2-363). In this case, you will lock your opponent's right arm.

If you desire to take him down, right after your lock, push upward against his upper chest while sweeping your left leg forward to make him fall (Figure 2-364). You may use your left hand to strike upward to his nose (Figure 2-365) or downward to his groin (Figure 2-366).

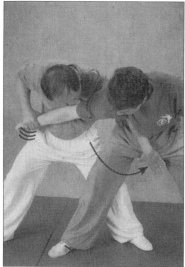

Figure 2–366

Theory:

Misplacing the Bone (elbow). When this technique is used, your opponent can only be controlled for a short time. In fact, often this technique is only used as set up for a nose and/or groin attack.

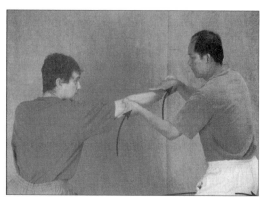

Figure 2–367

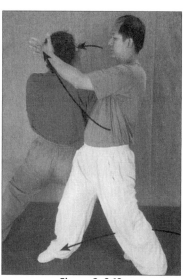

Figure 2–368

Technique #10: Twist the Neck to Kill a Chicken

(Sha Ji Niu Jing) 殺雞扭頸

In this technique, again use your right forearm to repel your opponent's punch to your right and grab his right wrist, while placing your left hand on his right elbow (Figure 2-367). When you intercept, you should also step your right leg backward. Next, step your right leg behind his right leg, and at the same time place your left hand behind his head and right hand on his chin (Figure 2-368). Finally, twist his head to his left and upward to lock his neck (Figure 2-369).

If you desire to take him down, simply sweep your right leg backward while pushing his chin backward (Figure 2-370). If necessary, you may jerk both of your hands diagonally, breaking his neck (Figure 2-371).

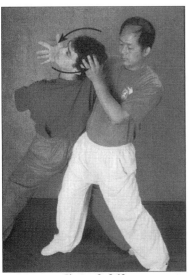

Figure 2–369

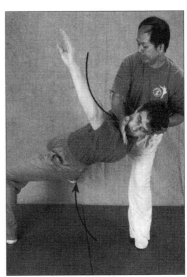

Figure 2–370

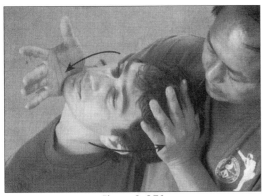

Figure 2–371

Theory:

Misplacing the Bone (neck). In order to prevent your opponent from striking you with his right elbow, your actions must be quick. That means that you must lock your opponent's neck and push his head backward diagonally in a short time. Once you have put him in this position, he will not have good balance and root to generate power for his elbow to attack you.

Technique #11: Force the Bow

(Qiang Po Jiu Gong) 強迫鞠躬

This is a neck locking technique. Right after you have repelled your opponent's right punch with your right hand, grab his wrist and pluck it down immediately (Figure 2-372). Next, step your left leg behind him while inserting your left arm under his left armpit (Figure 2-373). Immediately release your right hand's grabbing and place your right hand on his head, and use both of your hands to push his head downward to lock his neck tightly (Figure 2-374).

If necessary, you may use your knee to kick his *Changqiang* cavity (Gv-1)(Figures 2-375 and 2-376).

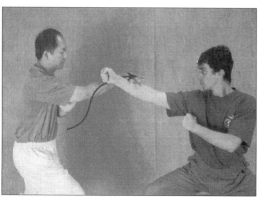

Figure 2–372

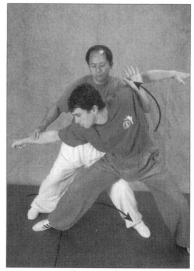

Figure 2–373

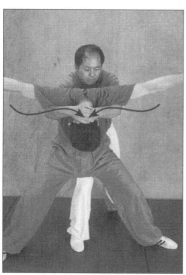

Figure 2–374

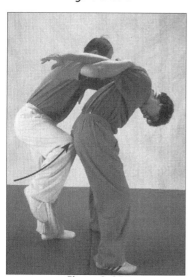

Figure 2–376

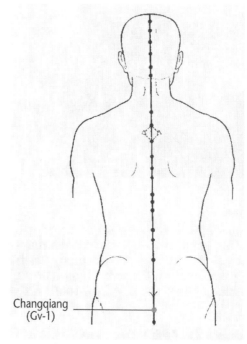

Changqiang
(Gv-1)

Figure 2–375, Changqiang cavity (Gv-1)

Theory:

Misplacing the Bone (neck) and Cavity Press (*Changqiang* cavity). The leverage generated from your elbows and hands is very important. If you do not have good leverage and lock his neck tightly, your opponent can easily slip out by raising both of arms. If your locking is correct, he should not be able to raise his arms and escape. In this Qin Na, you should also beware of a back kick to your shin or groin from his legs. Generally, if you place your right leg or left leg on his Changqiang cavity, his kicking will not be effective.

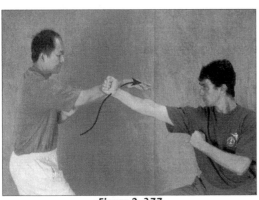

Figure 2–377

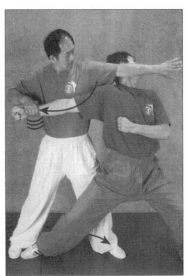

Figure 2–378

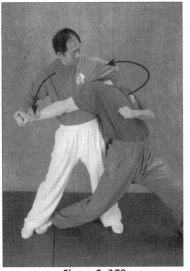

Figure 2–379

Technique #12: Arm Wraps Around the Dragon's Neck

(Bi Chan Long Jing) 臂纏龍頸

In this technique, first use your right forearm to repel his right hand punch (Figure 2-377). Next, step your left leg behind his right leg, while plucking your right hand down to grab his wrist and placing your left arm on his neck (Figure 2-378). Finally, circle your left arm around his neck and bend his body backward (Figure 2-379). In this case, you have locked your opponent's neck.

If you want to take your opponent down, simply sweep his right leg forward with your left leg while pushing his upper body down with your left arm. If necessary, you may increase the locking power on your left arm, and this will cut off the oxygen supply to your opponent and seal his breath. However, you should not do so unless it is a life and death situation.

Theory:

Sealing the Breath (neck). To prevent your opponent from struggling strongly, bend his body backward with your left arm. This will destroy his balance and also his capability for resisting.

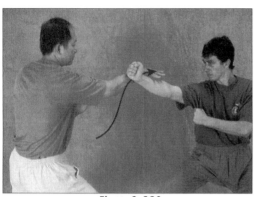

Figure 2–380

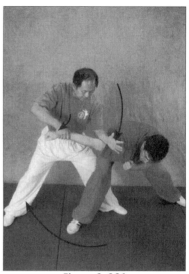

Figure 2–381

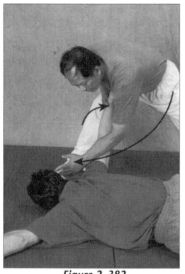

Figure 2–382

Technique #13: White Tiger Turns Its Body

(Bai Hu Zhuan Shen) 白虎轉身

In this technique, right after you intercept your opponent's right hand punch, grab his wrist (Figure 2-380). Immediately step your right leg backward while placing your left forearm on the tendon of his rear upper-arm (Figure 2-381). Finally, through the leverage of both of your hands and the body's rotating power, you may throw him down easily (Figure 2-382).

Theory:

Pressing the Tendon (back side of upper-arm). On the rear side of your upper-arm, there is a big tendon which is usually exposed for pressing. If you press on the correct location, the pain generated is very significant. This will allow you to circle your opponent down easily.

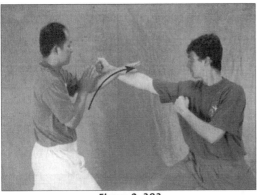

Figure 2–383

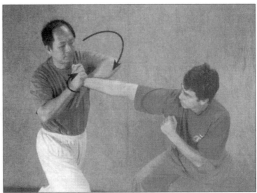

Figure 2–384

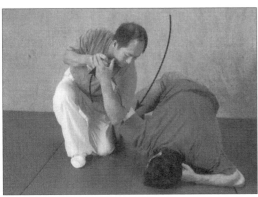

Figure 2–385

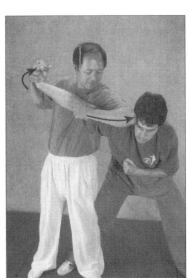

Figure 2–386

B. REPELLING TO THE LEFT WITH THE LEFT HAND

Technique #1: Old Man Promoted to General

(Lao Han Bai Jiang) 老漢拜將

When your opponent punches you with his right fist, first use your left forearm to repel his punch to your left (Figure 2-383). Then, immediately circle your left elbow around his left forearm, while using your right hand to grab his right hand (Figure 2-384). Finally, place his elbow under your left armpit, and use the leverage of your right hand and left shoulder to press him down (Figure 2-385). As you do this, you should also lower your left knee down. This will provide you with a better position for your control.

Another option for this control is to use your left elbow to strike his face or temple (Figure 2-386).

Theory:

Misplacing the Bone (elbow). When you press your opponent down, you should keep his arm straight and the pressing should be straight on the rear side of his elbow. If you jerk your power, you may easily break his elbow.

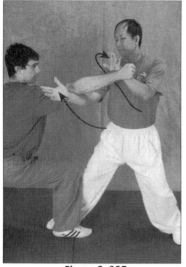

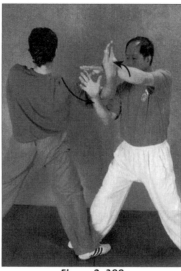

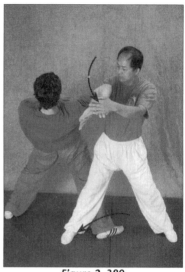

Figure 2–387

Figure 2–388

Figure 2–389

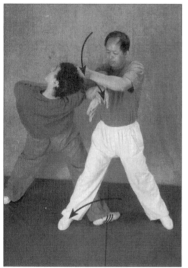

Figure 2–390

Technique #2: Twist the Wing with Both Hands or Forward Upward Turning

(Shuang Shou Ban Chi or Qian Shang Fan)
雙手扳翅，前上翻

When your opponent punches you with his right fist, first repel the strike with your left forearm while placing your right arm under his elbow (Figure 2-387). Next, pull his elbow toward you with your right forearm, while pushing his wrist forward with your left forearm (Figure 2-388). Finally, reposition your right leg behind his right leg, and at the same time lock his arm (Figure 2-389). You may use your right arm to lock his right arm while pulling his hair downward with your left hand (Figure 2-390). You may also use your right leg to sweep your opponent's right leg and make him fall. It is very important that you stand on the right side your opponent's body to avoid his left hand's strike.

Theory:
Misplacing the Bone (elbow). When you apply this technique, your opponent's arm may be stiff. This makes it harder for you to bend his arm. The key to making his arm bend is to use the wrist area on the thumb side to hook downward, while pushing your left arm upward. This will offer you good leverage to bend his arm. In this technique, if you jerk your power suddenly, you may pop out your opponent's elbow.

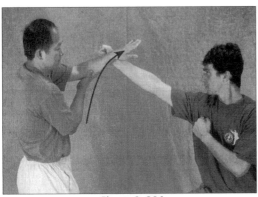

Figure 2–391

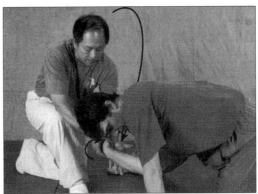

Figure 2–392

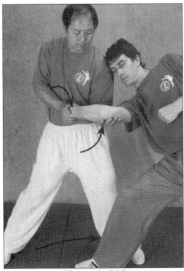

Figure 2–393

Technique #3: Push the Boat to Follow the Stream

(Shun Shui Tui Zhou) 順水推舟

When your opponent punches at your chest with his right fist, again use your left forearm to repel the punch. Then, immediately cover his hand downward and at the same time use your right hand to grab his right hand (Figure 2-391). Finally, use the momentum of the body's rotation to lock your opponent's arm to the ground (Figure 2-392).

Alternatively, when you turn, you may simply use your left hand to lock his right elbow and push it upward while twisting his right wrist with your right hand (Figure 2-393).

Theory:
Dividing the Muscle/Tendon (wrist); In the alternative technique, also included is a Misplacing the Bone (elbow). The hardest part of this technique is to hook downward with your left hand and grab his wrist with your right hand right after your repelling. You must practice until it becomes smooth.

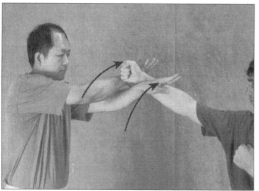

Figure 2–394

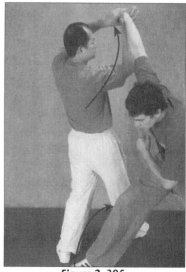

Figure 2–395

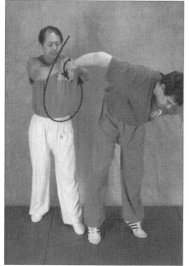

Figure 2–396

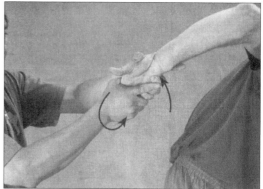

Figure 2–397

Technique #4: Send the Devil to Heaven

(Song Mo Shang Tian) 送魔上天

When your opponent punches at your chest with his right fist, first repel the punch with your left forearm while at the same time placing your right hand on his right wrist (Figure 2-394). Next, grab his right wrist with both of your hands, while stepping your right leg to his right and using your entire body to rotate and twist his right arm (Figure 2-395). Finally, use both of your hands to twist the hand and bend it downward (Figure 2-396). You should increase your twisting and bending pressure until your opponent's heels are off the ground.

To make the control more effective, you may use your left hand to grab and twist his wrist while using your right hand to grab his fingers and pressing them downward (Figure 2-397).

Theory:

Dividing the Muscle/Tendon (wrist). An important point is that, when you have locked your opponent in the final position, you should emphasize the pinkie lock by twisting, which is more efficient and effective.

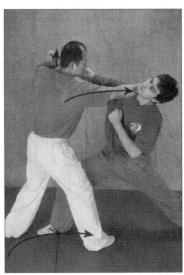

Figure 2-398

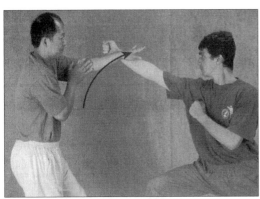

Figure 2-399

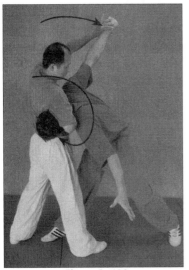

Figure 2-400

Technique #5: The Hand Seizes the Dragon's Head

(Shou Kou Long Tou) 手扣龍頭

When your opponent strikes you with his right fist, first repel his attack with your left forearm, while also repositioning yourself to his right hand side to avoid his left hand attack (Figure 2-398). Next, step your right leg in next to his right leg, while grabbing his right wrist with your left hand and placing your right arm on his neck (Figure 2-399). Finally, circle your right arm around his neck and lock him (Figure 2-400). If you squeeze tightly on the sides of his neck, you may seal his oxygen supply. In just a minute or so, he will begin to lose consciousness. You should not do this unless it is absolutely necessary. This is because if you do not know how to revive your victim, he can die due to lack of oxygen to his brain. Alternatively, you may lift your right forearm and press upward to choke his throat, also sealing his oxygen supply.

Theory:

Sealing the Breath (neck). The position where you stand is very important. Otherwise, you may be attacked by your opponent's left hand.

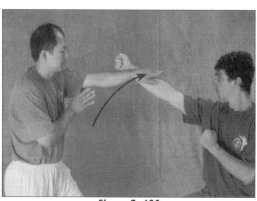

Figure 2–401

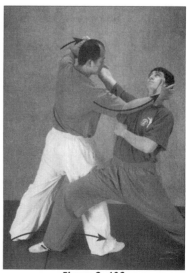

Figure 2–402

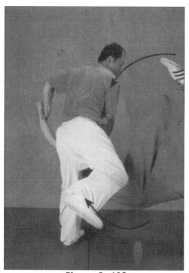

Figure 2–403

Technique #6: The Lame Man Shows His Courtesy
(Bo Zi You Li) 跛子有禮

When your opponent uses his right hand to punch at your chest, use your left forearm to repel his punch to your left (Figure 2-401). Next, step your right leg behind his right leg and use your right arm to push his neck (Figure 2-402). Finally, sweep your right leg backward while pressing your right arm forward to make your opponent fall (Figure 2-403).

Theory:
Taking Down. To prevent your opponent from grabbing you with his right hand while falling, right after your interception, try to grab his right arm or shoulder, or even push it forward.

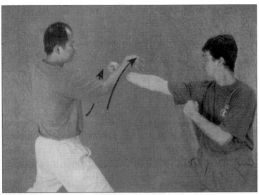

Figure 2-404

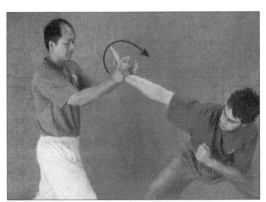

Figure 2-405

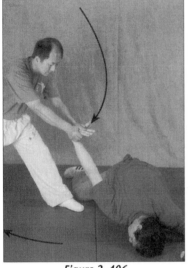

Figure 2-406

C. COVERING TO THE LEFT WITH THE RIGHT HAND

Technique #1: Wild Chicken Spreads Its Wings

(Ye Ji Zhan Chi) 野雞展翅

In this technique, when your opponent punches your chest with his right fist, use your right hand to cover his right wrist while clamping your left hand to grab it (Figure 2-404). Immediately after the grab, turn your opponent's wrist clockwise (Figure 2-405). Finally, step your right leg backward and use both of your hands to press his wrist down (Figure 2-406). You should press him down until his elbow touches the ground.

Theory:

Dividing the Muscle/Tendon (wrist). When you grab, use the entirety of both of your hands to grab, and when you turn your opponent's hand clockwise, you should use your entire body instead of just your arms. When you press your opponent down, the power is generated from the leverage of your pinkies and thumbs. Keep trying until the most effective angle and leverage are found.

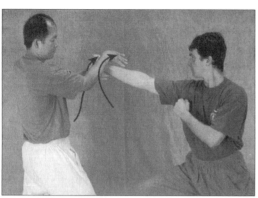

Figure 2–407

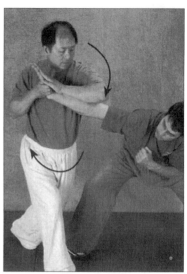

Figure 2–408

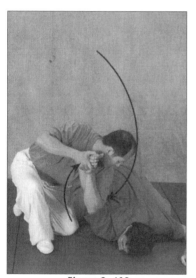

Figure 2–409

Technique #2: Old Man Promoted to General

(Lao Han Bai Jiang) 老漢拜將

When your opponent punches your chest with his right hand, use your right hand to cover the punch while also using your left hand to clamp upward to his wrist and grab it (Figure 2-407). Immediately after grabbing his right wrist with both of your hands, turn your body to your right, while circling your left elbow above his right elbow and placing it under your armpit (Figure 2-408). Finally, use the leverage of both of your hands and left shoulder to press him down to the ground (Figure 2-409).

Theory:

Misplacing the Bone (elbow). When you press your opponent down, you should keep his arm straight and the pressing should be straight on the rear side of his elbow. If you jerk your power, you can easily break his elbow.

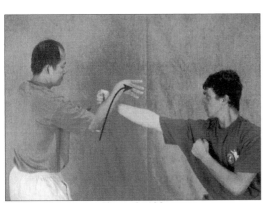

Figure 2–410

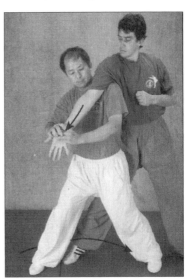

Figure 2–411

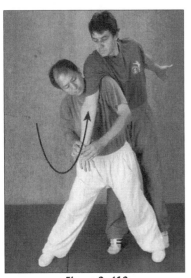

Figure 2–412

Technique #3: One Post to Support the Heavens

(Yi Zhu Ding Tian) 一柱頂天

In this technique, again use your right forearm to cover your opponent's punch (Figure 2-410). Next, step your left leg to the front of his right leg, circle your right hand around his forearm and grab his wrist with both of your hands, while also placing your left shoulder under his upper-arm (Figure 2-411). Finally, lift his arm straight upward against his shoulder (Figure 2-412). Through the leverage of your right hand and left shoulder, you may lock him up until his heels are off the ground.

Theory:

Misplacing the Bone (shoulder). In order to increase the pain, you may place your shoulder against his rear upper-arm tendons.

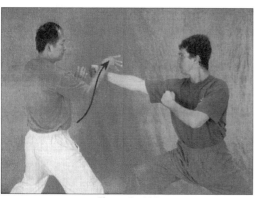

Figure 2–413

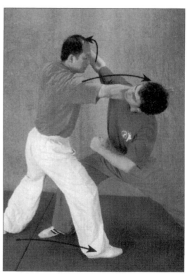

Figure 2–414

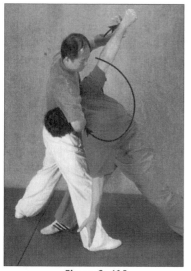

Figure 2–415

Technique #4: The Hand Seizes the Dragon's Head

(Shou Kou Long Tou) 手扣龍頭

When your opponent strikes you with his right fist, first cover his attack with your right forearm while also repositioning yourself to his right side to avoid his left hand attack (Figure 2-413). Next, immediately use your left hand to grab his right wrist, while placing your right arm on his neck (Figure 2-414). Finally, circle your right arm around his neck and squeeze the side of his neck (Figure 2-415). If you squeeze tightly on the sides of his neck, you may seal the oxygen supply to his brain. In just a minute or so, you may make him lose consciousness. You should not do this unless it is necessary. This is because, if you do not know how to revive your victim, he can die due to lack of oxygen to his brain. Alternatively, you can lift your right forearm up, and press upward to choke the front side of his neck, thus sealing his oxygen supply.

Theory:

Sealing the Breath (neck). The position where you stand is very important. Otherwise, you may be attacked by his left hand.

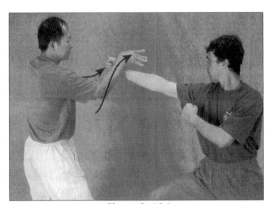

Figure 2-416

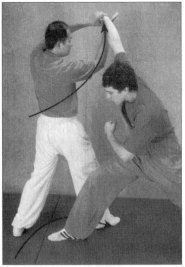

Figure 2-417

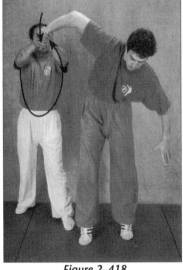

Figure 2-418

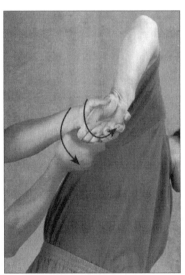

Figure 2-419

Technique #5: Send the Devil to Heaven

(Song Mo Shang Tian) 送魔上天

When your opponent punches at your chest with his right fist, first cover the punch with your right forearm while also using your left hand to grab his right hand (Figure 2-416). Then, use both of your hands to grab his right wrist and hand, step your right leg to his right, and use your entire body to rotate and twist your opponent's arm (Figure 2-417). Finally, use your left hand to twist his wrist, pinkie and entire right hand and bend the fingers downward (Figure 2-418). You should increase your twisting pressure until his heels are off the ground.

Theory:

Dividing the Muscle/Tendon (wrist) and Misplacing the Bone (shoulder). An important point for this technique is that, when you have locked your opponent in the final position, you should emphasize the pinkie twisting with your left hand and bend the fingers downward with your right hand (Figure 2-419).

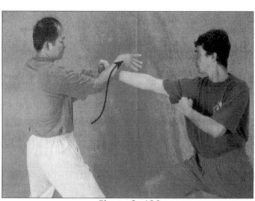

Figure 2–420

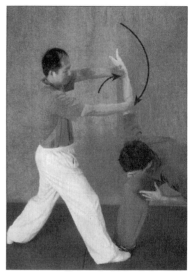

Figure 2–421

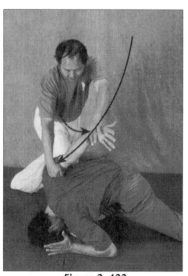

Figure 2–422

Technique #6: Phoenix Spreads Its Wings

(Feng Huang Zhan Chi) 鳳凰展翅

When your opponent punches at you with his right fist, again use your right hand to cover his attack (Figure 2-420). Then, immediately slide your right hand to his elbow, while using your left hand to grab his wrist. Using the leverage of pulling your right hand toward you and your left hand forward, you may easily break your opponent's elbow (Figure 2-421). Alternatively, you may also place your right hand on his shoulder and use it as a leverage point (Figure 2-422).

Theory:

Misplacing the Bone (elbow or shoulder). In order to break your opponent's elbow, you must use a jerking power. Naturally, where you position yourself is very important. A good position will prevent your opponent from attacking you and also offer you a good angle and leverage for your locking.

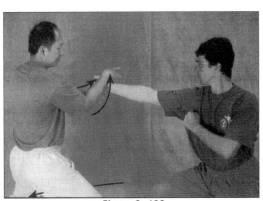

Figure 2–423

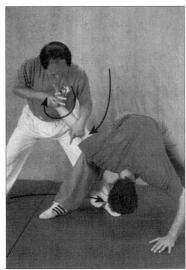

Figure 2–424

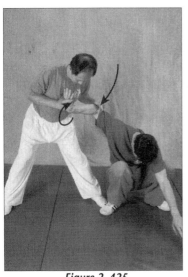

Figure 2–425

Technique #7: White Ape Breaks the Branch

(Bai Yuan Ban Zhi) 白猿扳枝

When your opponent punches at your chest with his right fist, again step your left leg backward, using your right hand to cover the punch while clamping your left hand upward (Figure 2-423). Next, step your left leg behind his right leg, using your right hand to grab his right hand and twisting it clockwise, while placing your left forearm on his elbow and pressing it downward to lock him (Figure 2-424). Alternatively, you may also use your left hand to press his elbow while twisting his right wrist (Figure 2-425).

Theory:

Dividing the Muscle/Tendon (wrist) and Misplacing the Bone (elbow). The key to locking is in the right hand's wrist twisting and the left hand's elbow locking. With good leverage, you should be able to lock him effectively.

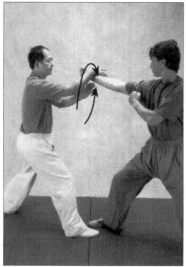
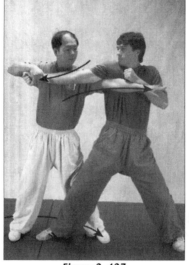
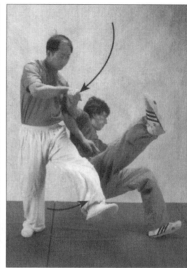

| *Figure 2–426* | *Figure 2–427* | *Figure 2–428* |

Technique #8. Foot Slip the Drunk Fellow

(Jiao Ban Zui Han) 腳拌醉漢

When your opponent attacks you with his right fist, again use your right hand to cover his punch (Figure 2-426). Next, step your left leg in behind his right leg, while moving your left arm under his right arm to reach his neck or upper chest (Figure 2-427). At this time, you should also circle your right hand around his forearm and grab his wrist. Finally, push your left hand backward and downward, while sweeping your left leg forward (Figure 2-428). This will make your opponent fall.

Theory:

Taking Down. Before you step in your left leg, you should have generated sufficient pressure from your left arm push to make your opponent lean backward and destroy his balance. Only then is it safe for you to step in your left leg. If your opponent still has his balance while you are stepping in, he can use his right hand to hook your neck or attack you easily.

Technique #9: Fisherman Spreads his Fishing Net

(Yu Fu Sa Wang) 漁夫撒網

In the last technique, after you have pushed your opponent's upper body backward (Figure 2-429), you may use your right forearm to hook his right knee upward (Figure 2-430) and then use your body's rotation power to throw him to your left (Figure 2-431).

Theory:

Taking Down. Before you step in your left leg, you should have generated sufficient pressure from your left arm push to make your opponent lean backward and destroy his balance. Only then is it safe for you to step in your left leg. If your opponent still has his balance while you are stepping in, he can easily use his right hand to hook your neck or attack you.

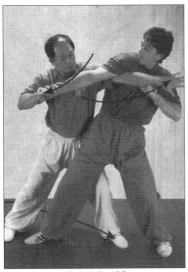

Figure 2–429

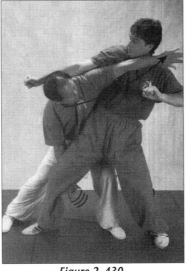

Figure 2–430

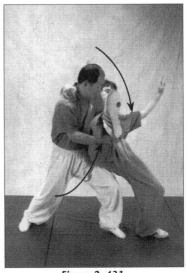

Figure 2–431

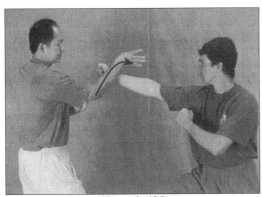

Figure 2–432

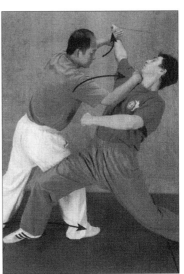

Figure 2–433

Technique #10: The Lame Man Shows His Courtesy

(Bo Zi You Li) 跛子有禮

In this technique, again use your right forearm to cover your opponent's right fist punch (Figure 2-432). Next, step your right leg behind his right leg, while using your left hand to grab your opponent's wrist and moving your right forearm to his upper chest (Figure 2-433). Finally, press your right forearm forward, while sweeping your right leg backward to make your opponent fall (Figure 2-434).

Theory:

Taking Down. Before you step in your right leg, you should have generated sufficient pressure from your right arm's push to make your opponent lean back. Only then is it safe for you to step in your right leg. If your opponent still has his balance, he can easily use his right hand to push you or attack you.

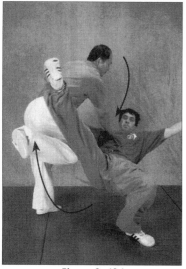

Figure 2–434

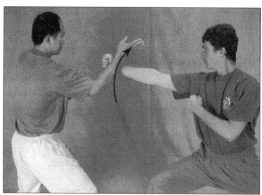

Figure 2–435

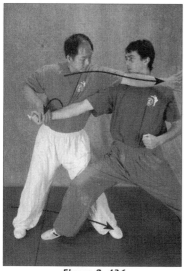

Figure 2–436

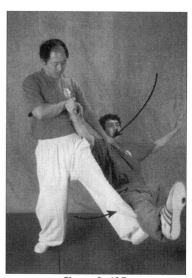

Figure 2–437

Technique #11: Face the Heavens and Fall Down

(Yang Tian Fan Die) 仰天翻跌

In this technique, immediately after your right arm's covering (Figure 2-435), step your left leg behind your opponent's right leg, while circling your right hand to grab his wrist and placing your left forearm on his neck (Figure 2-436). Finally, press your left arm backward while sweeping your left leg forward to make your opponent fall (Figure 2-437).

Theory:

Taking Down. In this technique, you should position yourself on your opponent's right side. This will prevent him from attacking you with his left hand. When you sweep, you should sweep your opponent low and behind, at a forty-five degree angle to his center line. The leverage generated from your right hand and right leg sweep is the main key for power. In addition, while you are sweeping, if you also lift his right arm upward with your left hand, you can destroy his balance much more easily.

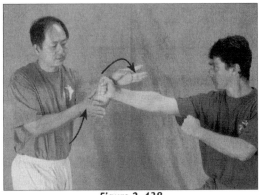

Figure 2–438

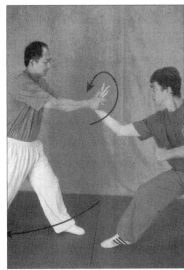

Figure 2–439

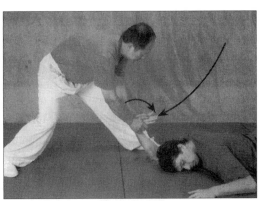

Figure 2–440

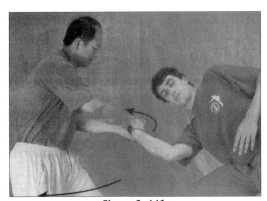

Figure 2–441

D. COVERING TO THE RIGHT WITH THE LEFT HAND

Technique #1: White Ape Worships the Buddha or Reverse Wrist Press

(Bai Yuan Bai Fo or Fan Ya Wan) 白猿拜佛，反壓腕

When your opponent punches at you with his right fist, first use your left forearm to cover his attack while also clamping your right hand upward (Figure 2-438). Next, step your right leg backward, while rotating your opponent's wrist counterclockwise (Figure 2-439) and finally pressing him down (Figure 2-440). You should continue your pressing strength until your opponent's elbow touches the ground. You may also bend and twist his hand to his left for your locking (Figure 2-441).

In this technique, if your opponent tenses his wrist, it will be very difficult for you to control him. In this case, you should use your right hand to attack his eyes first to move his attention away from his wrist (Figure 2-442), then immediately apply the technique. Alternatively, you may also use your right hand to hook his neck (Figure 2-443) and then kick his chest with your right knee (Figure 2-444).

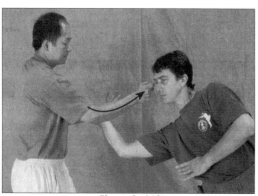
Figure 2–442

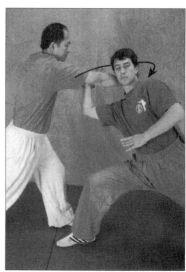
Figure 2–443

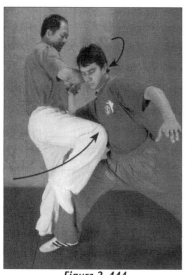
Figure 2–444

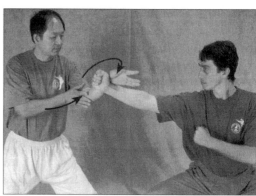
Figure 2–445

Theory:

Dividing the Muscle/Tendon (wrist). The key to control is to use the entirety of both of your hands to generate the pressing pressure instead of just using the thumbs.

Technique #2: White Tiger Turns Its Head or Upward Elbow Wrap

(Bai Hu Fan Shou or Shang Chan Zhou) 白虎返首 ，上纏肘

In this technique, first step your right leg backward and use your left forearm to cover your opponent's right punch, while using your right hand to clamp his wrist upward (Figure 2-445). Next, circle his wrist counterclockwise while twisting his hand with both of your hands (Figure 2-446). Finally, reposition yourself by stepping your left leg behind his right leg, while using your right hand to push his elbow upward and twisting his left hand with your left hand (Figure 2-447). With the leverage of the left and right hands, if you

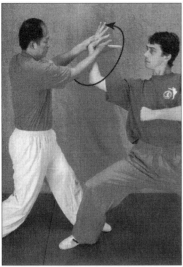

Figure 2–446

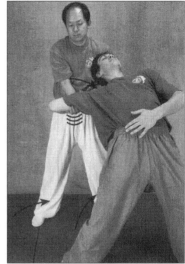

Figure 2–447

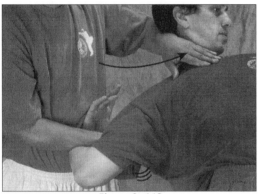

Figure 2–448

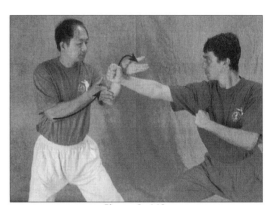

Figure 2–449

squeeze both sides in, you will be able to control him effectively. Alternatively, you may lock his right arm with your right arm and stomach, while pressing your left hand to his right neck to cause pain (Figure 2-448).

Theory:
Dividing the Muscle/Tendon (wrist) and Misplacing the Bone (elbow). In order to increase the control's effectiveness, your left hand must twist your opponent's hand strongly. With the leverage of the left and right hands, the pain generated will be significant. When you position your right hand, it should be on the upper-arm, as close as possible to the elbow. In addition, your right palm should be facing upward. When you circle both of your hands to lock him upward, you should use your entire body to generate power.

Technique #3: The Old Man Carries the Fish on His Back

(Lao Han Bei Yu) 老漢背魚

In this technique, again cover your opponent's punch with your left forearm while clamping your right hand upward to his wrist (Figure 2-449). Next, step your right leg to his back while turning your body to your right (Figure 2-450). As you do so, also place

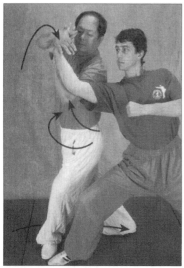

Figure 2–450

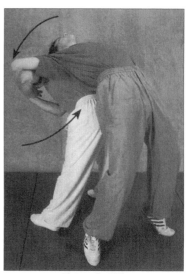

Figure 2–451

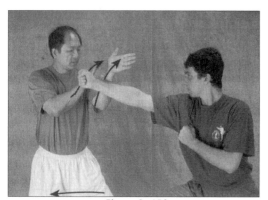

Figure 2–452

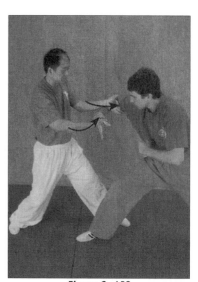

Figure 2–453

your opponent's right elbow on your upper-arm area. Finally, bow forward while pulling your hands downward (Figure 2-451).

Theory:

Misplacing the Bone (shoulder and elbow). The angle at which you control your opponent's arm is very important. If his arm is either too straight or too bent, the control will not be effective. With an accurate angle, you can generate great pain in your opponent's shoulder.

Technique #4: Spiritual Dragon Waves Its Tail or Reverse Elbow Wrap

(Shen Long Bai Wei or Fan Chan Zhou) 神龍擺尾，反纏肘

In this technique, first step your right leg backward and use your left forearm to cover your opponent's right punch (Figure 2-452). Next, grab his wrist with your right hand and push it until its arm is bent, while coiling your left arm around his right arm (Figure 2-453).

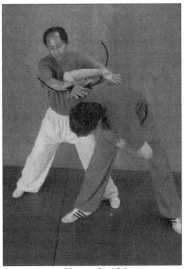
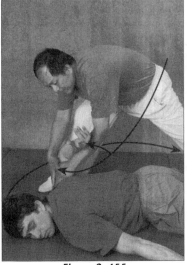
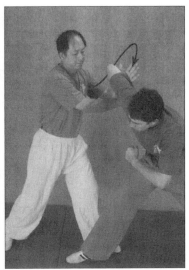

Figure 2–454   Figure 2–455   Figure 2–456

Then, place both of your hands on his upper-arm (Figure 2-454) and step your right leg backward, circling him down (Figure 2-455).

Theory:

Misplacing the Bone (shoulder and elbow). When applying this technique, you should keep your opponent's arm bent at all times. If he is able to straighten his arm, he will be able to get out. The trick to keeping his arm bent is through the help of your right hand and left upper-arm. Once your opponent is on the ground, if you continue your forward pressure, you may pop out his shoulder joint.

Technique #5: Pressing Shoulder with Single Finger and Extending the Neck for Water

(Yi Zhi Ding Jiang and Yin Jing Qiu Shui) 一指頂肩 ， 引頸求水

In the last technique, after you have locked your opponent's arm behind him, all of the tendons and ligaments in his shoulder will be very tense (Figure 2-456). In this situation, if you press your index finger into his *Jianneiling* cavity (M-UE-48), you will be able to generate great pain in his shoulder area (Figure 2-457). You should increase the pressing pressure on your index finger until your opponent's heels leave the floor. Alternatively, you may use your right hand to push his chin upward (Figure 2-458) or even grab his hair and pull it to his right (Figure 2-459). This will also cause great pain.

Theory:

Misplacing the Bone (shoulder), and Cavity Press (*Jianneiling* cavity). When you use your left arm to lock your opponent's right arm and lift it upward, you generate strain on his right shoulder's tendons and ligaments. This action also exposes his *Jianneiling* cavity for your cavity press attack. Without an accurate locking position for the shoulder, the cavity press will not be effective.

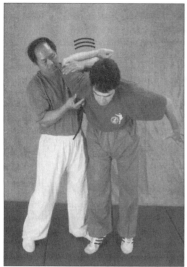

Figure 2–457

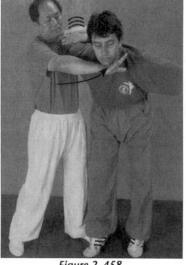

Figure 2–458

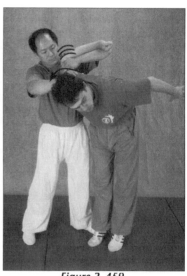

Figure 2–459

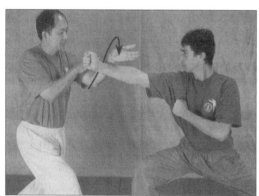

Figure 2–460

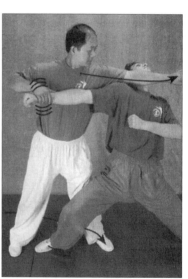

Figure 2–461

Technique #6: Face the Heavens and Fall Down

(Yang Tian Fan Die) 仰天翻跌

When your opponent attacks you with his right fist, again use your left hand to cover his punch (Figure 2-460). Next, step your left leg in behind his right leg and move your left arm to his neck, while also using your right hand to grab his right wrist (Figure 2-461). Finally, push your left arm backward and downward while sweeping your left leg forward (Figure 2-462). This will make your opponent fall.

Theory:

Taking Down. Before you step your left leg in, you should have generated sufficient pressure from your left arm push to make your opponent lean back and destroy his balance. Only then is it safe for you to step in your left leg. If your opponent still has his balance while you are stepping in, he can easily use his right hand to hook your neck or attack you.

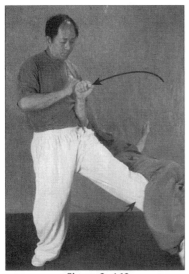

Figure 2–462

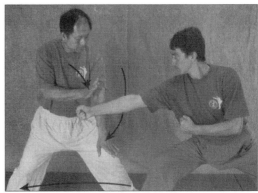

Figure 2–463

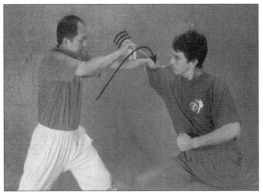

Figure 2–464

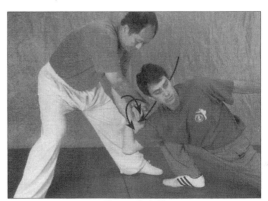

Figure 2–465

III. AGAINST ABDOMINAL PUNCH

A. Straight Punch

Technique #1: Low Outward Wrist Press

(Xia Wai Ya Wan) 下外壓腕

When your opponent punches your abdomen area with his right fist, first step your right leg backward while using your left forearm to repel his punch to your right (Figure 2-463). As you do so, also use your right hand to grab his right fist. Next, push his right hand toward him with your right hand and at the same time circle your left forearm around his right arm (Figure 2-464). Finally, push his elbow downward while increasing the pushing pressure of your right hand on his wrist (Figure 2-465). You should continue your pushing until his knee is down to the ground.

Occasionally, you will find this technique ineffective an opponent who is double jointed. Once you realize this, immediately place his right forearm under your left elbow area, and at the same time use both hands to lift his elbow upward to lock him (Figure 2-466).

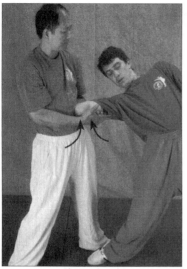

Figure 2–466

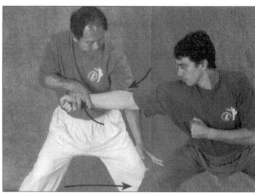

Figure 2–467

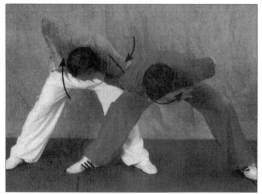

Figure 2–468

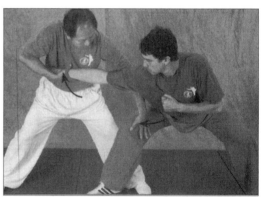

Figure 2–469

Theory:

Dividing the Muscle/Tendon (wrist). Misplacing the Bone (elbow and shoulder for the alternative technique). When you control your opponent's wrist, the pressure generated from the leverage of both hands is very important. With good leverage, the locking can be effective. However, if you have to use the alternative technique, the angle of lifting on the elbow is again important. With the correct angle, the pain generated can be significant. You should try and experiment with different angles until you find the most effective one.

Technique #2: Two Children Worship the Buddha

(Shuang Tong Bai Fo) 雙童拜佛

When your opponent uses his right fist to punch at your stomach area, first step your right leg backward and use your left forearm to repel it to your right (Figure 2-467). As you do so, also use your right hand to grab his wrist. Next, slide your left arm under his armpit and use your left upper-arm to press against the tendon behind his right upper-arm, then bow forward to increase the pressure on his upper-arm to generate pain (Figure 2-468).

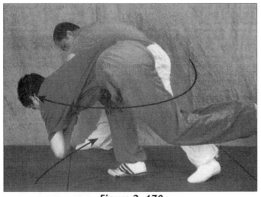

Figure 2–470

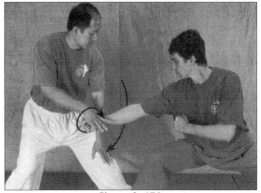

Figure 2–471

Theory:

Pressing the Tendon (upper-arm) and Misplacing the Bone (elbow). In order to effectively control your opponent, press your **left shoulder forward and pull your right hand backward**. The controlling leverage is generated from your left shoulder and your right hand. This technique can only temporarily control your opponent. It is very difficult to dislocate your opponent's elbow using this technique alone.

Technique #3: Tornado Wind Sweeps the Ground

(Xuan Feng Sao Di) 旋風掃地

In this technique, again use your left arm to repel the punch to your right and press your left hand on the internal side of his knee, while using your right hand to grab his wrist (Figure 2-469). Then, step your right leg backward and swing him off balance (Figure 2-470).

Theory:

Pressing the Tendon (upper-arm). In order to effectively control your opponent, you should press your left upper-arm forward and pull your right hand backward. When you press your left arm forward, you should press on the tendons on the back of his upper-arm. You should also press your left hand against the internal side of his knee to generate good leverage for your control. The entire controlling leverage is generated from your left upper-arm and your right hand. This technique is only to take him down.

Technique #4: Lion Worships the Buddha or Large Wrap Elbow

(Shi Zi Bai Fo or Da Chan Zhou) 獅子拜佛，大纏肘

In this technique, first use your left forearm to repel your opponent's punch to your right while using your right hand to grab his right wrist (Figure 2-471). Next, coil your right hand around his forearm, while using your left hand to grab his right wrist and push his arm until it is bent (Figure 2-472). Finally, reposition yourself and press your right hand on the upper-arm near the elbow area, forcing him down (Figure 2-473). If you continue to push his wrist forward with your left hand, you may dislocate his shoulder (Figure 2-474).

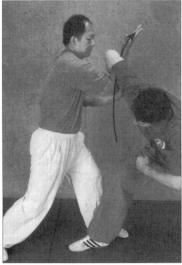

Figure 2–472

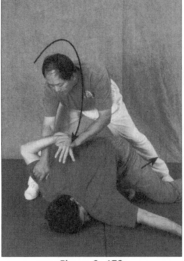

Figure 2–473

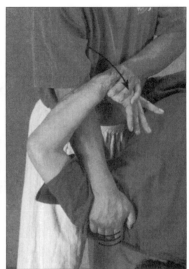

Figure 2–474

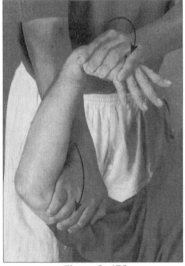

Figure 2–475

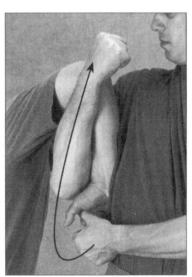

Figure 2–476

Theory:

Misplacing the Bone (shoulder) and Dividing the Muscle/Tendon (wrist). When you circle your right arm to lock your opponent's arm behind him, you should use the entire body's power instead of just the arm. In addition, in order to lock him efficiently, you should place your hand on his upper-arm near the elbow area instead of just on his shoulder (Figure 2-475). If you place your hand on his shoulder, because of the its strength, he may reverse the situation by simply circling his arm forward (Figure 2-476).

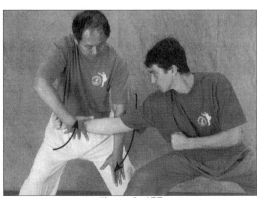

Figure 2–477

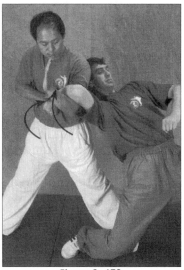

Figure 2–478

Technique #5: Feudal Lord Lifts the Tripod

(Ba Wang Tai Ding) 霸王抬鼎

When your opponent punches your abdominal area, again use your left forearm to repel the attack to your right while using your right hand to grab his right wrist (Figure 2-477). Next, twist his wrist counterclockwise and bend his elbow while lifting your left arm to lock his right arm in place (Figure 2-478).

Theory:

Misplacing the Bone (elbow). In order to make your opponent's elbow bend, the twisting of your right hand and the pressing of your left forearm against his elbow are very important. With good coordination, you may easily bend it.

B. Uppercut Punches to the Stomach

As mentioned earlier, because of the ribs' protection and the awkward punching angle, the chest area is not a common target for uppercut punching attacks. Normally, the uppercut punch is aimed at the stomach area or the chin. Here we will introduce techniques which can be used against uppercut punches to the stomach area.

Technique #1: Feudal Lord Lifts the Tripod

(Ba Wang Tai Ding) 霸王抬鼎

When your opponent throws an uppercut punch at your stomach with his right fist, first step your right leg backward and use your left forearm to intercept the elbow, while using your right arm to intercept his forearm near the wrist area (Figure 2-479). Then, immediately push your left forearm forward, while rotating your right arm backward and locking him in position (Figure 2-480).

Theory:

Misplacing the Bone (elbow). In this technique, if you turn your body to your right, you can change the lock into "The Old Man Carries the Fish on His Back" technique. In this case, you are locking both the elbow and the shoulder.

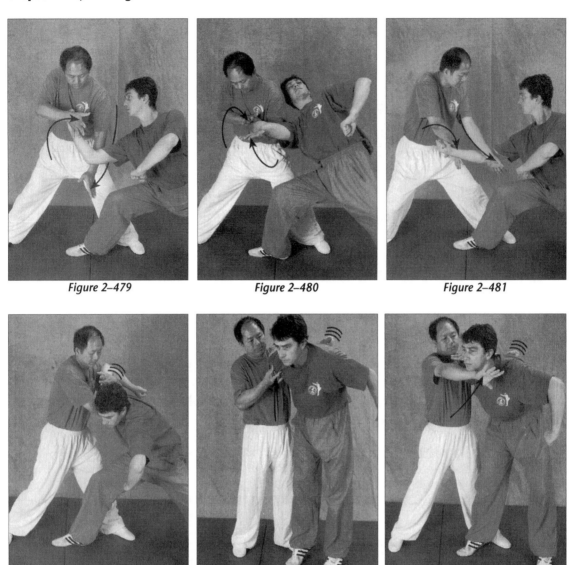

Figure 2–479   *Figure 2–480*   *Figure 2–481*

Figure 2–482   *Figure 2–483*   *Figure 2–484*

Technique #2: Pressing Shoulder with Single Finger and Extending the Neck for Water

(Yi Zhi Ding Jiang and Yin Jing Qiu Shui) 一指頂肩，引頸求水

When your opponent uses his right hand to uppercut punch at your stomach, again use your right forearm to repel his punch to your right, and at the same time place your left hand on his elbow (Figure 2-481). Next, push your right forearm forward to keep his arm bent, while coiling your left hand up to his elbow to lock his arm behind him (Figure 2-482). Right after you have locked his arm, lift his arm up to increase the pain in his shoulder, while using your index finger to press the *Jianneiling* cavity (M-UE-48). This will cause significant pain in his shoulder area. You should increase the pressure on your index finger until your opponent's heels leave the floor (Figure 2-483). Alternatively, you may use your right hand to push his chin upward (Figure 2-484). This will also produce great pain.

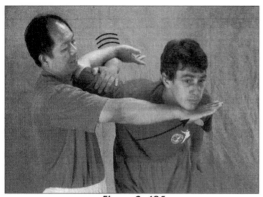

Figure 2–485

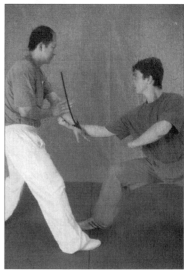

Figure 2–486

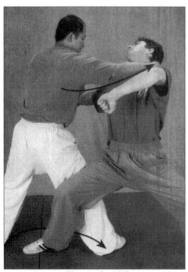

Figure 2–487

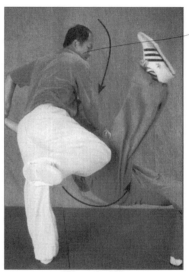

Figure 2–488

Theory:

Misplacing the Bone (shoulder), and Cavity Press (*Jianneiling* cavity). When you use your left arm to lock your opponent's right arm and lift it upward, you generate strain in his right shoulder's tendons and ligaments (Figure 2-485). This action also exposes his *Jianneiling* cavity for your cavity press attack. Without an accurate locking position for the shoulder, the cavity press will not be effective.

Technique #3: The Lame Man Shows His Courtesy

(Bo Zi You Li) 跛子有禮

When your opponent uses his right hand to uppercut punch your stomach, use your left forearm to block his punch to your left (Figure 2-486). Next, step your right leg behind his right leg while placing your right arm on his neck (Figure 2-487). Finally, sweep your right leg backward, while pressing your right arm forward to make your opponent fall (Figure 2-488).

Theory:

Taking Down. One of the most effective techniques against uppercut punches is to take down. The reason for this is that, when your opponent is executing an uppercut punch, the distance between you must be close. This allows you to reach his center and destroy his balance easily. To prevent your opponent from grabbing you with his right hand while falling, right after your left hand interception, try to grab his right arm or shoulder, or even push it forward.

■ Chapter 3 ■

QIN NA AGAINST
BLOCKING

3-1. Introduction

Often Qin Na techniques are applied following a feint, or fake attack. The feint is used to create an opportunity, or to set up the correct controlling angle for the Qin Na. Almost all of the Qin Na techniques are used as follow up techniques when your attacks are either blocked or intercepted.

Generally, when you attack your opponent, your opponent will intercept you with a block. Except for some martial styles such as White Crane, Eagle and Tiger, in which the fingers are commonly used to attack, the most common block uses the forearm to intercept with the fingers closed. Because of this, most of the techniques introduced in this chapter focus on control of the wrists, elbows, and shoulders. Techniques presented here are categorized according to the kind of blocking or intercepting used.

3-2. Qin Na Against Blocks to the Side

In order to prevent your attack reaching his body, your opponent can block or intercept either to the sides, upward, or downward. Therefore, we will divide the available Qin Na techniques according to these three categories.

Normally, blocks to the side are used against attacks to the chest or abdomen area. If the attacks are aimed at the chest area, this category again divides into four different types of blocking. These four include: your opponent blocks your right hand attack with his right hand to his right, or to his left, or he blocks your left hand attack to his right, or to his left.

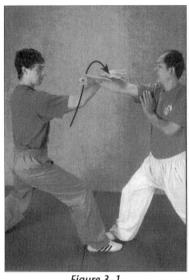
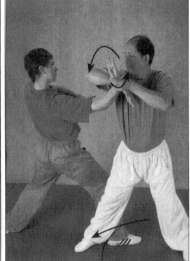
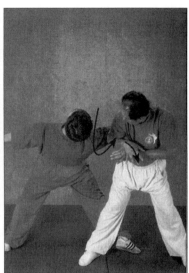

| Figure 3–1 | Figure 3–2 | Figure 3–3 |

We can subdivide the lower attacks into four groups as well. This again includes: your opponent blocks your right hand attack with his right hand to his right, or to his left, or he blocks your left hand attacks to his right, or to his left. Naturally, all of the above descriptions include the possibility that your opponent could use his left hand to block your right hand attacks either to his right or left.

I. ATTACKING THE CHEST

A. RIGHT ARM BLOCKS TO HIS RIGHT (RIGHT HAND ATTACKS)

Technique #1: Sparrow Hawk Shakes Its Wing or Backward Upward Turning

(Yao Zi Dou Chi or Hou Shang Fan) 鷂子抖翅，後上翻

When you attack your opponent with your right fist, if he blocks your punch with his right forearm to his right (Figure 3-1), use your left hand to grab his hand and twist it counterclockwise, while also using your right elbow to circle around his elbow (Figure 3-2). While you are doing so, you should step your right leg behind his right leg. Finally, bend his right wrist downward with your left hand while lifting your right elbow upward to lock his right elbow in position (Figure 3-3). If necessary, in order to increase the pain, you may use your right hand to bend your opponent's right pinkie backward (Figure 3-4).

Alternatively, you may continue your right arm's circling, locking his right arm with your stomach area and right forearm, while also using your left hand to push his chin to his left (Figure 3-5). You may also use your right hand to grab his throat while using left hand to push his head forward (Figure 3-6). When you do this, you should also step your left leg behind him. This will offer you a better angle for leverage.

Theory:
Dividing the Muscle/Tendon (wrist), Misplacing the Bones (elbow, pinkie, and shoulder), and Sealing the Breath (throat). Your stepping to his right is very important in order to prevent your opponent from striking you with his left hand.

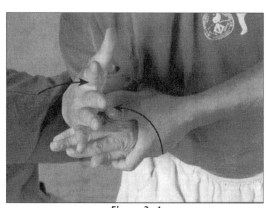

Figure 3–4

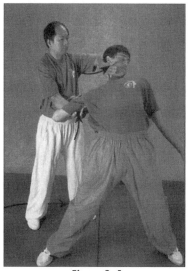

Figure 3–5

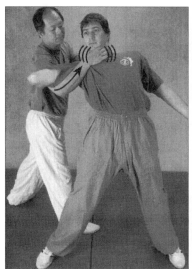

Figure 3–6

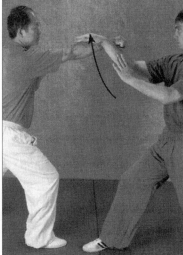

Figure 3–7

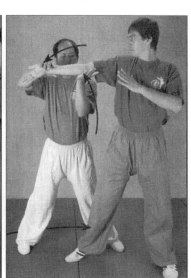

Figure 3–8

Technique #2: Heaven King Supports the Pagoda or Upward Elbow Press

(Tian Wang Tuo Ta or Shang Ya Zhou) 天王托塔 ， 上壓肘

Whenever your right fist attack has been blocked by your opponent's right forearm (Figure 3-7), immediately step your left leg behind his right leg, hook your right hand downward to grab your opponent's right wrist, and turn his wrist counterclockwise while placing your left hand on his elbow to keep his arm straight (Figure 3-8). Finally, using the leverage generated from both of your hands, lock your opponent upward until his heels are off the ground (Figure 3-9). If necessary, you may generate a jerking Jin to break his elbow.

Theory:

Misplacing the Bone (elbow). In order to make your opponent's right arm straight for your locking, you should step your left leg forward to create good pushing leverage for your left hand. With the coordination of both of your hands, you should be able to straighten it out.

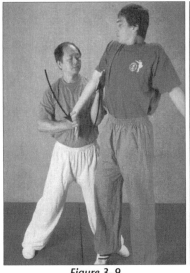

Figure 3–9

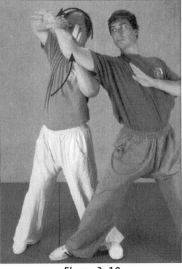

Figure 3–10

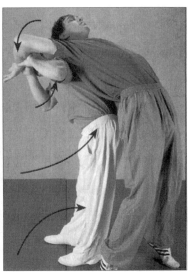

Figure 3–11

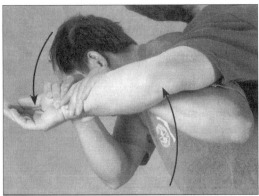

Figure 3–12

Technique #3: The Old Man Carries the Fish on His Back

(Lao Han Bei Yu) 老漢背魚

In the previous technique, if your opponent is very alert and immediately bends his elbow to prevent you from straightening it, you should immediately change your strategy and technique. First, you may simply push his elbow forward with your left hand while pulling his wrist back with your right hand to lock him up (Figure 3-10). Naturally, if you apply more power, you may pop his joint out of its socket.

You may also turn your body to your right and bow forward (Figure 3-11). This will lock his right arm on your left shoulder.

Theory:

Misplacing the Bone (shoulder and elbow). Normally, when your opponent senses that you are going to straighten his elbow, as in the last technique, his natural instinct is to bend his arm. Therefore, you may use the last technique to trick your opponent, and when he bends his arm, immediately use this technique to lock him in position. In order to generate strong power, your pushing and locking should come from your entire body instead of from your arms only. Always look for better leverage to do the job. The angle you set up at his elbow is very important (Figure 3-12). Too straight or too bent will make the technique ineffective.

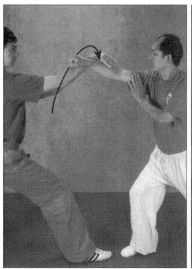

Figure 3–13

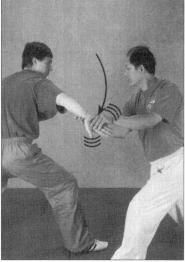

Figure 3–14

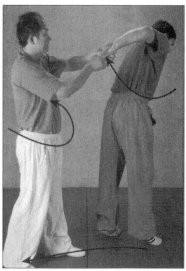

Figure 3–15

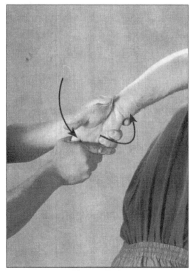

Figure 3–16

Technique #4: Send the Devil to Heaven

(Song Mo Shang Tian) 送魔上天

In the same situation, immediately after your opponent has blocked your right hand punch (Figure 3-13), step your left leg to the his right side and hook your right hand downward to grab his wrist, while also using your left hand to grab your opponent's wrist (Figure 3-14). Next, step your right leg behind him and use the body's turning momentum to twist his arm and wrist, locking his arm up behind his back (Figure 3-15). You should lock him up until his heels are off the ground.

To make the control more effective, use the leverage of your thumb and four fingers of your left hand to twist and bend his pinkie, while using your right hand to grab his fingers and bend them downward (Figure 3-16). This will generate significant pain in his pinkie and wrist area.

Theory:

Dividing the Muscle/Tendon (wrist) and Misplacing the Bone (shoulder). In order to lock your opponent upward, the leverage for twisting generated by your left thumb and pinkie is very important. This will put your opponent's pinkie tendon in a strained condition. If you use your right hand to bend his fingers downward, you can generate great pain. Only with good leverage can the technique be effective. In addition, the strength of your fingers is also important.

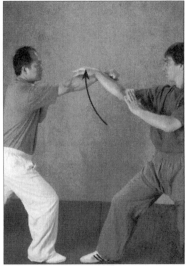

Figure 3–17

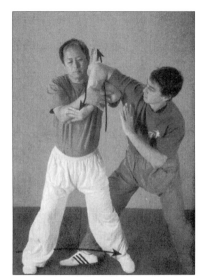

Figure 3–18

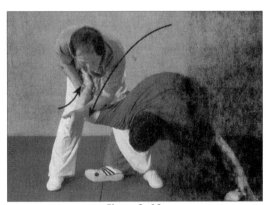

Figure 3–19

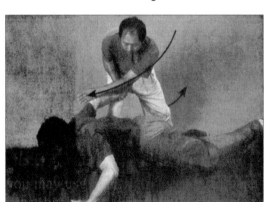

Figure 3–20

Technique #5: Luo Han Bows or Small Elbow Wrap

(Luo Han Xing Li or Xiao Chan Zhou) 羅漢行禮 , 小纏肘

In this technique, when you discover that your punch has been blocked (Figure 3-17), immediately change your strike into a grab and grasp your opponent's right wrist, placing your left forearm on your opponent's right elbow and stepping your left leg in front of his right leg (Figure 3-18). Finally, pull your opponent's right arm toward the front of your body to destroy his stability, while bowing (Figure 3-19). Immediately sweep your left leg backward to make him fall (Figure 3-20). When your opponent is on the ground, lock his arm behind his back with both of your knees, while pulling his hair to his right with your right hand (Figure 3-21).

Theory:

Misplacing the Bone (elbow and shoulder). In order to make your opponent fall, after you have locked him, pull him to your front to destroy his balance while sweeping your left leg backward. Once your opponent is on the ground, if necessary, you may rotate his arm toward his head and pop his shoulder out of joint.

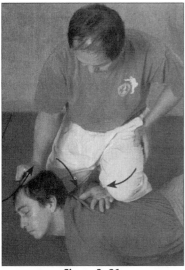

Figure 3–21

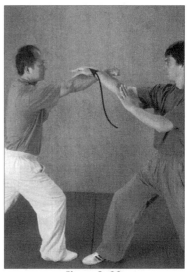

Figure 3–22

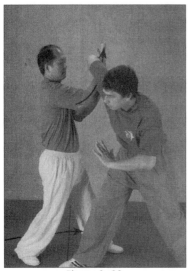

Figure 3–23

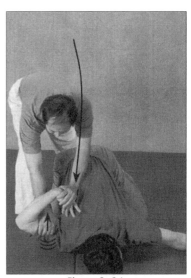

Figure 3–24

Technique #6: Lion Worships the Buddha or Large Elbow Wrap

(Shi Zi Bai Fo or Da Chan Zhou) 獅子拜佛，大纏肘

Immediately after your right hand punch has been blocked (Figure 3-22), hook your right hand down, and at the same time use your left hand to grab his wrist while coiling your right hand to his elbow area (Figure 3-23). While you are doing so, step your left leg behind his right leg. Finally, circle your right arm to lock him down to the ground (Figure 3-24).

Theory:

Misplacing the Bone (shoulder) and Dividing the Muscle/Tendon (wrist). When you circle your right arm to lock your opponent's arm behind him, use your entire body's power instead of just your arm. In addition, in order to lock him efficiently, place your hand on his upper-arm near the elbow area instead on his shoulder.

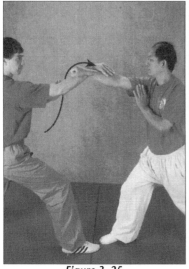

Figure 3–25

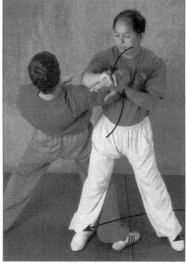

Figure 3–26

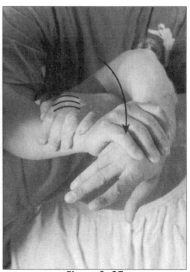

Figure 3–27

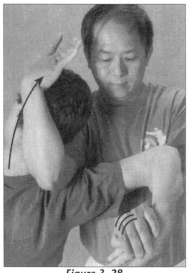

Figure 3–28

Technique #7: The Woodcutter Binds the Woods or Forward Turning Elbow

(Qiao Fu Kun Cai or Qian Fan Zhou)
樵夫捆材，前翻肘

Immediately after your right hand punch has been blocked (Figure 3-25), step your right leg behind his right leg, change your strike into a grab and grasp your opponent's right wrist, while placing your left hand on his elbow and pull it in to lock his arm in place (Figure 3-26). Locking both of your hands is very important to make this technique effective (Figure 3-27).

Alternatively, you may use your left hand to grab his right hand, while using your right forearm to push the back of his head forward (Figure 3-28). This will generate great tension and pain in his entire arm. If necessary, you may pop his arm out of joint easily.

Theory:
Misplacing the Bone (elbow). The position where you stand is very important. When you rotate your opponent's arm, rotate it to a right angle. If his arm is either too straight or too bent, the technique will not be effective.

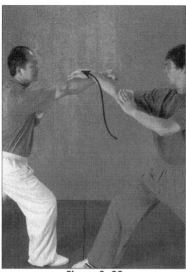 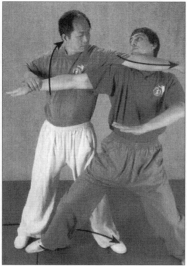 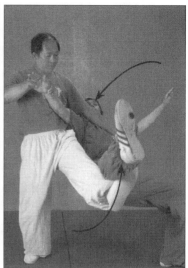

Figure 3–29   *Figure 3–30*   *Figure 3–31*

Technique #8: Face the Heavens and Fall Down

(Yang Tian Fan Die) 仰天翻跌

When your opponent blocks your right hand punch (Figure 4-29), immediately step your left leg behind his right leg, grab his right wrist with your right hand, press his right elbow against your chest, and place your left forearm against his neck (Figure 3-30). Finally, push your left hand backward and downward, while sweeping your left leg forward to make your opponent fall (Figure 3-31).

Theory:
Taking Down. When you step in, place his right elbow on your chest to lock his arm in place.

B. RIGHT ARM BLOCKS TO HIS LEFT (RIGHT HAND ATTACKS)

Technique #1: White Ape Worships the Buddha or Reverse Wrist Press

(Bai Yuan Bai Fo or Fan Ya Wan) 白猿拜佛，反壓腕

In this technique, when you discover that your punch has been intercepted by your opponent's right hand to his left (Figure 3-32), immediately use your left hand to grab his right wrist, and at the same time hook down your right hand while grabbing his right wrist (Figure 3-33). Finally, step your right leg back while pressing him down until his elbow touches the ground (Figure 3-34).

Alternatively, when you press him down, you may twist his hand slightly to the side, and then bend. This will generate more pressure on his wrist tendon and create more pain (Figure 3-35). You may also use your right hand to pull his pinkie backward to increase the pain (Figure 3-36). Naturally, you may use your right forearm to push his neck while twisting his right wrist to his right with your left hand (Figure 3-37). This can generate pain in his right arm.

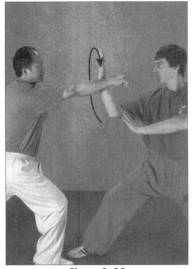

Figure 3–32

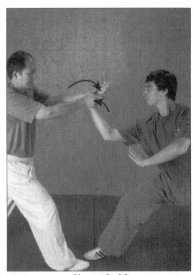

Figure 3–33

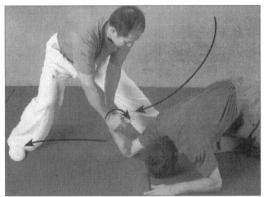

Figure 3–34

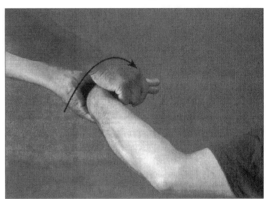

Figure 3–35

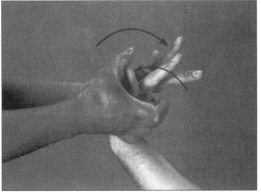

Figure 3–36

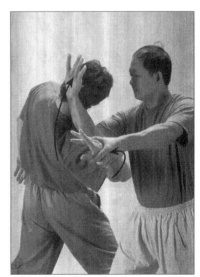

Figure 3–37

Theory:

Dividing the Muscle/Tendon (wrist). In the optional technique, Dividing the Muscle/Tendon (wrist and pinkie) and Misplacing the Bone (pinkie). To make the control effective, you must generate good leverage between your thumbs and pinkie. Once you have locked the hand, press downward with the entirety of both of your hands instead of just the thumbs.

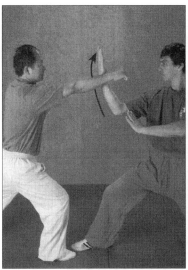 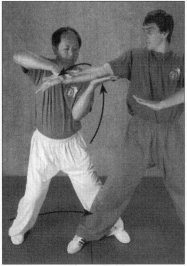 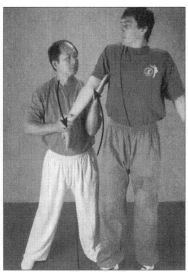

Figure 3–38   *Figure 3–39*   *Figure 3–40*

Technique #2: Heaven King Supports the Pagoda or Upward Elbow Press

(Tian Wang Tuo Ta or Shang Ya Zhou) 天王托塔 ，上壓肘

In the same situation, when you strike your opponent with your right fist and he blocks your attack with his right forearm (Figure 3-38), after you discover that your attack has been blocked, immediately change your right hand into a hook and hook downward so you may grab your opponent's right wrist with your right hand (Figure 3-39). While your right hand is grabbing your opponent's right wrist, also use your left hand to push his right elbow to make it straight, while also stepping your left leg behind his right leg. Finally, using the leverage generated from both of your hands, lock your opponent upward until his heels are off the ground (Figure 3-40). If necessary, you may generate a jerking Jin to break his elbow.

Theory:

Misplacing the Bone (elbow). In order to make your opponent's right arm straight for your locking, step your right leg forward to provide good leverage for your left hand's pushing. In addition, if your step your right leg to his right hand side, you will prevent him from attacking you with his left hand.

Technique #3: White Tiger Turns Its Head or Upward Elbow Wrap

(Bai Hu Fan Shou or Shang Chan Zhou) 白虎返首 ，上纏肘

In this technique, after you realize that your right hand punch has been blocked by your opponent's right hand (Figure 3-41), immediately use your left hand to grab his right hand, and circle your right hand back to his wrist while stepping your left leg behind his right leg (Figure 3-42). Finally, turn your left hand counterclockwise to twist his right wrist while lifting his elbow with your right hand (Figure 3-43). Your body should be behind your opponent's.

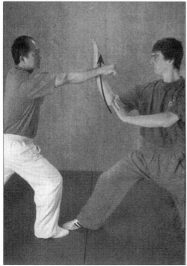

Figure 3–41

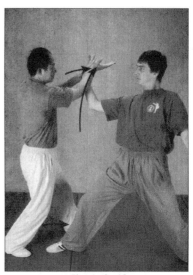

Figure 3–42

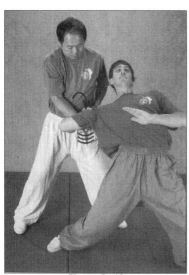

Figure 3–43

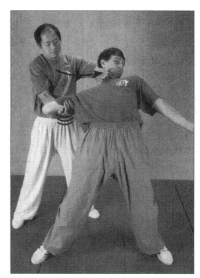

Figure 3–44

Alternatively, you may use your right arm to lock his right arm, while using your left forearm to push his neck (Figure 3-44). In this case, you can generate great pain in his entire right arm.

Theory:

Dividing the Muscle/Tendon (wrist) and Misplacing the Bone (elbow). When you rotate your arms to lock your opponent, use your entire body to direct the motion. Only then will your rotating power be strong. In order to increase the pain, use both of your hands to generate good leverage against your opponent's wrist and upper-arm.

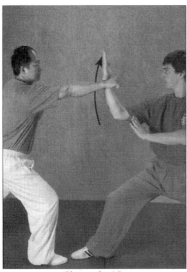

Figure 3–45

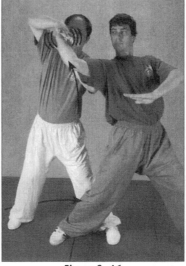

Figure 3–46

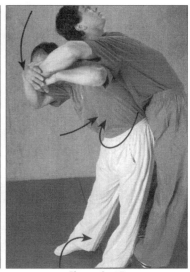

Figure 3–47

Technique #4: The Old Man Carries the Fish on His Back

(Lao Han Bei Yu) 老漢背魚

Again, when your right fist punch has been blocked by your opponent's right hand (Figure 3-45), use your left hand to grab his right wrist while also clamping your right hand backward to grab his right fist (Figure 3-46). When you do this, step your left leg behind his right leg and use your left elbow to push his elbow to his left to keep his elbow bent. Finally, turn your body to your right and bow forward to lock his right arm on your shoulder (Figure 3-47).

Theory:

Misplacing the Bone (shoulder and elbow). To make this technique effective, your opponent's arm should be neither too straight nor too bent. In order to generate strong power, your locking should be generated from your entire body's bowing. Always look for better leverage to do the job.

Technique #5: Send the Devil to Heaven

(Song Mo Shang Tian) 送魔上天

In the same situation, right after your opponent has blocked your right hand punch (Figure 3-48), immediately hook your right hand downward while using your left hand to clamp upward to grab your opponent's right wrist with both of your hands (Figure 3-49). Once you have grabbed his right wrist, immediately circle his right arm down and step your right leg beside his right leg, rotating your body (Figure 3-50). Finally, step your leg behind his body and use both of your hands to bend his wrist downward, locking him up until his heels are off the ground (Figure 3-51). The best control for the final position is to use your left hand to twist his hands clockwise, while using your right hand to grab his fingers and bend them downward (Figure 3-52).

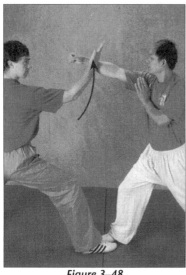
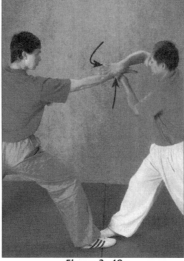
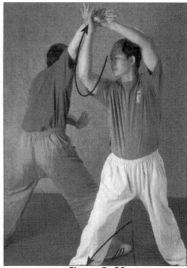

| Figure 3–48 | Figure 3–49 | Figure 3–50 |

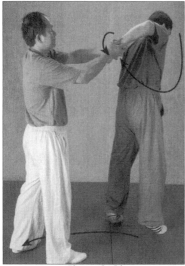
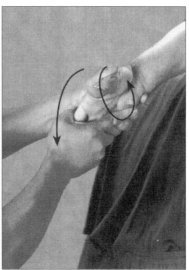

| Figure 3–51 | Figure 3–52 |

Theory:

Dividing the Muscle/Tendon (wrist) and Misplacing the Bone (shoulder). In order to lock your opponent upward, the leverage generated from the thumbs and index fingers of both of your hands is very important. Only with good leverage will the technique be effective. In addition, the strength of your fingers is very important. If you have weak finger strength and small hands, this technique will be very difficult for you.

Technique #6: The Lame Man Shows His Courtesy

(Bo Zi You Li) 跛子有禮

When your opponent uses his right hand to block your punch to his left (Figure 3-53), use your left hand to repel and grab his right hand, while stepping your right leg behind his right leg and using your right arm to circle his neck (Figure 3-54). Finally, sweep your right leg backward while pressing your right arm forward to make him fall (Figure 3-55).

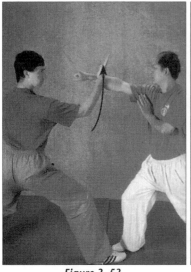

Figure 3-53

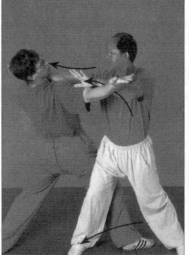

Figure 3-54

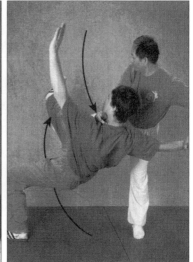

Figure 3-55

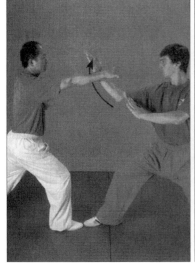

Figure 3-56

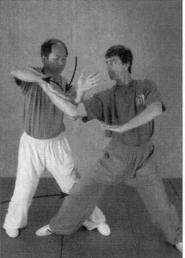

Figure 3-57

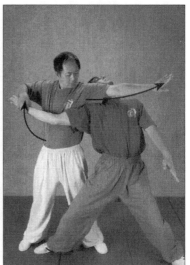

Figure 3-58

Theory:

Taking Down. In order to control your opponent's right arm more efficiently, use your left hand to grab his right hand and then twist it counterclockwise. This locking presents a good opportunity to step in and sweep your right leg.

Technique #7: Face the Heavens and Fall Down

(Yang Tian Fan Die) 仰 天 翻 跌

When your opponent has blocked your right hand punch to his left (Figure 3-56), immediately hook your right hand down and coil it around your opponent's wrist. Grab the wrist while stepping your left leg behind his right leg and pushing your left forearm against his right elbow (Figure 3-57). Next, lock his right arm against your chest while placing your left arm on his neck (Figure 3-58). Finally, push your left arm backward and downward, while sweeping your left leg forward (Figure 3-59). This will make your opponent fall.

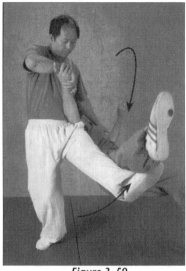

Figure 3–59

Theory:

Taking Down. When you step in, place his right elbow on your chest to lock his arm in place. His arm should be bent. Naturally, you may circle your left arm around his neck to seal his breath.

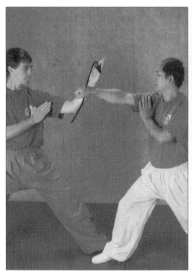

Figure 3–60

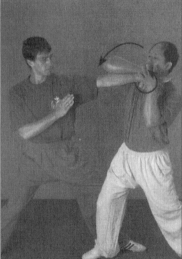

Figure 3–61

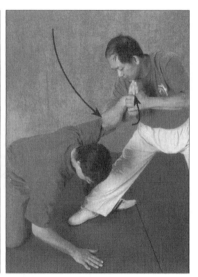

Figure 3–62

C. LEFT ARM BLOCKS TO HIS RIGHT (RIGHT HAND ATTACKS)

Technique #1: Forgive Me for not Going with You

(Shu Bu Tong Xing) 恕不同行

When your opponent intercepts your right hand punch to his right with his left arm (Figure 3-60), immediately use your left hand to grab his left hand, twisting it counterclockwise while placing your right arm over his left arm (Figure 3-61). Finally, use your right elbow to bend his left elbow, and bend your body to your right to lock him in position (Figure 3-62).

Theory:

Dividing the Muscle/Tendon (wrist). In order to lock your opponent effectively, your left hand grab must be firm and strong and your right arm should keep his arm bent. Only then will you generate great pain in your opponent's wrist when you bend to your right.

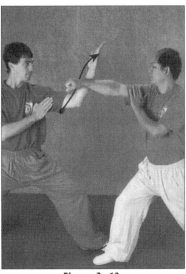
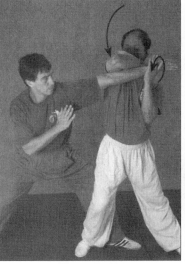
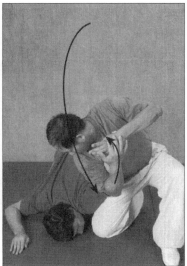

Figure 3–63   Figure 3–64   Figure 3–65

Technique #2: Old Man Promoted to General

(Lao Han Bai Jiang) 老漢拜將

When your opponent covers your right hand punch to his right with his left hand (Figure 3-63), again use your left hand to grab his left wrist, while placing your right armpit above his elbow (Figure 3-64). However, this time keep his elbow straight. Finally, use the leverage of your left hand and right shoulder to press him down (Figure 3-65). As you do this, also kneel down on your right leg; this will position you for better control.

Theory:

Misplacing the Bone (elbow) and Dividing the Muscle/Tendon (wrist). When you press your opponent down, keep his arm straight. The pressing should be straight on the back of his elbow. If you jerk your power, you may break his elbow easily.

Technique #3: Low Outward Wrist Press

(Xia Wai Ya Wan) 下外壓腕

When your opponent covers your right hand punch to his right with his left hand (Figure 3-66), again use your left hand to grab his left hand. Immediately circle your right forearm upward and then downward to coil around your opponent's forearm and reach his elbow (Figure 3-67). Then, use your right hand to push his elbow down until it is perpendicular to the ground, while using your left hand to press his hand downward to generate pain in his wrist (Figure 3-68).

Theory:

Dividing the Muscle/Tendon (wrist). In this technique, you do not generate any pain in your opponent's elbow. You right hand serves only to lock the arm in the correct position for your left hand's control. The actual pain originates in the wrist. The leverage for control is generated from the base of the palm, and the thumb and middle finger of your left hand, which is grabbing your opponent's wrist.

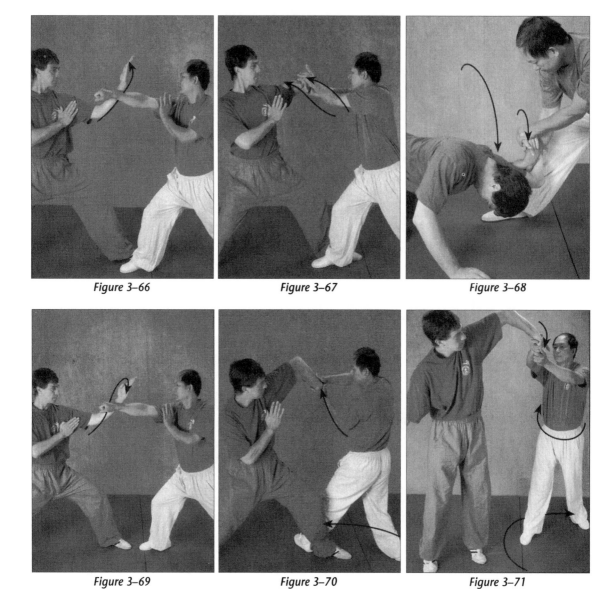

Figure 3–66   Figure 3–67   Figure 3–68

Figure 3–69   Figure 3–70   Figure 3–71

Technique #4: Send the Devil to Heaven

(Song Mo Shang Tian) 送魔上天

When your opponent covers your right hand punch to his right with his left hand (Figure 3-69), again use your left hand to grab his left hand while stepping your left leg beside his left leg (Figure 3-70). Finally, step your right leg again, turn your body clockwise and reposition yourself to his left hand side, while using both of your hands to twist his wrist and pinkie to lock him upward (Figure 3-71). You should increase your twisting and bending pressure until your opponent's heels are off the ground.

Theory:

Dividing the Muscle/Tendon (wrist) and Misplacing the Bone (shoulder). An important point to make this technique effective is that, when you have locked your opponent in the final position, emphasize the pinkie locking, which is more

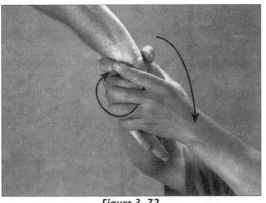

Figure 3–72

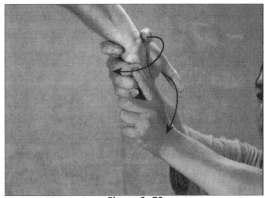

Figure 3–73

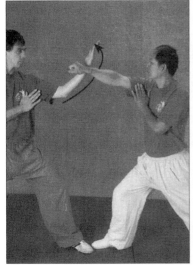

Figure 3–74

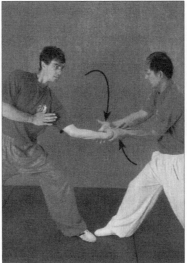

Figure 3–75

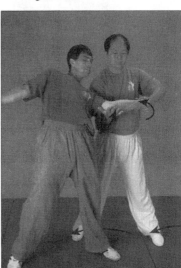

Figure 3–76

efficient and effective. With good pinkie twisting and wrist bending, your control can be effective (Figure 3-72). The most effective way to lock your opponent is to use your right hand to twist the pinkie to lock the hand, while using your left hand to grab the fingers and bend them downward (Figure 3-73).

Technique #5: Lion Shakes Its Head

(Shi Zi Yao Tou) 獅子搖頭

When your opponent has covered your right hand punch to his right with his left hand (Figure 3-74), immediately use your right hand to hook his forearm down and at the same time use your left hand to grab his left wrist (Figure 3-75). Finally, move your right hand to his elbow and push your right hand to your left and upward, while twisting his wrist with your left hand (Figure 3-76). In order to prevent him from attacking you with his right hand, step your right leg behind his left leg when you lock his elbow upward.

Theory:

Dividing the Muscle/Tendon (wrist) and Misplacing the Bone (elbow). The leverage generated from the left hand and the right hand is a very important key for this locking. Your left hand should twist his wrist strongly, and your right hand should generate good leverage for your left hand's twisting and bending.

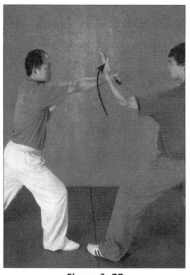

Figure 3–77

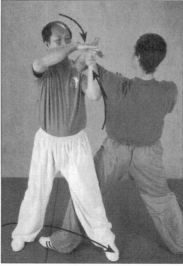

Figure 3–78

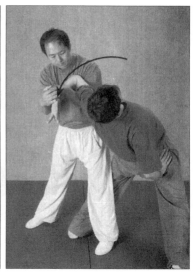

Figure 3–79

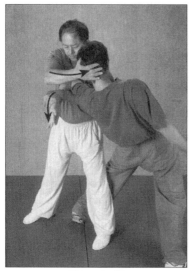

Figure 3–80

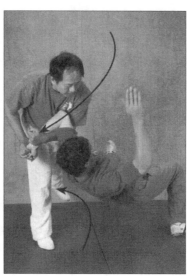

Figure 3–81

Technique #6: Twist the Wing with Both Hands or Forward Upward Turning

(Shuang Shou Ban Chi or Qian Shang Fan) 雙手扳翅，前上翻

When your right hand punch has been covered by your opponent's left forearm to his right (Figure 3-77), immediately use your right hand to hook down his left wrist, while also using your left hand to pull his left elbow toward you (Figure 3-78). As you do this, step your left leg behind his left leg. Finally, use both of your hands to bend his arm backward (Figure 3-79). In order to increase the pain, you may use your left hand to lock his arm while using your right hand to push his head forward (Figure 3-80). You may also sweep your left leg backward to make him fall (Figure 3-81).

Theory:

Misplacing the Bones (elbow and shoulder). In order to prevent your opponent from striking you with his right hand, your stepping to his left is very important. In addition, this stepping will offer you an additional option which allows your to sweep his leg and make him fall.

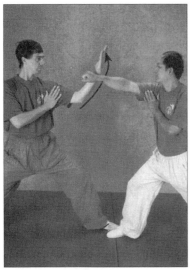

Figure 3–82

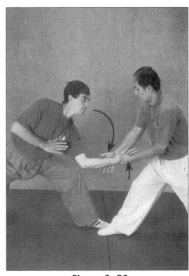

Figure 3–83

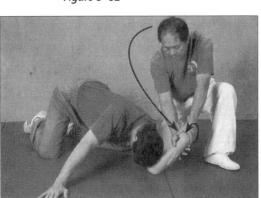

Figure 3–84

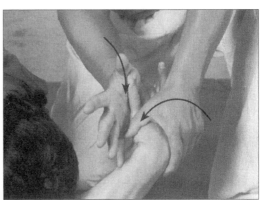

Figure 3–85

Technique #7: Push the Boat to Follow the Stream

(Shun Shui Tui Zhou) 順水推舟

Again, when your right hand punch has been intercepted by your opponent's left forearm to his right (Figure 3-82), immediately hook your right hand down and at the same time grab his left wrist with your left hand (Figure 3-83). Finally, squat down and turn your body to your left while swinging your arm down and lock him to the ground (Figure 3-84).

In order to increase the pain, after you have locked him down, you may use your right hand to push his pinkie backward (Figure 3-85). Alternatively, you may use your left hand to twist his left wrist, while using your right hand to push his neck to generate good leverage for his arm's locking (Figure 3-86).

Theory:

Dividing the Muscle/Tendon (wrist), Misplacing the Bone (pinkie in 1st option, elbow and shoulder in 2nd option). When you swing your opponent down to the ground, use your entire body's momentum instead of just using arms. Remember, good Qin Na techniques always use the body to generate power.

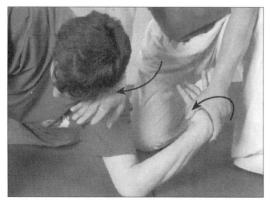

Figure 3–86

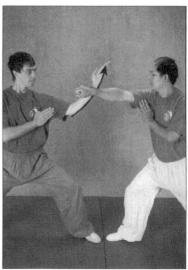

Figure 3–87

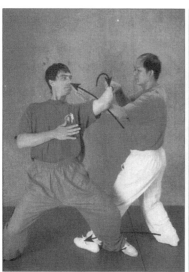

Figure 3–88

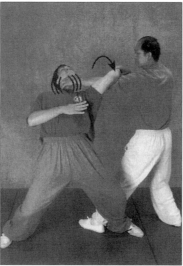

Figure 3–89

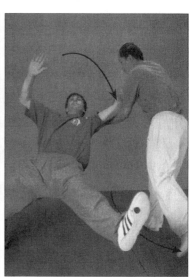

Figure 3–90

Technique #8: Eagle Claw to Seal the Throat

(Ying Zhua Suo Hou) 鷹爪鎖喉

When your opponent has covered your right hand punch with his left hand (Figure 3-87), immediately step your left leg behind his left leg and push his left hand backward, while using your left elbow to pull in his left elbow (Figure 3-88). Next, place your left hand on his throat to grab it (Figure 3-89). If you squeeze your left fingers tightly, you can choke your opponent's throat and seal his breath. This, however, might crush his windpipe, and should only be done if necessary.

Alternatively, you may use your left hand to push his neck, while sweeping your left leg backward to make your opponent fall (Figure 3-90).

Theory:

Sealing the Breath (throat) and Taking Down. In order to prevent your opponent from attacking you with his right hand, also push your left hand forward and make his body lean backward, destroying his balance.

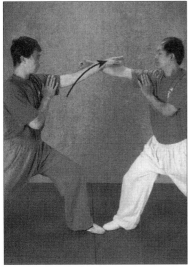

Figure 3–91

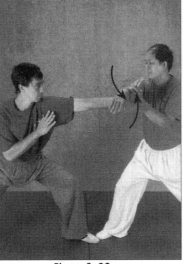

Figure 3–92

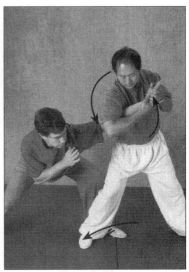

Figure 3–93

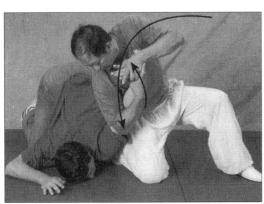

Figure 3–94

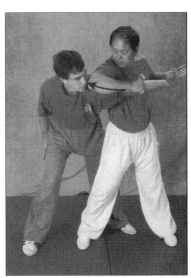

Figure 3–95

D. LEFT ARM BLOCKS TO HIS LEFT (RIGHT HAND ATTACKS)

Technique #1: Old Man Promoted to General

(Lao Han Bai Jiang) 老漢拜將

When your opponent repels your right hand punch with his left forearm to his left (Figure 3-91), immediately hook down your right hand and use your left hand to grab his left hand (Figure 3-92). Then, place your armpit on his elbow (Figure 3-93). Finally, use the leverage of your left hand and right shoulder to press him down (Figure 3-94). As you do this, kneel down on your right leg. This is a better position for control.

The option for this control is to use your right elbow to strike his face or temple (Figure 3-95). The other option is, when you have placed your right armpit on his elbow, if

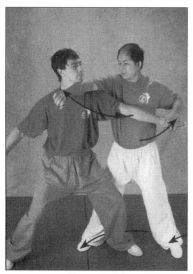

Figure 3–96

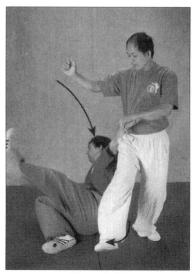

Figure 3–97

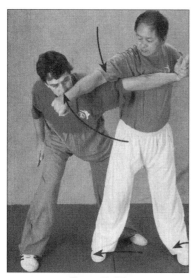

Figure 3–98

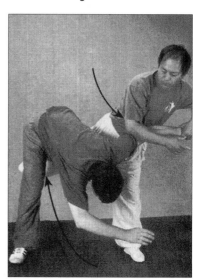

Figure 3–99

your right leg is behind his left leg (Figure 3-96), you may use your right forearm to push his neck while sweeping your right leg forward against his left leg (Figure 3-97). However, if your right leg is in the front of his left leg (Figure 3-98), simply press your right chest forward against his elbow while sweeping your right leg backward to make him fall (Figure 3-99).

Theory:

Misplacing the Bone (elbow). When you press your opponent down, keep his arm straight. The pressing should be directly on the rear side of his elbow. If you jerk your power, you may break his elbow easily.

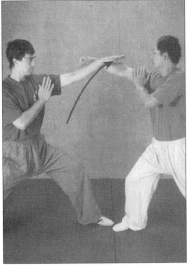
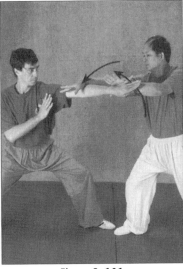
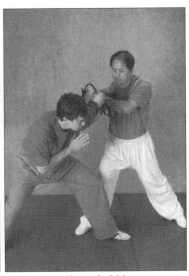

Figure 3–100   *Figure 3–101*   *Figure 3–102*

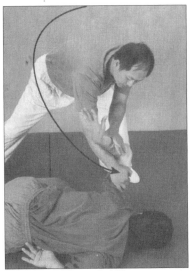

Figure 3–103

Technique #2: Spiritual Dragon Waves Its Tail or Reverse Elbow Wrap

(Shen Long Bai Wei or Fan Chan Zhou)

神龍擺尾，反纏肘

In this technique, when your punch has been repelled by your opponent's left forearm to his left (Figure 3-100), immediately use your left hand to grab his left wrist while coiling your right hand forward to reach his left elbow (Figure 3-101). Next, use your left hand to push his arm in and bend it while circling your right hand around his left arm to reach his upper-arm (Figure 3-102). Finally, release your left hand and continue to lock his left arm with your right arm while repositioning yourself behind his left leg, making a circle. Then press him down until his body reaches the ground (Figure 3-103). Once he is on the ground, immediately sit on his shoulder, pull his arm backward, and pull his hair upward to place his neck on your calf (Figure 3-104). In this case, you have locked both his left arm and his neck.

Theory:

Misplacing the Bone (shoulder and elbow) and also Sealing the Breathing (neck in option). When you apply this technique, keep your opponent's arm bent at all times. If he is able to straighten his arm, he will be able to get out. The trick to keeping his arm bent is to use the help of your left hand and right upper-arm to keep it bent. Once your opponent is on the ground, if you continue your pressure forward, you may pop his shoulder joint out of its socket easily.

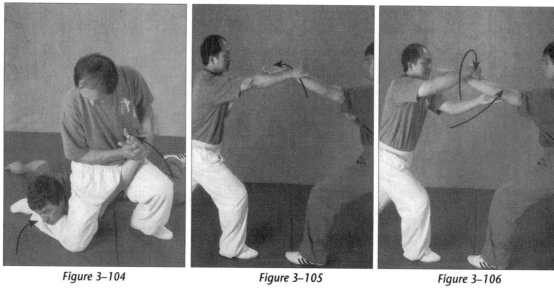

| Figure 3–104 | Figure 3–105 | Figure 3–106 |

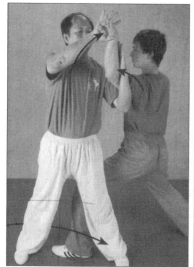
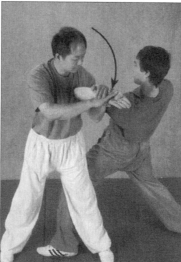
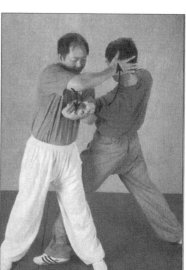

| Figure 3–107 | Figure 3–108 | Figure 3–109 |

Technique #3: The Woodcutter Binds the Wood or Forward Turning Elbow

(Qiao Fu Kun Cai or Qian Fan Zhou) 樵夫捆材，前翻肘

After your right hand punch has been repelled (Figure 3-105), immediately circle your right hand around his forearm and grab his wrist while placing your left hand on his elbow (Figure 3-106). Next, push his wrist forward, while pulling his elbow backward to bend his arm and stepping your left leg behind his left leg (Figure 3-107). Finally, use the leverage generated from both of your hands to lock his arm in place (Figure 3-108). In order to increase the locking efficiency, use your left hand to lock his arm while using your right hand to push his head forward (Figure 3-109). If you wish to take him down, sweep your left leg backward while rotating his left arm forward and downward.

Theory:

Misplacing the Bone (elbow). The position where you stand is very important. When you rotate your opponent's arm, rotate it at a right angle. If his arm is either too straight or too bent the technique will be ineffective.

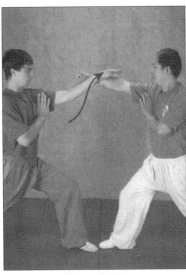
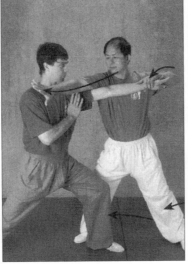
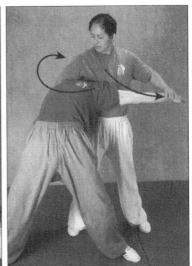

| Figure 3-110 | Figure 3-111 | Figure 3-112 |

Technique #4: Arm Wraps Around the Dragon's Neck

(Bi Chan Long Jing) 臂纏龍頸

In this technique, immediately after your punch has been repelled (Figure 3-110), push his left forearm to his right while using your left hand to grab his left wrist. Next, step your right leg behind his left leg, while pulling his left arm straight and placing your right arm on his neck (Figure 3-111). Finally, circle your right arm around his neck and bend his body backward (Figure 3-112). In this case, you have locked your opponent's neck.

If you want to take your opponent down, simply sweep your right leg forward while pushing his upper body down with your left arm. If necessary, you may increase your locking power on your right arm; this will seal the artery and cut off the oxygen supply to his brain. However, do not do so unless it is a life and death situation.

Theory:
Sealing the Breath (neck). To prevent your opponent from struggling strongly, simply bend his body backward with your right arm. This will destroy his balance and his capability for resisting.

Technique #5: Send the Devil to Heaven

(Song Mo Shang Tian) 送魔上天

When your opponent repels your right hand punch with his left forearm to his left (Figure 3-113), immediately step your left leg behind his left leg, hook your right hand down and grab his left wrist while also using your left hand to grab his left hand (Figure 3-114). Next, step your right leg behind him while using your entire body's turning momentum to twist and bend his wrist to lock him upward (Figure 3-115). You should increase your twisting and bending pressure until your opponent's heels are off the ground.

Theory:
Dividing the Muscle/Tendon (wrist) and Misplacing the Bone (shoulder). When you have locked your opponent in the final position, the trick to making this technique effective is to emphasize the pinkie's twisting and his wrist's bending.

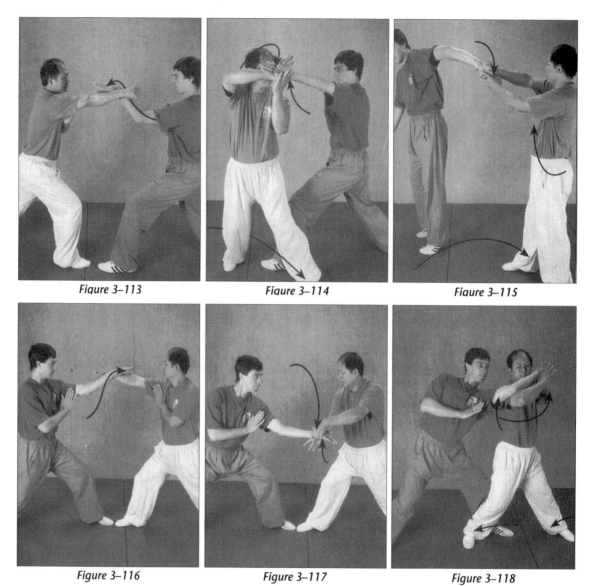

Figure 3–113　　　　　Figure 3–114　　　　　Figure 3–115

Figure 3–116　　　　　Figure 3–117　　　　　Figure 3–118

Technique #6: The Old Man Carries the Fish on His Back

(Lao Han Bei Yu) 老漢背魚

When your right hand punch has been repelled by your opponent's left hand (Figure 3-116), immediately use both of your hands to grab his left wrist (Figure 3-117). Next, step in your right leg to the front of his left leg and turn your body to your left, while using your right elbow to push his left elbow and keep it bent (Figure 3-118). Finally, pull his wrist down while bowing forward to generate pressure on his elbow and shoulder joints (Figure 3-119). If you increase your control pressure or jerk your controlling power suddenly, you may pull his shoulder out of its socket.

Theory:

Misplacing the Bone (shoulder and elbow). The angle you use to control your opponent's arm is very important. If you opponent's arm is either too straight or too bent, the control will not be effective. With an accurate angle, you may generate great pain in your opponent's shoulder.

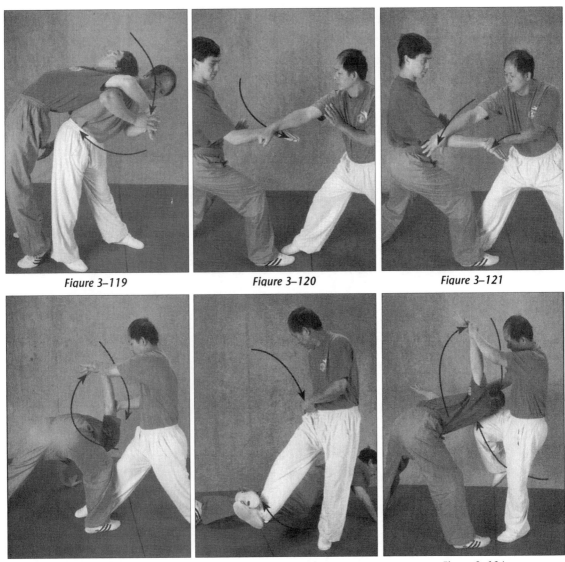

Figure 3–119　　　　　Figure 3–120　　　　　Figure 3–121

Figure 3–122　　　　　Figure 3–123　　　　　Figure 3–124

II. ATTACKING THE ABDOMEN

A. RIGHT ARM BLOCKS TO HIS RIGHT (RIGHT HAND ATTACKS)

Technique #1: Phoenix Spreads Its Wings

(Feng Huang Zhan Chi) 鳳凰展翅

When your opponent uses his right forearm to block your abdomen attack to his right (Figure 3-120), immediately use your left hand to grab his right wrist, while moving your right hand to his elbow or upper arm (Figure 3-121). Finally, use the leverage generated from both of your hands to lock his right arm up (Figure 3-122).

If you wish to take him down, simply sweep your right leg to his right leg while increasing the locking pressure on his right arm (Figure 3-123). Naturally, you can also use your right knee to kick his head or your foot to kick his groin (Figure 3-124).

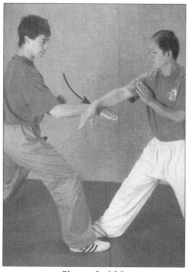
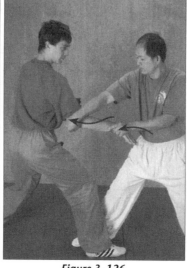
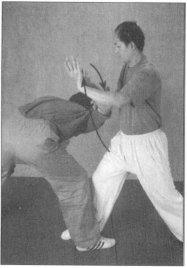

| Figure 3–125 | Figure 3–126 | Figure 3–127 |

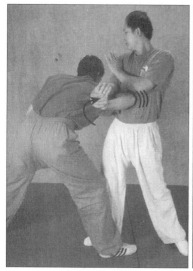
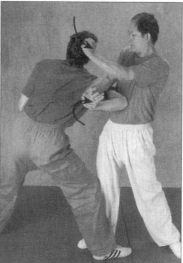

| Figure 3–128 | Figure 3–129 |

Theory:

Misplacing the Bone (shoulder and elbow). How you use the leverage to rotate, circle, and lock your opponent's right arm is very important to make this technique effective. When you lock your opponent's arm behind him, use your entire body's jerking power.

Technique #2: Hands Hold Panda

(Shou Bao Wan Xiong) 手抱浣熊

This technique is very similar to the last technique. When your abdominal attack has been repelled by your opponent's right hand to his right (Figure 3-125), use your left hand to grab his right wrist while placing your right hand on his elbow (Figure 3-126). Immediately, twist his arm and bend it behind his back (Figure 3-127). Finally, lock his right arm by your right hand and your stomach (Figure 3-128). In order to prevent him from attacking you with his left hand, you may simply use your left hand to grab his hair and pull it backward and downward (Figure 3-129).

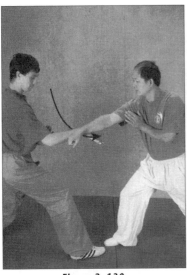

Figure 3–130

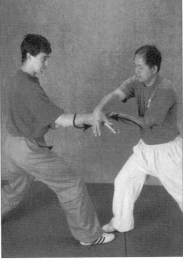

Figure 3–131

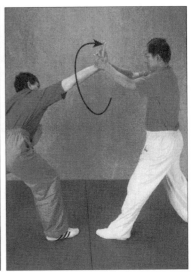

Figure 3–132

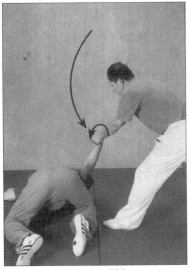

Figure 3–133

Theory:

Dividing the Muscle/Tendon (wrist). In order to make this technique effective, speed is very important. Without good speed, your opponent can sense what you intend to do and resist you easily.

Technique #3: Wild Chicken Spreads Its Wings

(Ye Ji Zhan Chi) 野雞展翅

In this technique, right after your punch has been blocked (Figure 3-130), immediately use your left hand to grab your opponent's right wrist, while also clamping your right hand down and grab the wrist as well (Figure 3-131). Right after the grab, immediately rotate his wrist clockwise (Figure 3-132). Finally, press him down until his left elbow touches the ground (Figure 3-133).

Theory:

Dividing the Muscle/Tendon (wrist). When you grab, use the entirety of both of your hands to grab, and when you turn your opponent's hand clockwise, use your entire body instead of just using arms. When you press your opponent down, the power is generated from the leverage of your pinkie and thumb areas. Keep trying until the most effective angle and leverage are found.

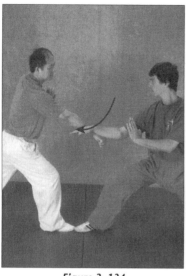
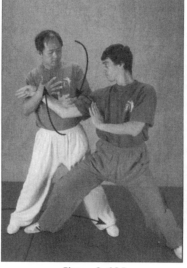
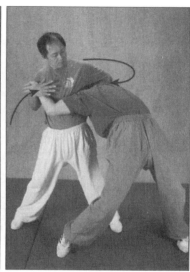

| Figure 3–134 | Figure 3–135 | Figure 3–136 |

Technique #4: Arm Wraps Around the Dragon's Neck

(Bi Chan Long Jing) 臂纏龍頸

When your abdominal punch has been repelled (Figure 3-134), immediately step your left leg behind his right leg, hooking your right arm up while pushing your left forearm against his elbow (Figure 3-135). Finally, circle your left arm around his neck while locking his right arm in front of your chest (Figure 3-136). If you squeeze tightly on the sides of his neck, you may seal the oxygen supply to his neck. In just a minute or so, you may make him lose consciousness. Naturally, do not so unless it is necessary. The reason is simply because if you do not know how to revive your victim, he will die due to lack of oxygen to his brain.

Theory:

Sealing the Artery (neck). The position where you stand is very important. Otherwise, you may be attacked by his left hand.

Technique #5: White Crane Breaks Its Wing

(Bai He Zhe Chi) 白鶴折翅

When your abdominal punch has been repelled (Figure 3-137), immediately use your left hand to grab his wrist while sliding your right hand to his elbow (Figure 3-138). Then use the leverage of both hands to bend and lock your opponent's right arm (Figure 3-139). If you find your opponent tries to attack you with his left hand, immediately kick his groin with your right leg.

Theory:

Dividing the Muscle/Tendon (wrist). The locking leverage is generated from your right hand and left hand's bending (Figure 3-140).

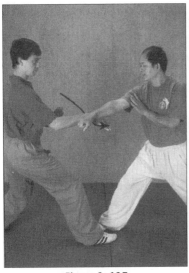

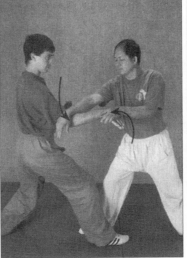

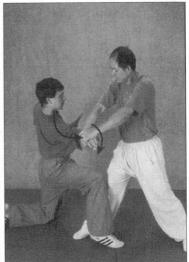

Figure 3–137   Figure 3–138   Figure 3–139

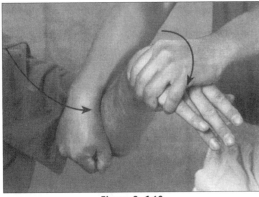

Figure 3–140

B. RIGHT ARM BLOCKS TO HIS LEFT (RIGHT HAND ATTACKS)

Technique #1: Lion Worships the Buddha or Large Elbow Wrap

(Shi Zi Bai Fo or Da Chan Zhou) 獅子拜佛，大纏肘

When your abdomen punch has been blocked by your opponent's right forearm (Figure 3-141), immediately step your left leg behind his right leg and use your left hand to grab his right wrist, while raising your right arm up to hook his elbow upward (Figure 3-142). Finally, press your right hand down while rotating your left hand toward his head (Figure 3-143).

Theory:

Misplacing the Bone (shoulder) and Dividing the Muscle/Tendon (wrist). When you circle your right arm to lock your opponent's arm behind him, use the entire body's power instead of just the arm. In addition, in order to lock him efficiently, place your hand on his upper-arm near the elbow area instead of on his shoulder. If you place your hand on his shoulder, because of its strength, he may reverse the situation by simply circling his arm forward.

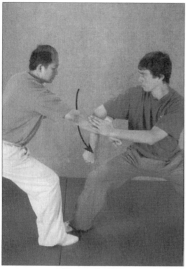
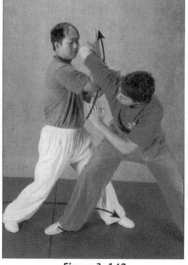
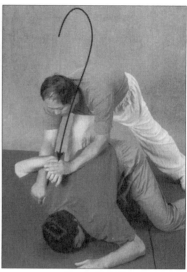

Figure 3–141   Figure 3–142   Figure 3–143

Technique #2: Pressing Shoulder with Single Finger and Extending the Neck for Water

(Yi Zhi Ding Jiang and Yin Jing Qiu Shui) 一 指 頂 肩 ， 引 頸 求 水

When your abdomen punch has been blocked by your opponent's right arm (Figure 3-144), immediately use your right hand to grab his right wrist while inserting your left arm under his elbow, reaching the back side of his upper-arm and locking his arm behind his back (Figure 3-145). Then, lift his arm up to increase the pain in his shoulder while using your index finger to press the *Jianneiling* cavity (M-UE-48)(Figure 3-146). This will cause significant pain in the shoulder area. You should increase the pressure on your index finger until your opponent's heels leave the floor. Alternatively, you may use your right hand to push his chin upward (Figure 3-147). This will also produce great pain.

Since your right hand is free, you may use it to attack anywhere on the front side of his body, such as grabbing the neck tendon (Figure 3-148), front tendon under the armpit (Figure 3-149), throat, groin, or attacking the solar plexus. Naturally, you may also use your right knee to kick his face while using your right hand to pull his head downward (Figure 3-150).

Theory:
Misplacing the Bone (shoulder), and Cavity Press (*Jianneiling* cavity). When using your left arm to lock your opponent's right arm and lift it upward, you generate a strain on his right shoulder's tendons and ligaments. This action also exposes his *Jianneiling* cavity for your cavity press attack. Without an accurate locking position for the shoulder, the cavity press will not be effective.

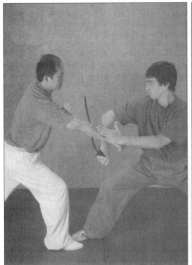

Figure 3–144

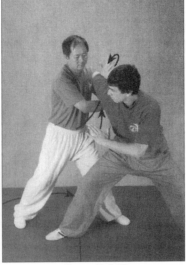

Figure 3–145

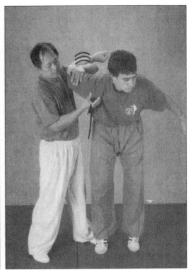

Figure 3–146

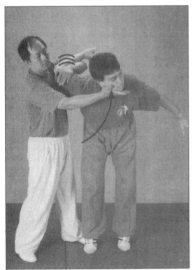

Figure 3–147

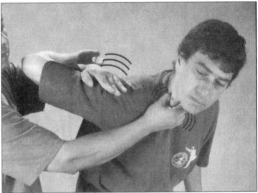

Figure 3–148

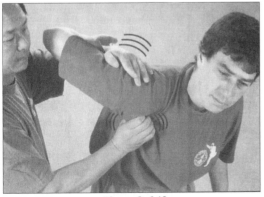

Figure 3–149

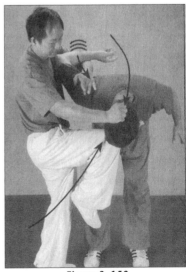

Figure 3–150

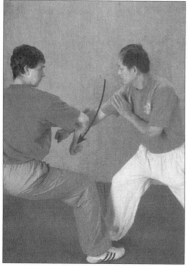

Figure 3–151

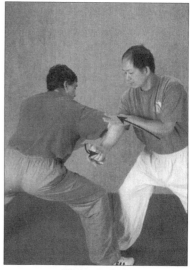

Figure 3–152

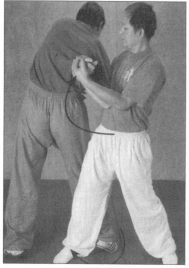

Figure 3–153

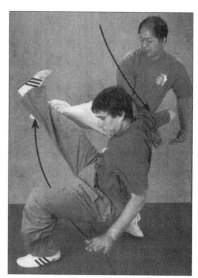

Figure 3–154

Technique #3: Hands Hold Panda

(Shou Bao Wan Xiong) 手抱浣熊

When your right hand's abdomen attack has been blocked by your opponent (Figure 3-151), use your right hand to grab his wrist while placing your left hand on his elbow (Figure 3-152). Then, use the leverage of both your hands to rotate his arm behind him and lock his arm in front of your chest (Figure 3-153). If you wish to take him down, simply sweep your right leg backward against his right leg, while pressing his upper body backward (Figure 3-154).

Theory:

Dividing the Muscle/Tendon (wrist). Your speed is very important to make this technique effective. If your opponent senses your intention, he can simply tighten up his arm to prevent you from locking him. In addition, beware of his left hand attack.

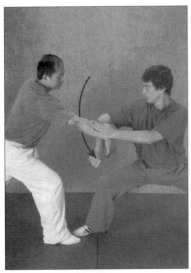

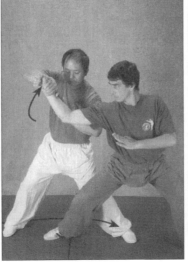

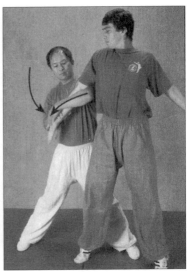

Figure 3–155   Figure 3–156   Figure 3–157

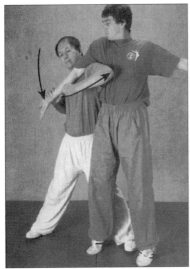

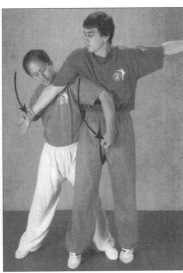

Figure 3–158   Figure 3–159

Technique #4: Hands Prop a Large Beam or Prop Up Elbow

(Shou Ban Da Liang, Shang Jia Zhou) 手扳大樑， 上架肘

When your opponent has blocked your abdomen punch with his right hand (Figure 3-155), immediately step your left leg behind his right leg, grab his wrist and rotate it until his palm is facing upward (Figure 3-156). As you do this, also place your left arm under his right elbow. Finally, using the leverage of the right hand and the left elbow, lock your opponent's right arm (Figure 3-157). You should continue your locking pressure until your opponent's heels leave the ground.

You may lock his arm by your left shoulder while using your left elbow to strike his chest (Figure 3-158) or use your left hand to grab his groin (Figure 3-159).

Theory:

Misplacing the Bone (elbow). Where you stand is very important. Wrong position-ing will offer your opponent an opportunity to attack you with his left hand.

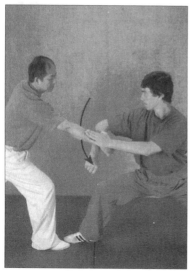

Figure 3–160

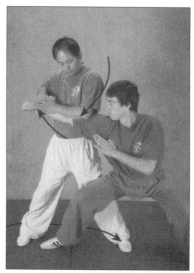

Figure 3–161

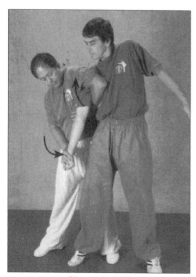

Figure 3–162

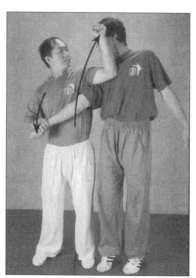

Figure 3–163

Technique #5: Hands Holding a Large Beam

(Shou Wo Da Liang) 手握大樑

When your abdominal attack has been blocked by your opponent (Figure 3-160), again step in your left leg behind his right leg, grab his wrist with your right hand, and at the same time circle your left arm around his arm to reach his upper-arm (Figure 3-161). Finally, push his wrist down with your right hand, while using your left forearm to press upward to his tendon and lock him (Figure 3-162).

If you find you cannot control your opponent easily, simply use your left fist to strike his face (Figure 3-163).

Theory:

Misplacing the Bone (elbow) and Pressing Tendon (upper-arm). In this technique, beware of your opponent's left hand attack. In addition, if you are shorter than your opponent, it will be harder for you to lock his upper-arm's tendon.

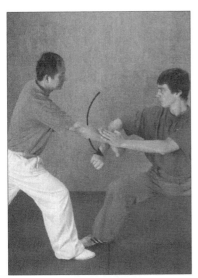

Figure 3–164

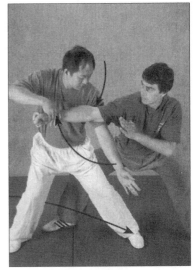

Figure 3–165

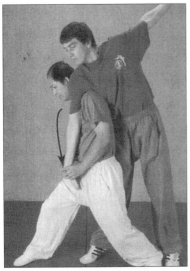

Figure 3–166

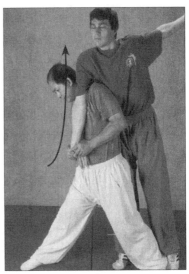

Figure 3–167

Technique #6: One Post to Support the Heavens

(Yi Zhu Ding Tian) 一柱頂天

When your abdominal attack has been blocked by your opponent (Figure 3-164), immediately step your left leg to the front of his right leg and grab his right wrist with your right hand, while using your left arm to push his elbow (Figure 3-165). Next, position your left shoulder under his right armpit while pulling his arm down to keep it straight with both of your hands (Figure 3-166). Finally, lift his entire arm upward to increase the pressure on his shoulder (Figure 3-167). You should continue lifting until his heels are off the ground. You should stand at the position from which it is hardest for your opponent to execute a left hand attack.

Theory:

Misplacing the Bone (elbow and shoulder). In this technique, you control the elbow to lock your opponent's arm in position, and lift the arm upward to tear off the ligaments of the shoulder.

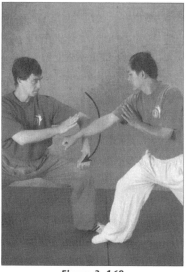

Figure 3–168

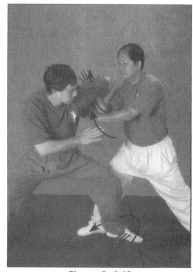

Figure 3–169

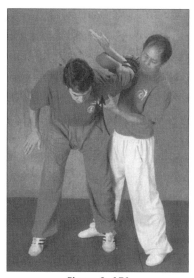

Figure 3–170

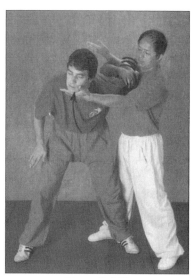

Figure 3–171

C. LEFT ARM BLOCKS TO HIS RIGHT (RIGHT HAND ATTACKS)

Technique #1: Pressing Shoulder with Single Finger and Extending the Neck for Water

(Yi Zhi Ding Jiang and Yin Jing Qiu Shui) 一指頂肩，引頸求水

When your abdominal punch has been blocked by your opponent's left arm (Figure 3-168), immediately use your left hand to grab his left wrist and push his arm into keep it bent, while inserting your right arm under his left elbow (Figure 3-169). As you do this, also step your right leg behind your opponent's left leg. Finally, lift his arm up to increase the pain in his shoulder while using your left index finger to press the *Jianneiling* cavity (Figure 3-170). Alternatively, you may use your left hand to push his chin upward to generate pain (Figure 3-171).

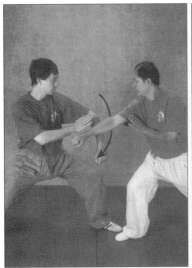
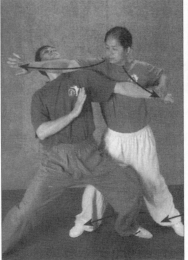
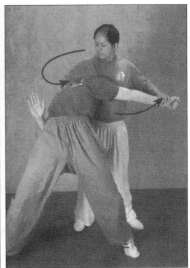

| *Figure 3–172* | *Figure 3–173* | *Figure 3–174* |

Theory:

Misplacing the Bone (shoulder), and Cavity Press (*Jianneiling* cavity). When you use your right arm to lock your opponent's right arm and lift it upward, you generate a strain on his right shoulder's tendons and ligaments. This action also exposes his *Jianneiling* cavity for your cavity press attack. Without an accurate locking position for the shoulder, the cavity press will not be effective.

Technique #2: Arm Wraps Around the Dragon's Neck

(Bi Chan Long Jing) 臂纏龍頸

In this technique, right after your punch has been repelled (Figure 3-172), immediately use your left hand to grab your opponent's left wrist, step your right leg behind his left leg, and place your right forearm against his neck (Figure 3-173). Finally, circle your right arm around his neck and bend his body backward (Figure 3-174).

If you want to take your opponent down, simply sweep your right leg forward while pushing his upper body down with your left arm. If necessary, you may increase the locking power of your right; this will seal the artery and cut off the oxygen supply to your opponent's brain. However, do not do this unless it is a life and death situation.

Theory:

Sealing the Breath (neck). To prevent your opponent from struggling strongly, simply bend his body backward with your right arm. This will destroy his balance and his capability to resist.

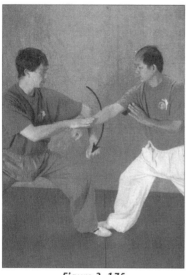
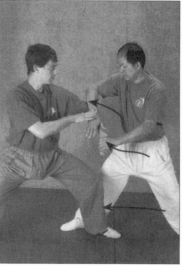
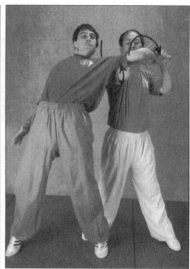

Figure 3–175 Figure 3–176 Figure 3–177

Technique #3: Daoist Greets with Hands

(Dao Zi Zuo Ji) 道子作揖

When your opponent uses his left forearm to repel your abdomen punch (Figure 3-175), immediately step your right leg behind his left leg, using your left hand to grab his left wrist while placing your right forearm on his left elbow (Figure 3-176). Next, use the rotation of your left hand and right elbow to lock him upward (Figure 3-177).

Theory:

Misplacing the Bone (elbow). When you rotate your left hand and right arm to lock your opponent upward, use your entire body's power.

Technique #4: Hands Holding a Large Beam

(Shou Wo Da Liang) 手握大樑

When your abdominal attack has been blocked by your opponent's left forearm (Figure 3-178), immediately step your right leg behind his left leg, grab his left wrist with your left hand, and circle your arm around his upper-arm (Figure 3-179). When you do this, keep his arm as straight as possible. Finally, push his wrist down with your left hand while using the right forearm to press upward to your opponent's upper-arm tendon and lock him there (Figure 3-180). Naturally, you must reposition yourself to avoid any attack from your opponent's left hand.

Theory:

Misplacing the Bone (elbow) and Pressing Tendon (upper-arm). In this technique, beware of your opponent's right hand attack. In addition, if you are shorter than your opponent, it will be harder for you to lock his upper-arm tendon.

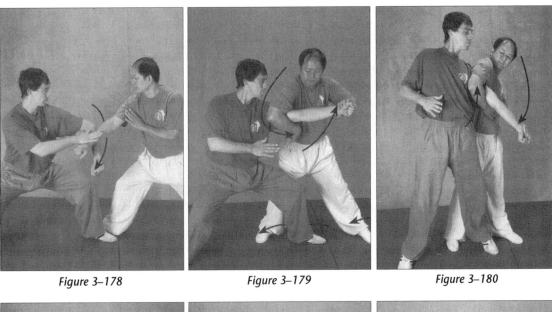

| Figure 3–178 | Figure 3–179 | Figure 3–180 |

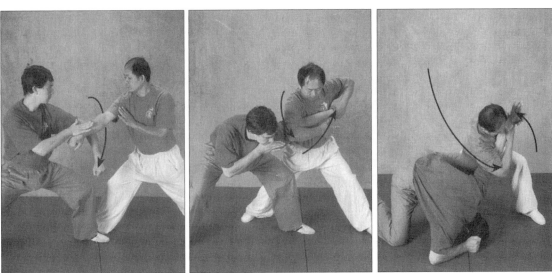

| Figure 3–181 | Figure 3–182 | Figure 3–183 |

Technique #5: Old Man Promoted to General

(Lao Han Bai Jiang) 老漢拜將

When your abdominal attack has been blocked (Figure 3-181), immediately use your left hand to grab your opponent's left wrist while placing your right armpit over his left elbow (Figure 3-182). Finally, use the leverage of your left hand and right shoulder to press him down (Figure 3-183). As you do this, kneel down on your right leg; this will provide a better position for your control.

Theory:

Misplacing the Bone (elbow). When you press your opponent down, keep his arm straight. The pressing should be straight on the back side of his elbow. If you jerk your power, you may break his elbow easily.

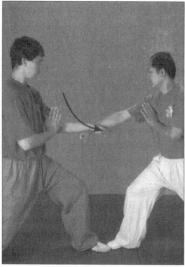

Figure 3-184

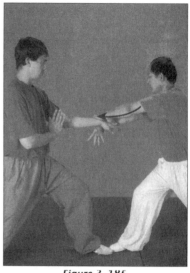

Figure 3-185

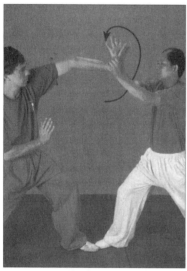

Figure 3-186

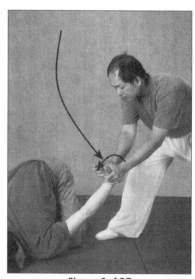

Figure 3-187

D. LEFT ARM BLOCKS TO HIS LEFT (RIGHT HAND ATTACKS)

Technique #1: Wild Chicken Spreads Its Wings

(Ye Ji Zhan Chi) 野雞展翅

When your abdominal punch has been repelled by your opponent's left forearm (Figure 3-184), immediately use your let hand to grab his left wrist (Figure 3-185). Rotate his arm counterclockwise while also using your right hand to grab his wrist (Figure 3-186). Finally, use both of your hands to press him down (Figure 3-187). You should press him down until his elbow touches the ground.

Theory:

Dividing the Muscle/Tendon (wrist). When you grab, you are using the entirety of both of your hands to grab, and when you turn your opponent's hand counterclockwise, use your entire body instead of just using your arms. When you press your opponent down, the power is generated from the leverage of your pinkie and thumb areas. Keep trying until the most effective angle and leverage are found.

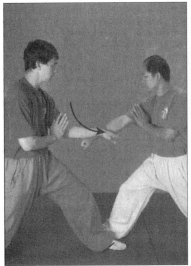
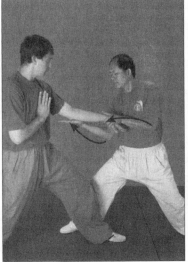
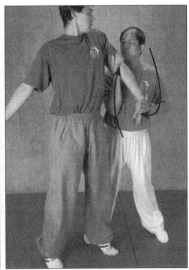

Figure 3–188   Figure 3–189   Figure 3–190

Technique #2: Heaven King Supports the Pagoda or Upward Elbow Press

(Tian Wang Tuo Ta or Shang Ya Zhou) 天王托塔，上壓肘

Once your abdominal attack has been blocked (Figure 3-188), immediately use your left hand to grab his left wrist and turn until his palm is facing upward, while also moving your right hand under his left elbow (Figure 3-189). Next, reposition yourself and press his wrist down with your left hand, while lifting his elbow upward with your right hand to lock him up (Figure 3-190). You should increase your controlling power until his heels are off the ground. You should keep yourself on the left hand side of your opponent. This will prevent him from attacking you with his right hand.

Theory:

Misplacing the Bone (elbow). The leverage generated from both of your hands is the key to the control. From the beginning, keep your opponent's elbow as straight as possible. If he has kept it bent, it would be difficult to lock him with this technique. However, if he bends his elbow before you have locked him in place, immediately push his elbow forward and upward while pulling his wrist inward. In this case, you will still be able to lock him.

Technique #3: Hands Prop a Large Beam or Prop Up Elbow

(Shou Ban Da Liang or Shang Jia Zhou) 手扳大樑， 上架肘

This technique is very similar to the last technique. Again, when your abdominal attack has been blocked by your opponent (Figure 3-191), immediately step your right leg in behind his left leg, grabbing his left wrist with your left hand while placing your right forearm under his elbow (Figure 3-192). Finally, use the leverage of your left hand and right elbow to lock him up (Figure 3-193).

Theory:

Misplacing the Bone (elbow). Again, pay attention to the position where you stand. Good positioning will prevent your opponent from attacking you with his left hand.

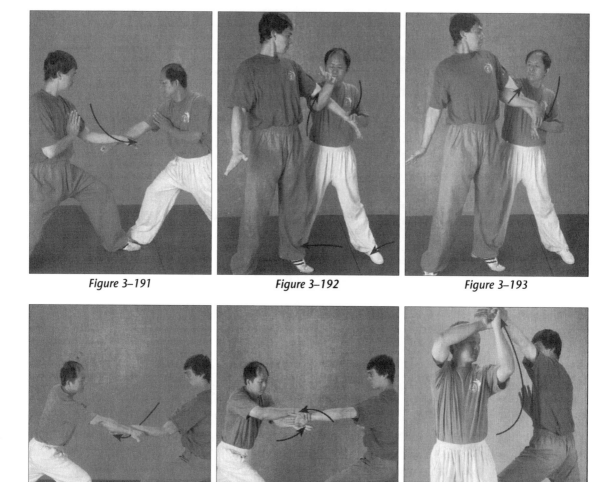

Figure 3–191　　　Figure 3–192　　　Figure 3–193

Figure 3–194　　　Figure 3–195　　　Figure 3–196

Technique #4: Send the Devil to Heaven

(Song Mo Shang Tian) 送魔上天

When your opponent has blocked your abdominal punch with his left arm (Figure 3-194), immediately use your left hand to grab his left wrist and also clamp your right hand on his left wrist (Figure 3-195). Next, step your left leg beside his left leg while swinging his left arm upward (Figure 3-196). Finally, step your right leg behind him and use both of your hands to bend his wrist downward (Figure 3-197). You should increase your twisting and bending pressure until your opponent's heels are off the ground. You may use your right hand to twist his wrist while using your left hand to grab his fingers and then bend them downward to generate pain.

Theory:

Dividing the Muscle/Tendon (wrist). The key point to execute this technique effectively is when you have locked your opponent in the final position, emphasize the pinkie lock.

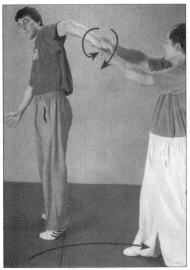

Figure 3–197

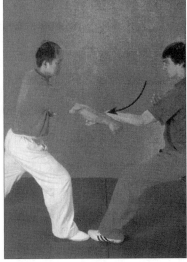

Figure 3–198

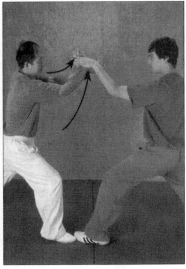

Figure 3–199

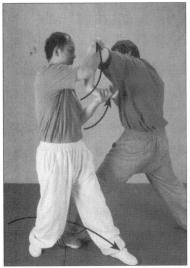

Figure 3–200

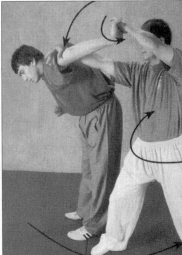

Figure 3–201

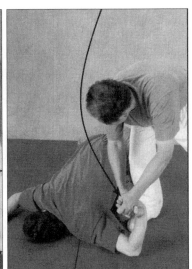

Figure 3–202

Technique #5: Large Python Turns Its Body

(Da Mang Fan Shen) 大蟒翻身

When your lower abdominal punch has been blocked (Figure 3-198), immediately use your right forearm to lift his left hand upward while using your left hand to grab his left fingers (Figure 3-199). Next, step your left leg behind his left leg while rotating his left arm with both of your hands (Figure 3-200). Then, continue turning your body to your right and twist and rotate his left arm (Figure 3-201). Finally, use the leverage generated from your right hand and left hand to press him down to the ground (Figure 3-202).

Theory:

Misplacing the Bone (shoulder and elbow). When you control your opponent and press him down, use your entire body's power instead of just using hands. In addition, when you press your opponent's elbow area with your right hand, press on the nerves located on the inside of the elbow.

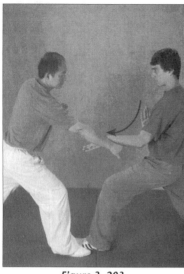 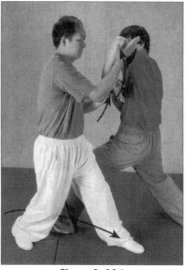 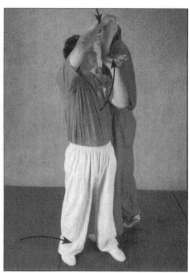

| Figure 3–203 | Figure 3–204 | Figure 3–205 |

Technique #6: Single Hand to Support the Heavens or Press the Wrist Up

(Zhi Shou Cheng Tian or Shang Ya Wan) 隻手撐天 ， 上壓腕

When your opponent has blocked your abdominal attack with his left hand (Figure 3-203), immediately step your left leg beside his left leg and use your left hand to grab his left wrist, while placing your right hand on his elbow (Figure 3-204). Next, press his left hand upward with your left hand and squeeze his elbow downward with your right hand (Figure 3-205). You must increase the upward pressing strength until his heels are off the ground. This can also prevent him from hitting you powerfully with his right hand.

Theory:
Dividing the Muscle/Tendon (wrist). In this technique, the major pain originates from the wrist. In order to increase the efficiency of the control, you may squeeze both of your hands against each other. You should position yourself on the left hand side of your opponent to prevent him from attacking you.

3-3. Qin Na Against Blocks Upward

A. SAME SIDE

Technique #1: Luo Han Bows or Small Elbow Wrap

(Luo Han Xing Li or Xiao Chan Zhou) 羅漢行禮 ， 小纏肘

When your right fist punch to your opponent's chest has been blocked upward by his left forearm (Figure 3-206), immediately use your left hand to grab his left wrist while placing your right forearm on his elbow (Figure 3-207). As you do this, also place your right leg in front of your left leg. Finally, pull your opponent's left arm toward the front of your

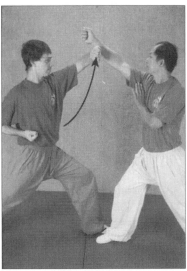

Figure 3–206

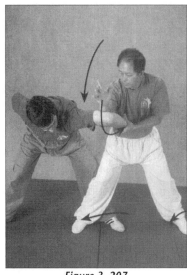

Figure 3–207

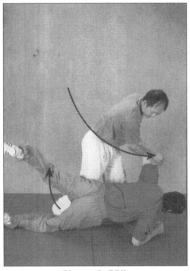

Figure 3–208

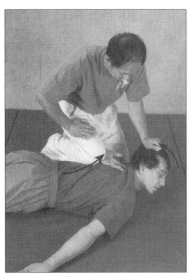

Figure 3–209

body to destroy his stability, while bowing and sweeping your right leg backward to make your opponent fall (Figure 3-208). When your opponent is on the ground, lock his arm behind his back and use your left hand to grab his hair and pull it to his left (Figure 3-209). With the help of both of your legs and left hand, you will be able to firmly lock him.

Theory:

Misplacing the Bone (elbow and shoulder). In order to make your opponent fall, after you have locked him, pull him to your front to destroy his balance while sweeping your right leg backward. Once your opponent is on the ground, if necessary you may rotate his arm toward his head and pop his shoulder out of joint.

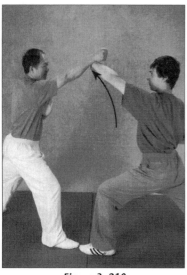 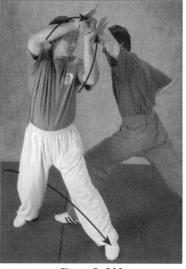 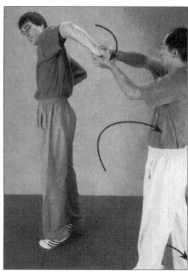

| *Figure 3–210* | *Figure 3–211* | *Figure 3–212* |

Technique #2: Send the Devil to Heaven

(Song Mo Shang Tian) 送魔上天

When you find out that your attack has been blocked upward by your opponent's left forearm (Figure 3-210), immediately step your left leg beside his left leg while grabbing his left wrist with both of your hands (Figure 3-211). Then, step your right leg behind him and turn your body clockwise, while using the body's momentum to twist his arm and wrist to lock him up (Figure 3-212). You should increase your twisting and bending pressure until his heels are off the ground.

Theory:
Dividing the Muscle/Tendon (wrist). The key point of executing this technique effectively is, when you have locked your opponent in the final position, emphasize the pinkie lock, which is more efficient and effective.

Technique #3: Pressing Shoulder with Single Finger and Extending the Neck for Water

(Yi Zhi Ding Jiang and Yin Jing Qiu Shui) 一指頂肩 ，引頸求水

When your attack has been blocked upward by your opponent's left arm (Figure 3-213), immediately use your left hand to grab his left wrist, while coiling your right hand around his left arm and reaching his elbow (Figure 3-214). Finally, raise his left arm up behind him with your right arm while using your index finger to press the *Jianneiling* cavity (M-UE-48) (Figure 3-215). This will cause significant pain in the shoulder area. You should increase the pressure on your index finger until your opponent's heels leave the floor. Alternatively, you may use your right hand to push his chin upward (Figure 3-216). This will also produce great pain.

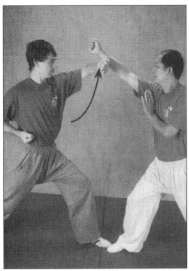

Figure 3-213

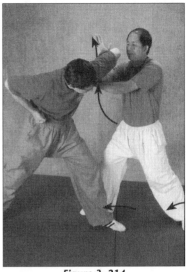

Figure 3-214

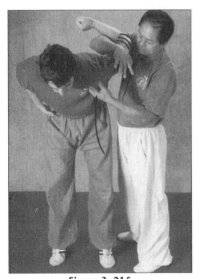

Figure 3-215

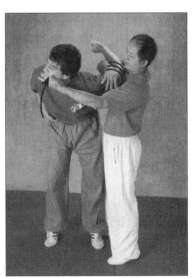

Figure 3-216

Theory:

Misplacing the Bone (shoulder), and Cavity Press (*Jianneiling* cavity). When you use your left arm to lock your opponent's left arm and lift it upward, you generate a strain on his left shoulder's tendons and ligaments. This action also exposes his *Jianneiling* cavity for your cavity press attack. Without an accurate locking position of the shoulder, the cavity press will not be effective.

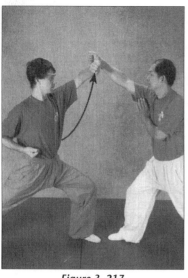
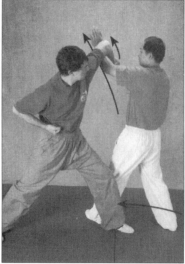
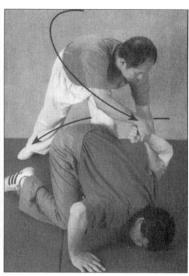

| *Figure 3–217* | *Figure 3–218* | *Figure 3–219* |

Technique #4: Lion Worships the Buddha or Large Elbow Wrap

(Shi Zi Bai Fo or Da Chan Zhou) 獅子拜佛，大纏肘

When your right fist punch has been blocked upward by your opponent's left forearm (Figure 3-217), immediately step your left leg to his left and open your right fist completely. Next, circle his wrist to the internal side and grab his left wrist (Figure 3-218). When you are doing so, also place your left forearm on his elbow. Finally, step your right leg forward, turn your body to your left, and use the body's turning momentum to lock his wrist and elbow until he is touching the ground (Figure 3-219).

Theory:

Misplacing the Bone (shoulder) and Dividing the Muscle/Tendon (wrist). When you circle your left arm to lock your opponent's arm behind him, use the entire body's power instead of just the arm. In addition, in order to lock him efficiently, place your hand on his upper-arm near the elbow area instead of on his shoulder.

Technique #5: The Woodcutter Binds the Wood or Forward Turning Elbow

(Qiao Fu Kun Cai or Qian Fan Zhou) 樵夫捆材，前翻肘

After your right hand's punch has been blocked upward by your opponent's left forearm (Figure 3-220), immediately step your left leg behind his left leg, coil your right hand around his wrist, and grab it from the inside while placing your left elbow under his left elbow (Figure 3-221). Finally, grab your own right wrist with your left hand and bend his left arm backward to lock his arm (Figure 3-222). Alternatively, you may use your left hand to grab his left wrist while using your right hand to push his head forward (Figure 3-223). If you wish to take him down, simply sweep your left leg backward while you are rotating his left arm forward.

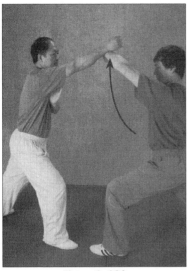

Figure 3–220

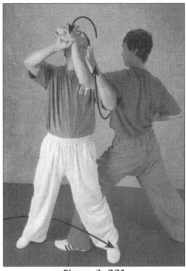

Figure 3–221

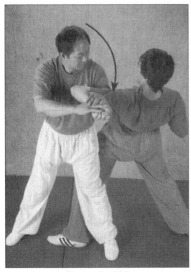

Figure 3–222

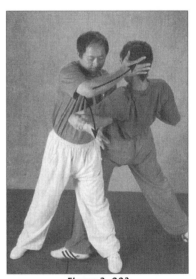

Figure 3–223

Theory:

Misplacing the Bone (elbow). The position where you stand is very important. When you rotate your opponent's arm, rotate it at the correct angle. Too straight or too bent is not effective.

Technique #6: Single Hand to Support the Heavens or Press the Wrist Up

(Zhi Shou Cheng Tian or Shang Ya Wan) 隻手撐天，上壓腕

When your right hand punch has been blocked upward by your opponent's left forearm (Figure 3-224), immediately use your left hand to grab his left wrist while also moving your right hand to his elbow (Figure 3-225). Next, step your left leg beside his left leg and press your left hand upward while squeezing your right hand downward, locking him up until his heels are off the ground (Figure 3-226).

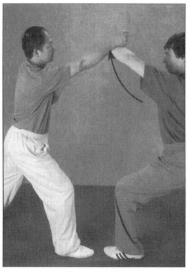

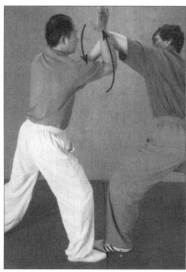

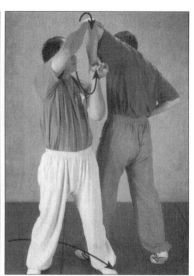

| Figure 3–224 | Figure 3–225 | Figure 3–226 |

Theory:
Dividing the Muscle/Tendon (wrist). The position where you stand is very important. In order to generate significant pain on your opponent's wrist, the positions for pressing on your left hand and the squeezing power from your right hand are very important.

B. OPPOSITE SIDE

Technique #1: Lion Worships the Buddha or Large Elbow Wrap
(Shi Zi Bai Fo or Da Chan Zhou) 獅子拜佛，大纏肘

When you punch your opponent with your right fist and he blocks it upward with his right forearm (Figure 3-227), immediately hook your right hand down on his forearm, and use your left hand to grab his right wrist and follow with coiling your right hand around his arm until it reaches your opponent's elbow (Figure 3-228). Finally, use the leverage of both of your hands to push your opponent down to the ground (Figure 3-229).

Theory:
Misplacing the Bone (shoulder) and Dividing the Muscle/Tendon (wrist). When you circle your right arm to lock your opponent's arm behind him, use the entire body's power instead of just the arm. In addition, in order to lock him efficiently, place your hand on his upper-arm near the elbow area instead of his shoulder.

Technique #2: Send the Devil to Heaven
(Song Mo Shang Tian) 送魔上天

When your chest attack has been blocked upward (Figure 3-230), immediately step your right leg to his right and hook your right hand down, while using your left hand to grab your opponent's wrist (Figure 3-231). Continue your body's rotation while stepping your left leg behind him and use both of your hands to lock his arm upward (Figure 3-232).

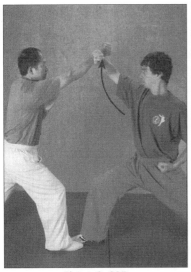

Figure 3–227

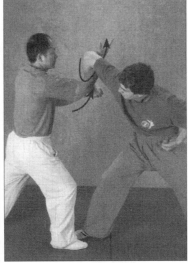

Figure 3–228

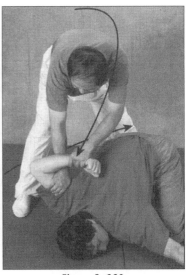

Figure 3–229

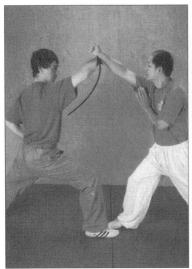

Figure 3–230

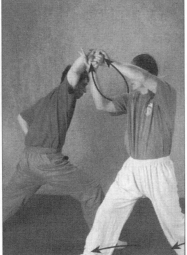

Figure 3–231

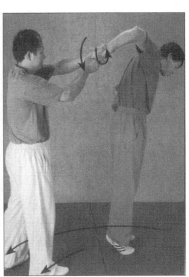

Figure 3–232

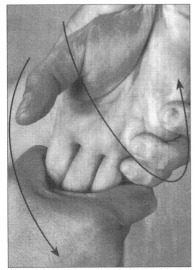

Figure 3–233

Theory:

Dividing the Muscle/Tendon (wrist) and Misplacing the Bone (shoulder). An important point in this technique is, when you have locked your opponent in the final position, emphasize the pinkie twisting, which is more efficient and effective. If you use your left hand to twist his pinkie while using your right hand to grab his fingers and bend them down, the technique can be even better (Figure 3-233).

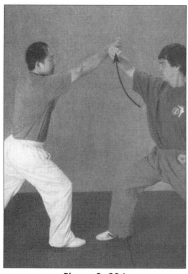

Figure 3–234

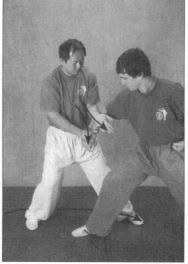

Figure 3–235

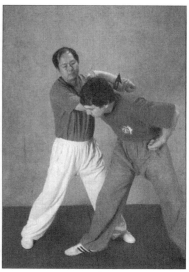

Figure 3–236

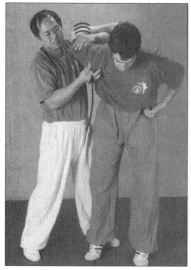

Figure 3–237

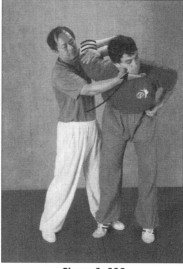

Figure 3–238

Technique #3: Pressing Shoulder with Single Finger and Extending the Neck for Water

(Yi Zhi Ding Jiang and Yin Jing Qiu Shui) 一指頂肩， 引頸求水

When your right hand attack has been blocked upward by your opponent's right arm (Figure 3-234), immediately step your left leg behind his right leg and hook down his forearm and grab his wrist with your right hand, while inserting your left hand under his right elbow (Figure 3-235). Next, lock his right arm behind his back and lift his arm up to increase the pain in his shoulder (Figure 3-236). Finally, use your right index finger to press his *Jianneiling* cavity (M-UE-48) (Figure 3-237). This will cause significant pain in the shoulder area. You should increase the pressure on your index finger until your opponent's heels leave the floor. Alternatively, you may use your right hand to push his chin upward (Figure 3-238). This will also produce great pain.

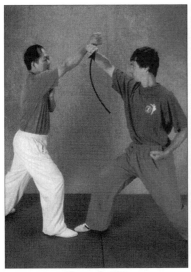 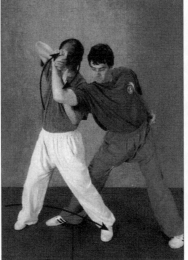 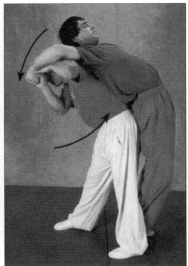

| *Figure 3–239* | *Figure 3–240* | *Figure 3–241* |

Theory:

Misplacing the Bone (shoulder), and Cavity Press (*Jianneiling* cavity). When use your left arm to lock your opponent's left arm and lift it upward, you generate a strain on his left shoulder's tendons and ligaments. This action also exposes his *Jianneiling* cavity for your cavity press attack. Without an accurate locking position of the shoulder, the cavity press will not be effective.

Technique #4: The Old Man Carries the Fish on His Back

(Lao Han Bei Yu) 老漢背魚

When your attack has been blocked upward by your opponent's right forearm (Figure 3-239), immediately step your left leg to the front of his right leg, hook your right hand down and grab his wrist, while using your left forearm to push his elbow (Figure 3-240). Finally, bend your body forward while pulling your hands downward to lock your opponent's entire arm in position (Figure 3-241).

Theory:

Misplacing the Bone (shoulder and elbow). In order to generate strong power, your pushing and locking should be generated from your entire body instead of from your arms only. Always look for better leverage to do the job. The angle of his elbow is very important; too straight or too bent will make the technique ineffective.

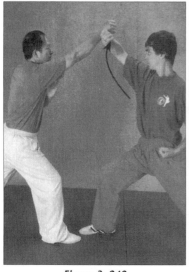

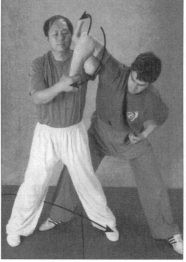

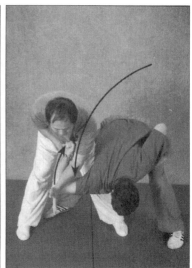

Figure 3–242   Figure 3–243   Figure 3–244

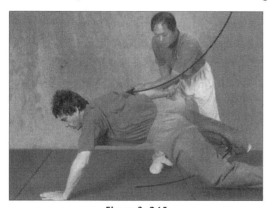

Figure 3–245

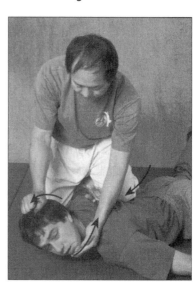

Figure 3–246

Technique #5: Luo Han Bows or Small Elbow Wrap

(Luo Han Xing Li or Xiao Chan Zhou) 羅漢行禮 ， 小纏肘

When your attack has been blocked upward by your opponent's right forearm (Figure 3-242), immediately step your left leg to the front of his right leg and hook down your right hand to grab his right wrist, while pushing your left forearm to his elbow (Figure 3-243). Next, pull your opponent's right arm toward the front of your body to destroy his stability, while bowing (Figure 3-244) and sweeping your left leg backward to make him fall (Figure 3-245). When your opponent is on the ground, lock his arm behind his back (Figure 3-246). You may also use both of your hands to twist his head to lock his neck. With the help of both of your legs, you will be able to firmly lock him.

Theory:

Misplacing the Bone (shoulder and neck). In order to make your opponent fall after you have locked him, pull him to your front to destroy his balance while sweeping your left leg backward. Once your opponent is on the ground, if necessary you may rotate his arm toward his head and pop his shoulder out of joint.

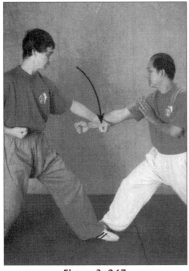

Figure 3–247

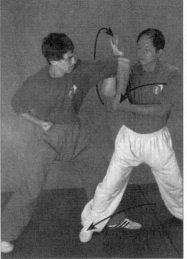

Figure 3–248

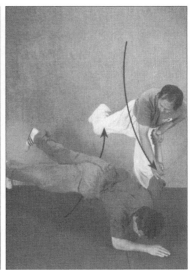

Figure 3–249

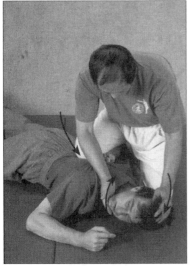

Figure 3–250

3-4. Qin Na Against Blocks Downward

A. SAME SIDE

Technique #1: Luo Han Bows or Small Elbow Wrap

(Luo Han Xing Li or Xiao Chan Zhou)
羅漢行禮，小纏肘

This technique is the same as the last one, except the way of setting up is different. In this technique, right after your right hand abdominal attack has been blocked downward by your opponent's left forearm (Figure 3-247), immediately step your right leg to the front of his left leg and use your left hand to grab his left wrist, while placing your right forearm on his elbow area (Figure 3-248). Finally, pull your opponent's left arm toward the front of your body to destroy his stability, while bowing and sweeping your right leg backward to make him fall (Figure 3-249). When your opponent is on the ground, lock his arm behind his back (Figure 3-250). With the help your both legs, you will be able to lock him there firmly. Naturally, as in the last technique, you may again use both of your hands to lock his neck.

Theory:

Misplacing the Bone (shoulder and neck). In order to make your opponent fall, after you have locked him, pull him to your front to destroy his balance while sweeping your right leg backward. Once your opponent is on the ground, if necessary you may rotate his arm toward his head and pop his shoulder out of joint.

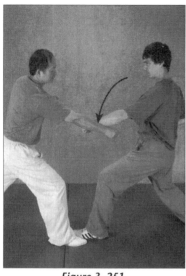

Figure 3–251

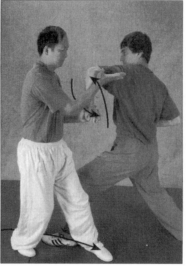

Figure 3–252

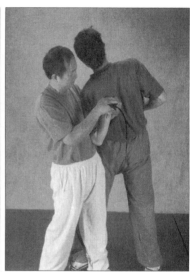

Figure 3–253

Technique #2: Hands Hold Panda

(Shou Bao Wan Xiong) 手抱浣熊

When your abdominal attack has been blocked downward (Figure 3-251), immediately step your left leg behind his left leg and use your left hand to grab his left wrist, while placing your right hand on his left elbow (Figure 3-252). Next, pull your right hand in while pushing your left hand forward to position his arm behind his back. Finally, lock his arm between both of your hands and your left chest (Figure 3-253). To prevent him from struggling, use your right hand to grab his hair and pull it downward.

Theory:

Dividing the Muscle/Tendon (wrist). Speed is very important to make this technique effective. If your opponent senses your intention, he can simply tighten up his arm to prevent you from locking him. In addition, beware of his right hand attack.

Technique #3: The Woodcutter Binds the Woods or Forward Turning Elbow

(Qiao Fu Kun Cai or Qian Fan Zhou) 樵夫捆材 ，前翻肘

When your right hand's abdominal punch has been blocked downward by your opponent's left forearm (Figure 3-254), immediately step your left leg behind his left leg and use your right forearm to push his forearm upward, while placing your left elbow on his left elbow (Figure 3-255). Finally, grab your own right wrist with your left hand and bend his left arm backward to lock his arm (Figure 3-256). If you wish to take him down, simply sweep your left leg backward while you are rotating his left arm forward.

Theory:

Misplacing the Bone (elbow). The position where you stand is very important. When you rotate your opponent's arm, rotate it at the correct angle. Too straight or too bent is not effective.

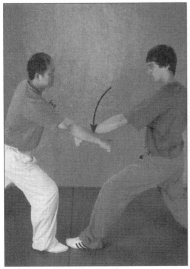

Figure 3–254

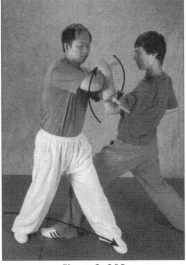

Figure 3–255

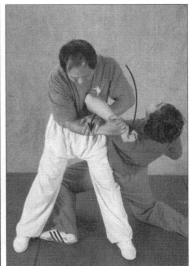

Figure 3–256

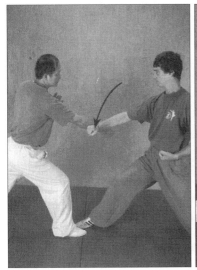

Figure 3–257

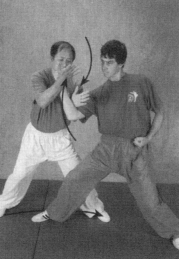

Figure 3–258

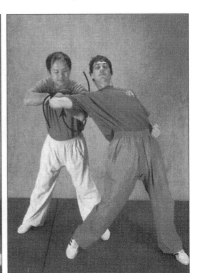

Figure 3–259

B. OPPOSITE SIDE

Technique #1: Daoist Greets with Hands

(Dao Zi Zuo Ji) 道子作揖

When your opponent has blocked your right hand's abdominal attack downward with his right forearm (Figure 3-257), immediately step your left leg behind his right leg and hook your right hand upward, while using your left forearm to push his elbow forward to bend his right arm (Figure 3-258). Continue to bend his arm backward until you lock it firmly (Figure 3-259).

Theory:

Misplacing the Bone (elbow). In this technique, if you turn your body, you can change the lock into "The Old Man Carries the Fish on His Back" technique. In this case, you are locking both the elbow and the shoulder.

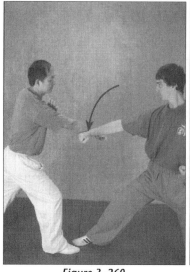

Figure 3–260

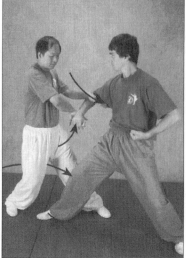

Figure 3–261

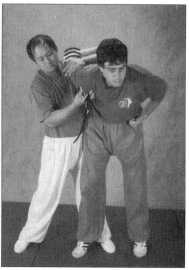

Figure 3–262

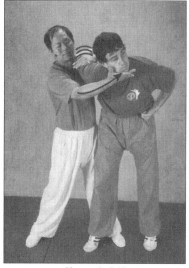

Figure 3–263

Technique #2: Pressing Shoulder with Single Finger and Extending the Neck for Water

(Yi Zhi Ding Jiang and Yin Jing Qiu Shui)
一指頂肩，引頸求水

When your right hand abdominal attack has been blocked downward by your opponent's right hand (Figure 3-260), immediately step your left leg behind his right leg and turn your hand upward, while inserting your left hand into your opponent's right elbow area (Figure 3-261). Next, use the leverage generated from your left hand and elbow to lock your opponent's arm while using your index finger to press the *Jianneiling* cavity (Figure 3-262). Alternatively, you may use your right hand to push his chin sideways and upward (Figure 3-263). This will also produce great pain.

Theory:

Misplacing the Bone (shoulder), and Cavity Press (*Jianneiling* cavity). When you use your left arm to lock your opponent's right arm and lift it upward, you generate a strain on his right shoulder's tendons and ligaments. This action also exposes his *Jianneiling* cavity for your cavity press attack. Without an accurate locking position of the shoulder, the cavity press will not be effective.

▪ Chapter 4 ▪

QIN NA AGAINST KICKING

4-1. Introduction

Applications of Qin Na against kicking are much harder than for those against hand attacks. There are several reasons for this. First, because the legs are more powerful than are the hands, it is much harder to use the hands to control them. Secondly, since the joints of the ankles, knees, and hips are much bigger that those of the arms, it is very difficult to lock them efficiently. Not only that, it is impossible for your hands to control your opponent's toes in the way you can control the fingers. This is simply because his toes are much shorter and are almost always protected by shoes. Third, more than half of the effective kicking techniques focus on kicking the lower body. Because of this, it is harder to use your hands to intercept and further control these lower kicks. Furthermore, when you use your hands to block these low kicks, you may also expose the vital areas of your upper body for your opponent's attack. Finally, many of the Chinese martial arts kicks are double kicks. When these double kicks are executed, they are fast, one after the other, and very powerful. Therefore, unless you have very special training, it is almost impossible to execute any Qin Na techniques.

From the above explanation, you can see why, compared to Qin Na techniques against hand attacks, there are fewer Qin Na techniques against legs. In this chapter, we will introduce those Qin Na techniques which can be used against kicks. In the next section, we will first introduce those techniques against high kicks to the face area. Then, in Section 4-3, techniques against kicking to the stomach area will be discussed. In Section 4-4, several Qin Na techniques against lower kicks will be summarized. Finally, in Section 4-5, some leg Qin Na techniques which can be used against stationary stances will be introduced.

4-2. Qin Na Against High Kicks to the Face

It was explained earlier that, intercepting or blocking kicks — especially double high kicks — is very difficult. Normally the best defense against single high kicks is attacking the groin area. The reason for this is simply that, whenever your opponent is executing a single high kick, his groin area must be exposed. Not only that, whenever your opponent is kicking high, his root will not be as strong as when he stands on two legs. Due to this reason, take-down Qin Na techniques are very effective against these high kicks.

However, if your opponent uses double kicks to attack you, since they are powerful and fast, it is almost impossible to use any Qin Na techniques. Furthermore, when he uses double kicks, the groin area is not as exposed, and there is no root for you to destroy. Consequently, both strategies against the single high kicks are ineffective. Therefore, the best strategy against double high kicks is to dodge or to keep a safe distance. Wait until your opponent lands and tries to regain his balance and root, then immediately attack. Since this strategy is not classified as Qin Na technique, we will discuss it no further here.

I. SIDEWAYS HIGH KICKS

The best way of defending against a sideways high kick is to reposition yourself at a disadvantageous position for your opponent's kicking. For example, if your opponent kicks your face with his right leg (Figure 4-1), if you move to his left, you will immediately put him in a poor angle to execute his kick effectively (Figure 4-2). Once you have repositioned yourself in this way, you will be able to punch his face or kick his groin area easily.

Technique #1: Single Horse Thrusts Forward

(Dan Ma Zhi Chong) 單馬直衝

As your opponent is kicking your left face sideways with his right leg, immediately reposition yourself to his left empty door (Figure 4-3). Right before he regains his stability, step your left leg in beside his left leg and at the same time use your left hand to circle around his neck (Figure 4-4). Finally, sweep your left leg forward while pressing your left arm downward to take him down (Figure 4-5). If you can act very fast, you need not reposition yourself to avoid his kick first, and may simply step in your left leg beside his left leg, and circle your left arm around his neck and sweep him down.

Theory:

Taking Down. Other than kicking your opponent's groin, the two effective strategies to defending against a single high kick is to step backward and keep a safe distance, or to step into short range. This will make your opponent's kicks ineffective. When you step into short range, you also set up techniques to take your opponent down. Effective take-down techniques destroy his root and balance.

Technique #2: The Hands Push Hua Mountain

(Shou Tui Hua Shan) 手推華山

When your opponent kicks at the left side of your face with his right leg, immediately readjust your legs to his left hand side to avoid his kicks (Figure 4-6). Then, immediately step in your left leg and at the same time use both of your hands to push his upper chest to make him fall (Figure 4-7). If you are too slow and your opponent has already regained his balance before you push him, then you should strike his face and withdraw.

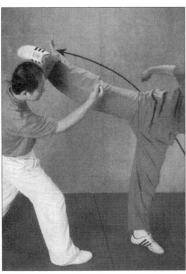

Figure 4–1

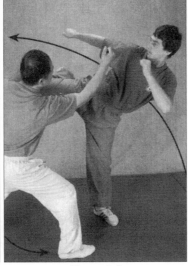

Figure 4–2

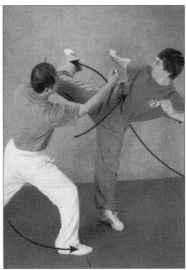

Figure 4–3

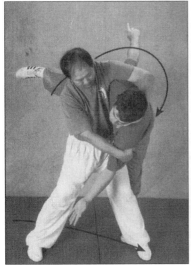

Figure 4–4

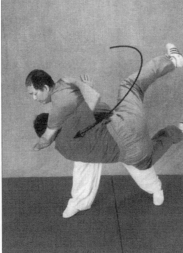

Figure 4–5

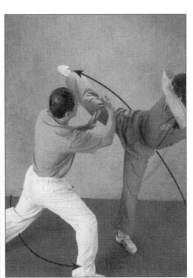

Figure 4–6

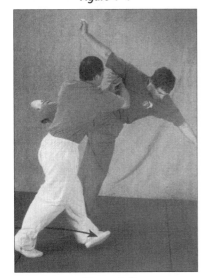

Figure 4–7

Theory:

Taking Down. When you step in to your opponent's left hand side, his right leg kick will not be effective. Not only that, if you can take this opportunity to push him before he regains his balance and root on both legs, you may bounce him off. This will offer you an opportunity for further attack.

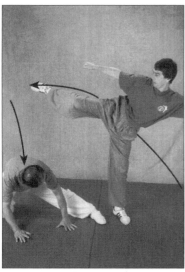
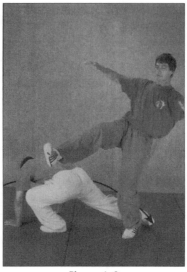
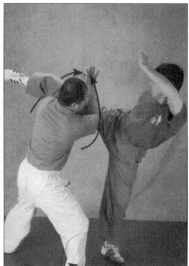

| Figure 4–8 | Figure 4–9 | Figure 4–10 |

Technique #3: Leg Sweeps with a Thousand Pounds

(Tui Sao Qian Jun) 腿掃千鈞

When your opponent kicks the left side of your face with his right leg, immediately squat down to avoid the kick (Figure 4-8), then immediately sweep your right leg to the back side of his left leg to make him fall (Figure 4-9).

Theory:

Taking Down. The timing to make this technique effective is very important. Naturally, it is also very risky to execute this technique. When you squat your body down, you must immediately use this momentum to sweep your right leg. Without this momentum, your sweeping will be slow and weak.

Technique #4: Left Lift and Right Press

(Zhou Ti You Tui) 左提右推

When your opponent kicks the left side of your face with his right leg, immediately readjust your position to your opponent's left (Figure 4-10). As you do this, also use your left forearm to lift his right leg upward on the knee area, and use your right forearm to push his thigh or upper body to make him fall (Figure 4-11).

Theory:

Taking Down. Again, you must reposition yourself to change out of the angle which is most advantageous for your opponent. As you do this, also use your left arm to prevent his right leg from returning to the ground and use your right forearm to push him off balance. Alternatively, you may circle your body to your left and throw him down by stepping your left leg backward.

II. STRAIGHT HIGH KICKS

If your opponent kicks at your upper body straight, you may treat it in the same way as your defense against sideways high kicks. That is, reposition yourself to his empty door or the standing leg side, and attack his groin. Alternatively, you may squat down and

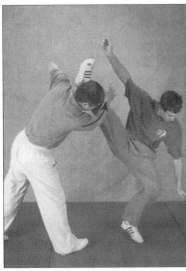

Figure 4–11

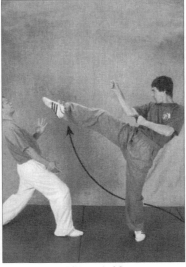

Figure 4–12

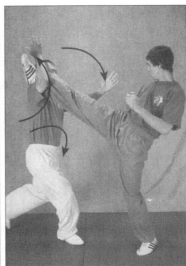

Figure 4–13

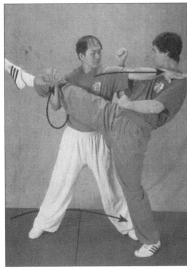

Figure 4–14

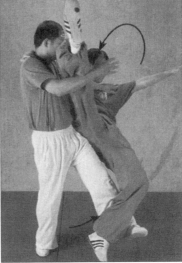

Figure 4–15

sweep his standing leg to make him fall. Here, we will introduce three techniques which can be used to defend against straight high kicks. Naturally, you must practice for a long time until you can catch the right timing and correctly execute the techniques.

Technique #1: Lift the Leg and Push the Neck

(Tai Jiao Tui Jing) 抬 腳 推 頸

When your opponent kicks your upper body with his right leg (Figure 4-12), immediately reposition yourself to his right hand side and hook your right arm up to stop him from dropping his leg (Figure 4-13). Next, step your left leg in and use your left arm to press his upper body (Figure 4-14). Finally, push your left hand backward and downward while sweeping your left leg forward (Figure 4-15). This will make your opponent fall.

Theory:

Taking Down. The coordination of your left hand push and left leg sweeping is very important. With good coordination, you may make your opponent fall easily.

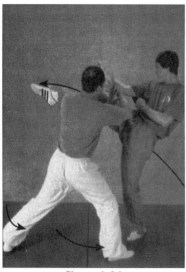
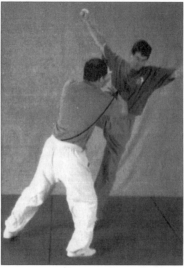
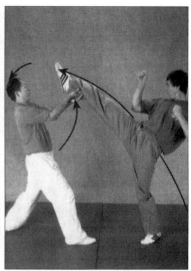

| *Figure 4–16* | *Figure 4–17* | *Figure 4–18* |

Technique #2: The Hands Push Hua Mountain

(Shou Tui Hua Shan) 手推華山

When your opponent kicks your upper body with his right leg, immediately readjust both of your legs to his left hand side to avoid his kicks (Figure 4-16). While you are doing this, also press both of your hands against his upper chest and then push him off balance (Figure 4-17).

Theory:

Taking Down. When you step in to your opponent's left hand side, his right leg kick will not be effective. Not only that, if you can take this opportunity to push him before he regains his balance and root on both legs, you may bounce him off. This will offer you an opportunity for further attack.

Technique #3: Two Hands Lift the Leg

(Shuang Shou Tai Jiao) 雙手抬腳

Again, if your opponent kicks your upper body with his right leg, you may lean your upper body backward and use both of your hands to lift his right leg upward at the ankle area (Figure 4-18). After you have trapped his leg, continue to lift upward until he falls. Alternatively, right after lifting, you may simply use your right leg to kick his groin (Figure 4-19).

Theory:

Taking Down. When you lift both of your hands to trap your opponent's leg, the timing and the speed must be right. With the right timing, you may use his upward kicking momentum to destroy his root easily. Naturally, this requires a lot of practice.

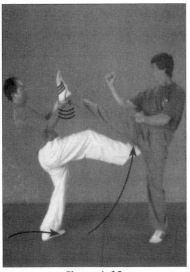

Figure 4–19

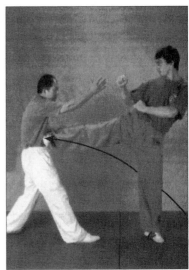

Figure 4–20

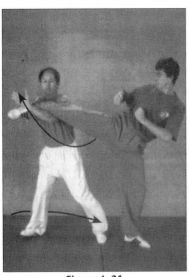

Figure 4–21

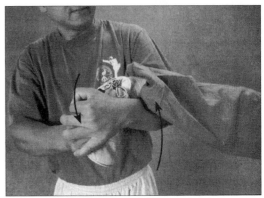

Figure 4–22

4-3. Qin Na Against Kicks to the Middle Body

Kicks to the middle section of the body are more practical and faster than high kicks. The reason for this is simply because, if you kick your opponent's mid-section, your groin will not be as exposed for your opponent's attack as during high kicks. Because of this, middle body kicking is used more often than high kicks.

Technique #1: The Arms Lift Up the Large Beam

(Shou Tai Da Liang) 手抬大樑

When your opponent kicks your stomach area with his right leg (Figure 4-20), turn your body to your right and step your left leg beside his right hand side, while hooking your left forearm upward to trap his right leg on the calf or ankle area (Figure 4-21). Once you have trapped his leg, use both of your hands to twist his ankle to lock his leg up (Figure 4-22). If you continue to raise up your left arm, you may easily make him fall.

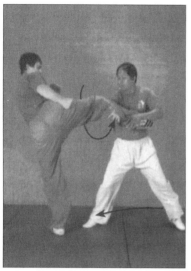

Figure 4–23

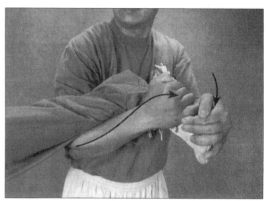

Figure 4–24

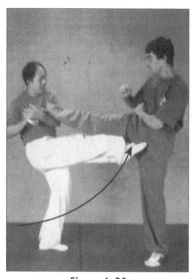

Figure 4–25

Naturally, you may also adjust your body to his left and use your right forearm to hook his right leg upward (Figure 4-23). Again, use both of your hands to twist his ankle and lock his leg up (Figure 4-24). However, it is more dangerous to execute your technique on this side simply because your opponent is able to attack you with his left hand .

If you decide to injure him instead of only making him fall, use your right leg to kick his groin (Figure 4-25).

Theory:

When you execute this technique, both the distance and angle between you and your opponent are very important. With a safe distance and correct angle, through practice, you may execute this technique skillfully and easily.

Technique #2: Upward to Press the Dragon Tendon

(Shang Ya Long Jin) 上壓龍筋

In the last technique, once you have locked your opponent's right leg, use your left forearm to press his middle rear calf area, while using your right hand to grab and push his foot downward (Figure 4-26). In this case, the tendons on the rear side of his calf will be pressed and generate great pain.

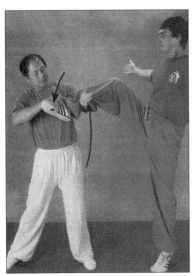

Figure 4–26

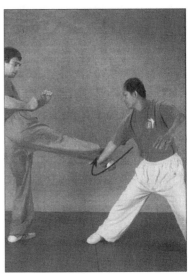

Figure 4–27

Theory:

Pressing the Tendons on the rear side of the calf. The location where you press your left arm is very important. With correct pressing, and with the help of the right hand, good leverage can be generated for the control.

Technique #3: White Crane Spreads Its Wings

(Bai He Liang Chi) 白鶴亮翅

This technique is commonly used in Taijiquan. When your opponent kicks the middle section of your body, step your left leg to the side, while using your right arm to repel the kick and also lift his leg upward (Figure 4-27). If you catch the right timing, you may make him fall easily.

Theory:

Taking Down. Again, the timing, distance, and speed are the keys to making this technique successful. If you can catch the correct timing, you may use your opponent's forward kicking momentum against him.

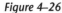

4-4. Qin Na Against Kicking to the Lower Body

There are a few common places which your opponent can kick you on the lower part of your body. These places include the Lower *Dan Tian* (about one to two inches under the navel), groin, knees, or shins. Relatively speaking, the lower the kick, the harder it can be to intercept with the hands. That means it is very difficult to apply Qin Na techniques against low kicks to the knees and shin. However, in order to execute these kicks effectively, your opponent must keep the distance between you and him short. This implies that as long as you keep a good distance between you and your opponent, it will not be easy for him to execute his techniques successfully.

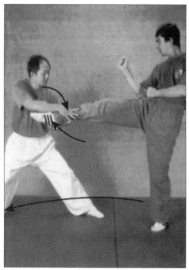

Figure 4–28

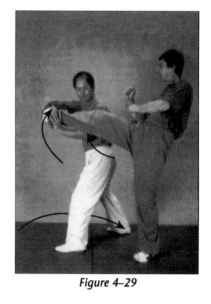

Figure 4–29

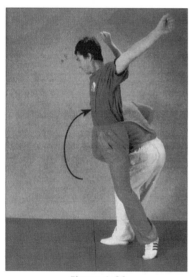

Figure 4–30

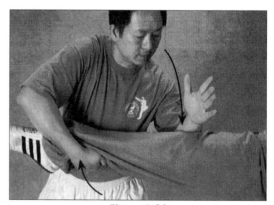

Figure 4–31

Technique #1: The Hands Drag the Cow's Leg

(Shou Tuo Niu Tui) 手拖牛腿

When your opponent uses his right leg to kick your lower body, step your right leg backward, while scooping up your left hand to grab his ankle area and clamping your right hand downward to grab his ankle (Figure 4-28). Once you have successfully grabbed his right leg, immediately step your right leg backward while using your left upper-arm to press his right thigh (Figure 4-29). Finally, swing him down (Figure 4-30).

Theory:

Taking Down. Because your opponent is kicking low, you must posture yourself low in order to catch his leg. It is because your opponent's kicking is very power-ful that you must use both of your hands to handle the job. Right after you have grabbed his leg, immediately pull to keep a safe distance between you and him to avoid further attack from his hands. When you swing him down, you may also use your forearm to press the tendons on his thigh and then swing him down (Figure 4-31). Naturally, if you know how to use the entire body's momentum, you can make 'he whole technique much easier.

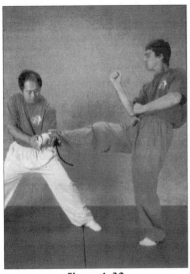

Figure 4–32

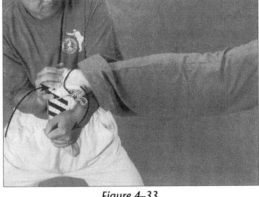

Figure 4–33

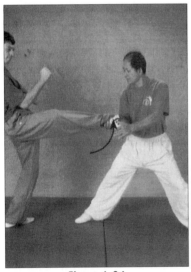

Figure 4–34

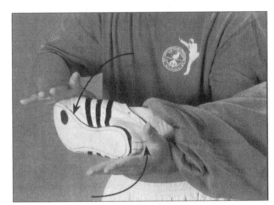

Figure 4–35

Technique #2: Grab the Ankle and Twist

(Zhua Hua Niu Jiao) 抓踝扭脚

Again, when your opponent kicks your lower body, use both of your hands to grab his ankle from his right (Figure 4-32) and then immediately twist his ankle clockwise (Figure 4-33). Alternatively, you may grab his ankle from his left (Figure 4-34) and then twist his ankle counterclockwise (Figure 4-35).

Theory:

Dividing the Muscle/Tendon (ankle) and Misplacing the Bone (knee). When you twist your opponent's ankle, use the entire body's power instead of just using hands. Again, the safe distance between you and your opponent is very important.

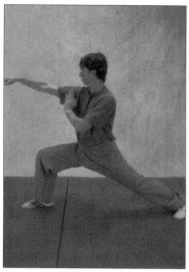
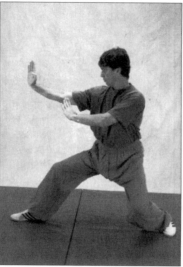
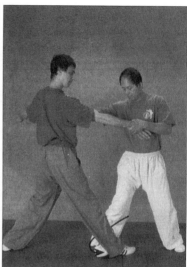

| Figure 4–36 | Figure 4–37 | Figure 4–38 |

4-5. Qin Na Against a Firm Stance

Instead of defense, the techniques introduced in this section are offensive and used to lock your opponent's leg while he is standing stationary. Normally, in order to make the techniques successful, the distance between you and your opponent must be in the short range. Therefore, these techniques are normally used right after you have intercepted your opponent's hand attack.

Technique #1: Leg Wraps Around the Dragon's Leg

(Jiao Chan Long Tui) 腳 纏 龍 腿

This technique can be used against two common stances in martial arts: Bow-Arrow Stance (or Mountain Climbing Stance)(Figure 4-36) and Four-Six Stance (Figure 4-37). When your opponent uses his right hand to punch you with the Bow and Arrow or Four-Six stance, use your left hand to repel and grab his right wrist, while placing your right leg behind his right ankle (Figure 4-38). Finally, twist his leg to make him fall (Figure 4-39).

Theory:

Misplacing the Bone (knee). Although most of the time this technique is used to make your opponent fall, if you jerk your knee while your opponent's leg is locked, you may pop his knee joint out of joint.

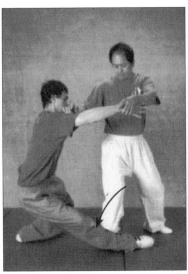
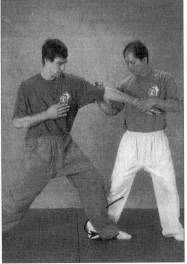
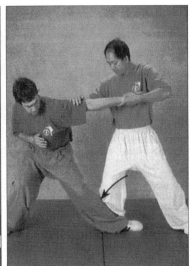

| *Figure 4-39* | *Figure 4-40* | *Figure 4-41* |

Technique #2: Leg Presses the Dragon's Leg

(Tui Ya Long Tui) 腿 壓 龍 腿

This technique is also commonly used against the same two stances discussed in the last technique. The only difference is that you are using your right leg to lock your opponent's left leg instead of his right leg.

When your opponent attacks you with his left hand, repel it to your right with your left forearm and grab his wrist (Figure 4-40). As you do this, also step your right leg behind his left ankle. Finally, press your upper calf toward the side of his upper calf and force him down to the ground (Figure 4-41).

Theory:

Pressing the Muscles (side of upper calf) and Misplacing the Bone (knee). When you execute this technique, the angle of pressing is very important. With the correct angle, you may press your opponent down without too much effort. Also providing the correct locking angle, if you jerk your knee, you may seriously injure the ligament in his knee area.

▪ Chapter **5** ▪

QIN NA AGAINST
KNIFE ATTACKS

5-1. Introduction

Because there were many kinds of weapons used in ancient times, there are many Qin Na techniques specifically created to fight against these weapons. However, in modern society, other than knives and guns, many weapons are seldom seen in public. Therefore, we will only discuss those Qin Na techniques which can be used against knife attacks.

Defending against a knife attack is usually harder and much more dangerous than defending against a barehand attack, so speed is extremely important. You must also perform your techniques firmly and accurately.

At this point, I would like to remind you that if your opponent has a gun and keeps a good distance away from you, then you should **not** try to fight back unless you are absolutely sure that he will shoot you anyway. If it is only a question of money, then give it to him. A bullet is much faster than you are, and your money isn't worth the risk to your life. However, if your opponent is quite a distance away from you, you may have a chance to run and find something to hide behind. If the distance is very short and you can reach the gun without stepping, then you may also have a chance to counter and disarm your opponent. However, you must be very proficient to do this. Otherwise, you are taking an enormous risk.

Before discussing the Qin Na against the knife attacks, in the next section we will first introduce some basic training for use against knife attacks. This will offer you a foundation to understand the Qin Na techniques described in the third section.

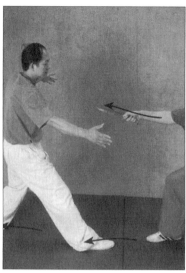
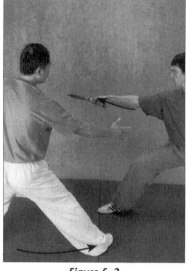
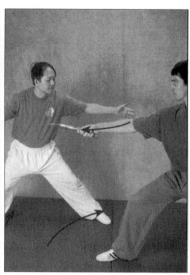

Figure 5–1   Figure 5–2   Figure 5–3

5-2. Basic Training

To defend against a knife attack, in addition to speed, accuracy, and power, you also need to train specific drills. For example, the distance, the angle at which you face your opponent, the timing, and the accuracy of your interception are extremely important. Any mistake can get you hurt. In this section, therefore, we will first focus on escaping from or intercepting an attack. It is best if you practice with a training partner, and still better if you have several partners so that you can get used to a variety of body types and personalities.

Start by having your partner attack you with a rubber knife, so that you can practice escaping from the attacks any way you can. Once you can do this easily, practice intercepting the attack by pushing the wrist or hand.

Once you have learned how to escape, have your partner attack you any way he likes, while you practice avoiding the attack by changing the distance and angle to him. For example, if your partner stabs at you with his right hand, you can dodge backward (Figure 5-1), to his left (Figure 5-2), or to his right (Figure 5-3). Dodging backward is not as good as dodging to the side because the attacker can easily hop forward and continue his attack (Figure 5-4). In addition, if you keep dodging backward, you may be forced into a corner or against a wall. Dodging to the side gives you a chance to circle him or even enter his empty door for an attack.

Once you can escape easily, then you must learn how to intercept the attack. If you get attacked in an area where there is not enough room to keep retreating or dodging, you will have to intercept the attack skillfully. If you know how to intercept, you will not need too much space to defend yourself. To learn how to intercept a knife attack, again have your partner attack you any way he likes, while you practice intercepting with your hands. How you intercept an attack depends on the actual situation, and also on how your opponent is holding the knife. For example, if your opponent thrusts the knife at you with the tip of the knife pointing at you, use your right hand to slap his right wrist while dodging to his left (Figure 5-5). Alternatively, you may use your left hand to slap his right wrist while dodging to his right (Figure 5-6).

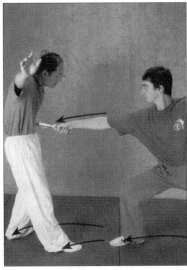

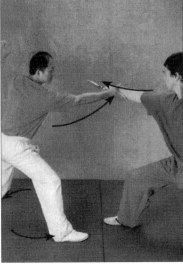

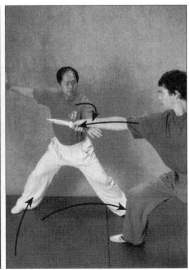

| Figure 5–4 | Figure 5–5 | Figure 5–6 |

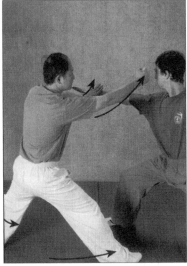

Figure 5–7

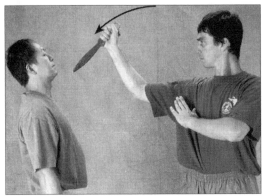

Figure 5–8

Again, retreating backward is not as good as dodging to the sides, because your opponent can hop forward faster than you can retreat and stab you. Furthermore, if you only retreat backward, you will find it difficult to get close enough to him to counterattack. When you dodge to the side, however, it is much easier to close the distance between you (Figure 5-7).

When your opponent, however, holds the knife with the blade projecting from the little finger side of his hand, his reach is relatively shorter, and his choice of techniques is also limited. For example, he can stab you (Figure 5-8) or slice you (Figure 5-9). Usually this grip is used only by professional martial artists who have trained how to use the knife in coordination with kicks and body movement. For untrained people, however, the first grip is easier and more common.

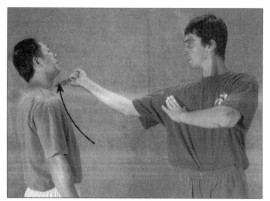

Figure 5–9

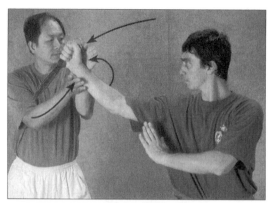

Figure 5–10

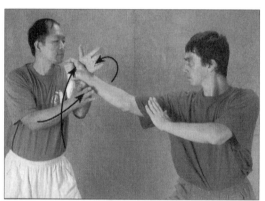

Figure 5–11

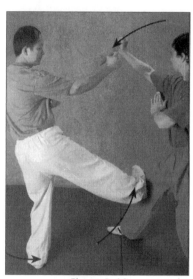

Figure 5–12

To intercept a stabbing attack with the knife held this way, step backward or dodge to the side, and at the same time cover his wrist with your hand (Figure 5-10). If he tries to slice you, use the same covering technique to prevent him from attacking you again (Figure 5-11). However, one of the best ways to defend against an attacker who is holding the knife this way is to kick him, since your leg is probably longer than his arm and knife (Figure 5-12). In fact, use your legs as much as possible. To practice, have your partner attack you any way he likes while using this grip. Practice stepping backward or to the sides while also kicking his shin, knee, abdomen, or groin (Figures 5-13 and 5-14).

Next, learn how to use a belt, clothes, or even shoes to intercept an attack. First have your partner attack you so that you can practice using an article of clothing to intercept. Hold the end of the article in one hand and wrap the material around your forearm (Figure 5-15). Practice intercepting with this arm until you can skillfully push the attack to the side (Figures 5-16 and 5-17) or downward (Figure 5-18).

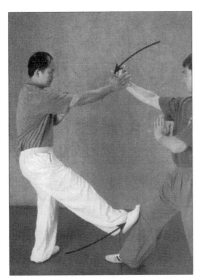

Figure 5–13

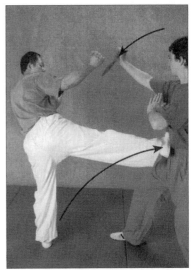

Figure 5–14

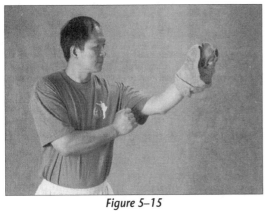

Figure 5–15

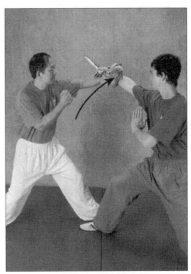

Figure 5–16

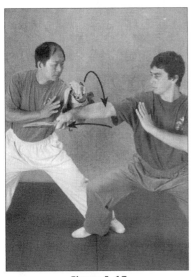

Figure 5–17

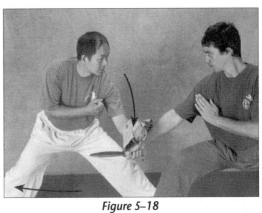

Figure 5–18

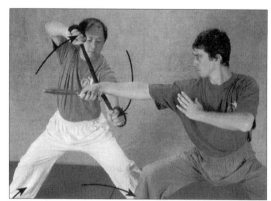

Figure 5–19

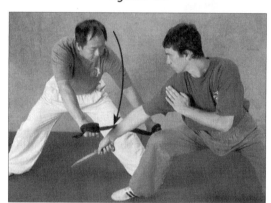

Figure 5–20

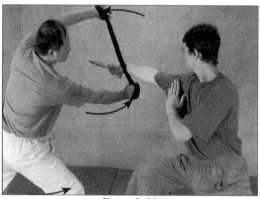

Figure 5–21

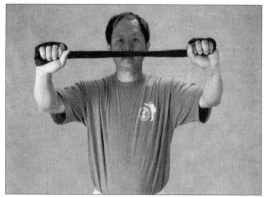

Figure 5–22

You should then also learn how to use a belt to intercept an attack. Wrap an end of the belt around each hand (Figure 5-19). When your partner attacks, intercept with the center part of the belt. When you dodge to your left, have your right hand on top and your left hand on the bottom (Figure 5-20), and when you dodge to your right, have your left hand on the top and your right hand on the bottom (Figure 5-21). You can also push the attack downward (Figure 5-22). Once you have blocked the attack, you may be able to punch with either hand. An article of clothing can also be used to block this way.

Once you have mastered the footwork and dodging tactics, learn how to snap the belt. First practice holding the end with the buckle, and learn how to snap the belt so that it hits the target and bounces back quickly (Figure 5-23). Once you can do this comfortably, practice holding the belt by the other end, and snap the end with the buckle at the target. You can do a lot more damage to your opponent that way.

Finally, you can also practice intercepting with shoes. Put your hands inside the shoes to protect them (Figure 5-24), and then practice blocking your partners attacks without losing your shoes (Figure 5-25).

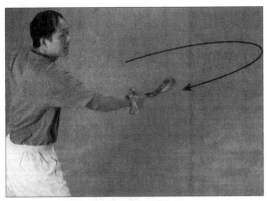

Figure 5-23

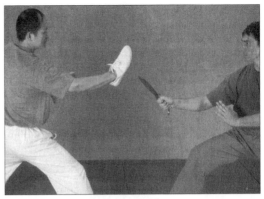

Figure 5-24

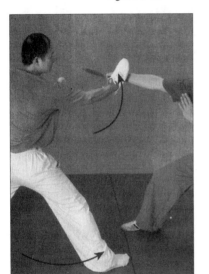

Figure 5-25

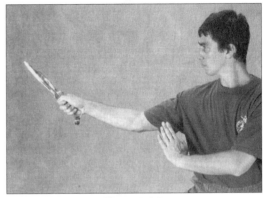

Figure 5-26

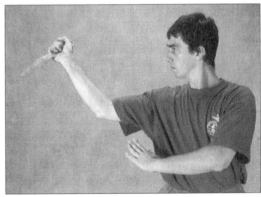

Figure 5-27

5-3. Qin Na Against Knife Attacks

Using Qin Na against a knife attack is very dangerous unless you are quite proficient. Generally speaking, punching and kicking your opponent to injure him is easier than seizing and controlling him. Before you can use Qin Na efficiently, practice until you are very skillful, fast, and accurate in every technique.

In this section we will introduce Qin Na techniques which can be used against knife attacks. The intercepting techniques you use varies depending upon whether your opponent is holding the knife with the point on the thumb-side (point-out) (Figure 5-26) or on the little finger side of the hand (point-in or point-down) (Figure 5-27). If you are interested in learning how to use the belt, brick, or shoes for the same purpose, please refer to *How to Defend Yourself*, by YMAA.

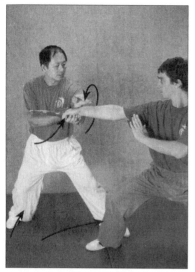

Figure 5–28

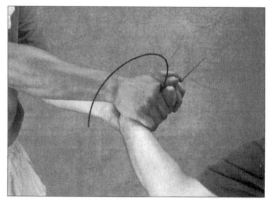

Figure 5–29

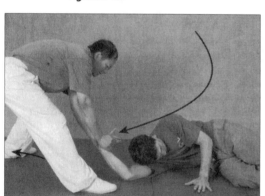

Figure 5–30

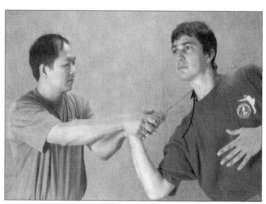

Figure 5–31

I. AGAINST A KNIFE HELD POINT-OUT

A. STABBING THE UPPER BODY

Technique #1: White Ape Worships the Buddha or Reverse Wrist Press

(Bai Yuan Bai Fo or Fan Ya Wan) 白猿拜佛 ，反壓腕

If your opponent stabs at your chest, cover the attack with your left hand on his wrist while simultaneously clamping upward with your right hand (Figure 5-28). When you are doing so, reposition yourself to the right hand side of your opponent. Turn both hands counterclockwise to twist his wrist (Figure 5-29), then press downward with both hands until his elbow touches the ground or he is lying on the ground (Figure 5-30). When you control him, the knife should be pointing at his face or neck. If necessary, move his hands so that he cuts or stabs himself with his own knife (Figure 5-31).

If you cannot control your opponent easily, immediately punch him in the nose with your right hand (Figure 5-32).

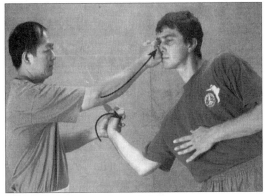

Figure 5–32

Theory:

Dividing the Muscle/Tendon (wrist). To defend against a knife attack, always remember that you must first control his wrist which holds the knife and also keep the tip of knife pointing at him. In this case, your opponent's mind will be on defending instead of attacking. In addition, reposition yourself into an advantageous position for your action.

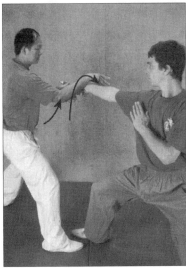

Figure 5–33

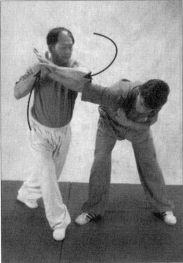

Figure 5–34

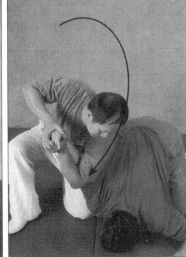

Figure 5–35

Technique #2: Old Man Promoted to General

(Lao Han Bai Jiang) 老漢拜將

If your opponent stabs your chest, cover the attack with your right hand and clamp his wrist with your left hand (Figure 5-33), then immediately turn your body to your right while moving your left elbow over his elbow to lock it under your armpit (Figure 5-34). Keep his arm straight and press downward with your shoulder while bending your left knee to the ground (Figure 5-35). Apply pressure until your opponent's face touches the ground.

If you find that you are losing control of his wrist, immediately kick his groin with your right leg (Figure 5-36).

Theory:

Misplacing the Bone (elbow) and Dividing the Muscle/Tendon (wrist). When you press your oppo-

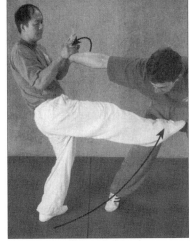

Figure 5–36

nent down, use the entire body's twisting and lowering momentum. The leverage generated from your hands and armpit area is very important. If you jerk your shoulder against your opponent's elbow, you may break his elbow easily.

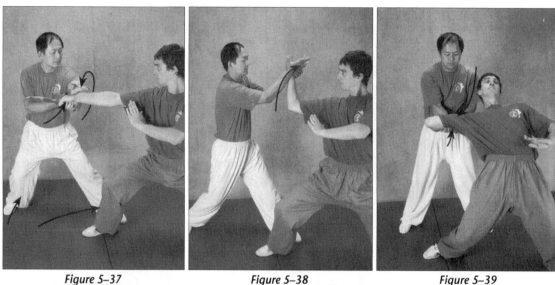

| Figure 5–37 | Figure 5–38 | Figure 5–39 |

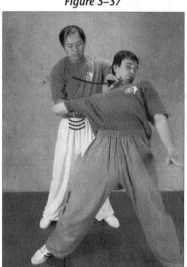 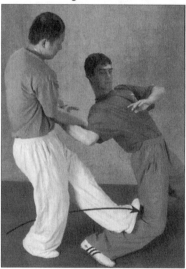

| Figure 5–40 | Figure 5–41 |

Technique #3: White Tiger Turns Its Head or Upward Elbow Wrap

(Bai Hu Fan Shou or Shang Chan Zhou) 白虎返首 ， 上纏肘

If your opponent stabs your chest, cover the attack with your left hand and clamp upward with your right hand (Figure 5-37). As you do this, reposition yourself to his right hand side. Move his forearm counterclockwise while locking his wrist with your left hand (Figure 5-38). Finally, twist his wrist counterclockwise with your left hand and push his elbow upward with your right hand to lock him in place (Figure 5-39). When you are controlling your opponent, keep the knife pointing at his neck so that you can cut or stab him with it. Alternatively, you may lock his right arm with your right hand and your stomach area, while pushing his right neck with your left hand to generate pain on his right arm (Figure 5-40). While you are doing this technique, you may kick the back of his right knee with your right leg to bring him down (Figure 5-41).

Theory:

Misplacing the Bone (elbow) and Dividing the Muscle/Tendon (wrist). The key to control is generated from the wrist twisting. With the wrist's twisting and right hand's pulling, you can generate great pain in his wrist.

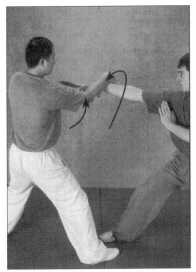

Figure 5–42

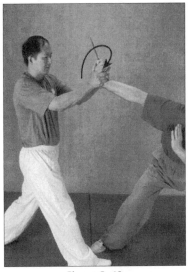

Figure 5–43

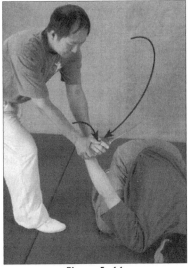

Figure 5–44

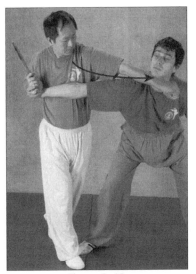

Figure 5–45

Technique #4: Wild Chicken Spreads Its Wings

(Ye Ji Zhan Chi) 野雞展翅

If your opponent stabs at you, cover his attack with your right hand and clamp upward with your left hand (Figure 5-42). Twist his arm clockwise while holding on tightly to his wrist with both hands (Figure 5-43), and then press down on his wrist to push him down (Figure 5-44).

Right after you have turned his hand to your right, you may immediately strike his throat with your forearm (Figure 5-45).

Theory:

Dividing the Muscle/Tendon (wrist). In order to make the control effective, keep his arm as straight as possible. When you control his wrist, use the entire body's momentum to turn and to press his wrist.

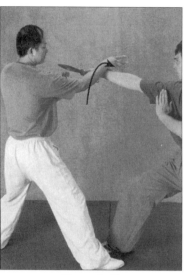

Figure 5–46

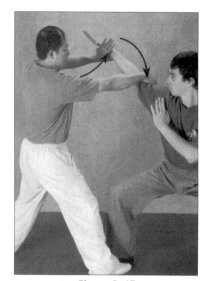

Figure 5–47

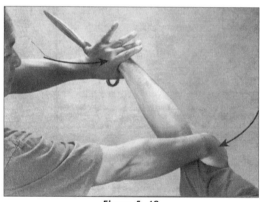

Figure 5–48

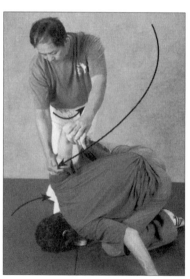

Figure 5–49

Technique #5: Phoenix Spreads Its Wings

(Feng Huang Zhan Chi) 鳳凰展翅

If your opponent stabs at your chest with his right hand, first cover the attack with your right hand while clamping upward with your left hand (Figure 5-46). Immediately move your right hand to his elbow or upper post arm and hook it while using your left hand to grab his right wrist (Figures 5-47 and 5-48). If you use the leverage of both hands, you can break his elbow very easily or bring him down (Figure 5-49).

You may also move your right hand along his arm to grab his hair (or hook his neck) and pull his head downward so that you can knee his face, chest, or groin (Figure 5-50). Alternatively, you may sweep his right leg and make him fall (Figure 5-51). Once you have locked his arm, there are many other techniques which you may use.

Theory:

Misplacing the Bone (elbow). If you would like to bring him down, move your right hand to his shoulder area and this will offer you better leverage for locking.

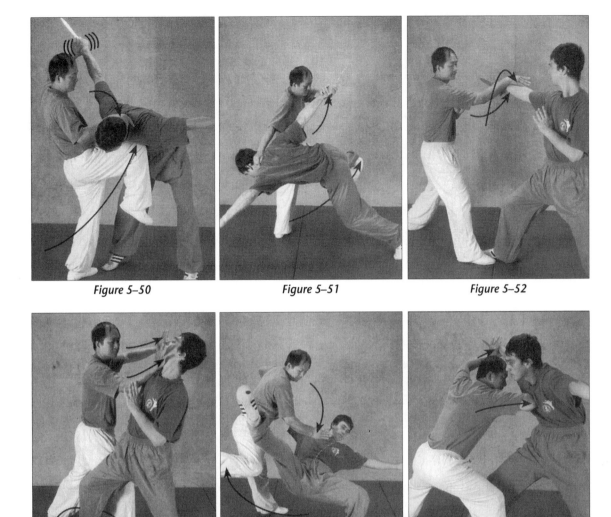

Figure 5-50   Figure 5-51   Figure 5-52

Figure 5-53   Figure 5-54   Figure 5-55

Technique #6: The Lame Man Shows His Courtesy

(Bo Zi You Li) 跛子有禮

When your opponent stabs at you with the knife in his right hand, again use your right hand to cover his wrist (Figure 5-52). Then grab his wrist with your left hand and grab his throat or push his chin with your right hand, while stepping your right leg behind his right leg (Figure 5-53). Sweep your right leg backward while pressing your right arm downward against his throat to make him fall (Figure 5-54).

Right after your left hand has immobilized his right arm, you may use your right hand to strike his temple or poke his eyes, or you may strike him in the chest with your elbow (Figure 5-55).

Theory:
Taking Down. When you place your right leg behind his right leg, position your leg on his rear knee area. This will offer you a better and more powerful sweeping. Good coordination of your right hand push and the right leg sweeping is an important key for executing this technique effectively.

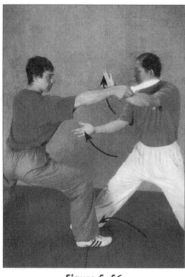
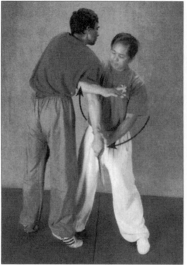
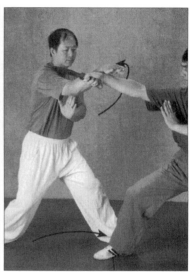

| Figure 5-56 | Figure 5-57 | Figure 5-58 |

Technique #7: Hands Holding a Large Beam

(Shou Wo Da Liang) 手握大樑

When your opponent stabs you, dodge slightly to your right while using your left hand to repel his wrist (Figure 5-56). Right after the repelling, immediately grab his wrist with your left hand while placing your right forearm under his elbow or upper-arm to lock him upward (Figure 5-57). When you control his elbow, if you use the leverage of both of your hands, you can easily break his elbow.

Theory:

Misplacing the Bone (elbow) or Pressing the Tendons (upper-arm). In this technique, right after you have locked your opponent's elbow, do not hesitate to increase your locking pressure until his heel is up. This will prevent him from striking you powerfully with his left hand. Naturally, position yourself to his right as much as possible. If you jerk your right arm, you may break his joint easily.

Technique #8: Embrace the Moon in the Chest

(Huai Zhong Bao Yue) 懷中抱月

Similar in theory to the previous technique, you may also dodge slightly to your left and repel the attack with your right hand while stepping your left leg behind his right leg (Figure 5-58). Then grab his wrist with your right hand and lock his elbow upward with your left arm (Figure 5-59). You may break his elbow from this position if necessary. If you feel that your arm is too weak to lock his elbow, use your shoulder instead (Figure 5-60). It is also very easy for you to strike his lower ribs with your left elbow (Figure 5-61).

Theory:

Misplacing the Bone (elbow). The leverage generated from both of your hands and your left elbow is the key to the control.

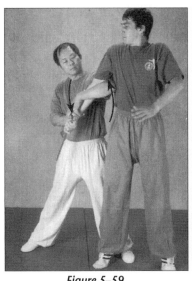

Figure 5–59

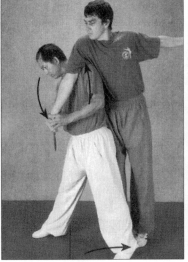

Figure 5–60

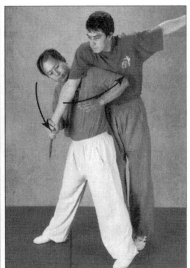

Figure 5–61

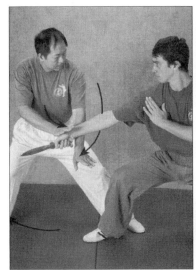

Figure 5–62

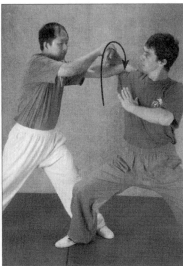

Figure 5–63

B. STABBING THE LOWER BODY

Technique #1: Low Outward Wrist Press

(Xia Wai Ya Wan) 下 外 壓 腕

If your opponent stabs to your lower body, step your right leg backward and repel the attack to your right with your left forearm, while grabbing his wrist with your right hand (Figure 5-62). Circle your left arm counterclockwise upward and then downward (Figures 5-63 and 5-64), and lock his wrist and elbow in position (Figure 5-65).

Theory:

Dividing the Muscle/Tendon (wrist). In this technique, the pain is generated from the control of the wrist. Your left hand serves only to lock your opponent's arm in position.

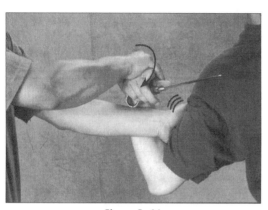

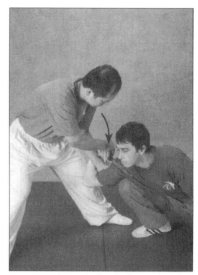

Figure 5–64

Figure 5–65

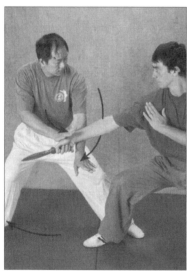

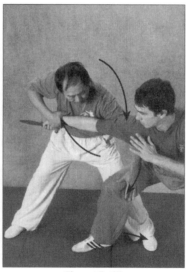

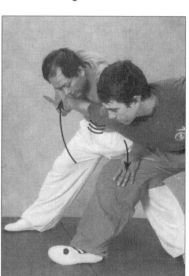

Figure 5–66

Figure 5–67

Figure 5–68

Technique #2: Two Children Worship the Buddha

(Shuang Tong Bai Fo) 雙童拜佛

If your opponent stabs to your lower body, again step your right leg backward and repel the attack to your right with your left forearm, while grabbing his wrist with your right hand (Figure 5-66). Immediately slide your left leg in against his right knee, while inserting your left arm under his right arm and either place it on his right thigh or stomach area (Figure 5-67). Finally, bow your body forward, the left hand pressing his thigh down, and pulling your right hand backward while thrusting your left shoulder against his right shoulder to lock him (Figure 5-68).

Alternatively, right after you have intercepted the attack and grabbed his wrist, you may step back with your right leg and swing your opponent to the ground in an arc (Figure 5-69). You have to use the leverage of both arms to move him easily.

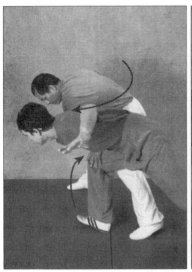
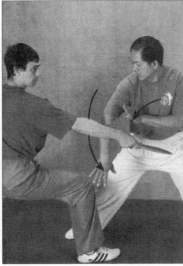
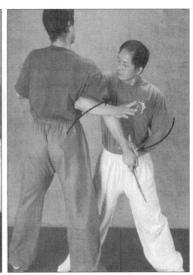

Figure 5–69   Figure 5–70   Figure 5–71

Theory:

Dividing the Muscle/Tendon (wrist). In this technique, the pain is generated from the control of the wrist. Your left hand serves only to lock your opponent's arm in position

Technique #3: Embrace the Moon in the Chest

(Huai Zhong Bao Yue) 懷 中 抱 月

When your opponent stabs you, use your right forearm to repel his attack to your left while using your left hand to grab his right wrist (Figure 5-70). Immediately after the repelling, place your right forearm under his elbow or upper-arm to lock him upward (Figure 5-71). When you control his elbow, if you use the leverage of both of your hands, you can easily break his elbow.

Theory:

Misplacing the Bone (elbow) or Pressing the Tendons (upper-arm). In this technique, right after you have locked your opponent's elbow, do not hesitate to increase your locking pressure until his heels are up. This will prevent him from striking you powerfully with his left hand. Naturally, position yourself to his right as much as possible. If you jerk your right arm, you may break his joint easily.

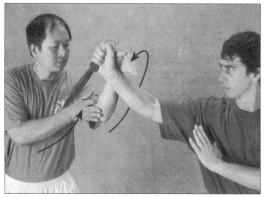

Figure 5–72

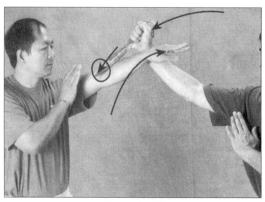

Figure 5–73

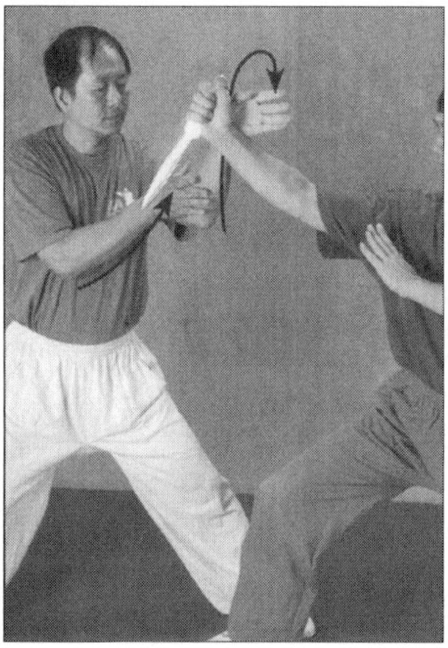

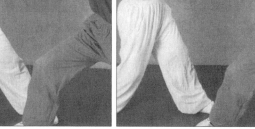

Figure 5–74

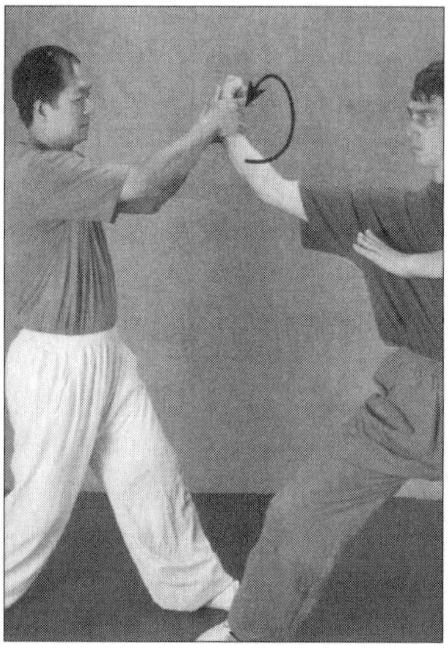

Figure 5–75

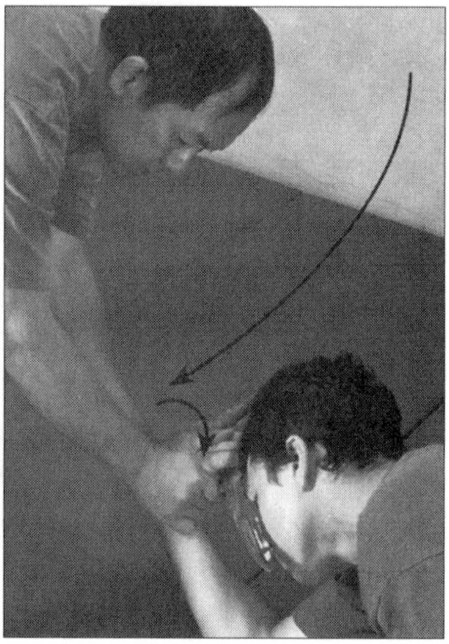

Figure 5–76

II. AGAINST A KNIFE HELD POINT-IN OR POINT-DOWN

When your opponent holds his knife with the point on the little finger side of the hand, only use covering techniques to intercept (Figure 5-72). If you intercept by repelling, your forearm can be cut easily (Figure 5-73).

Technique #1: White Ape Worships the Buddha or Reverse Wrist Press

(Bai Yuan Bai Fo or Fan Ya Wan) 白猿拜佛 ， 反壓腕

If your opponent stabs at you with the knife in his right hand, cover his wrist with your left hand while clamping upward with your right hand (Figure 5-74). As you do this, reposition yourself to your opponent's right hand side. Twist his wrist counterclockwise (Figure 5-75) and press his hand forward to generate pain. You should push until his elbow touches the ground or he is lying on the ground (Figure 5-76).

Theory:

Dividing the Muscle/Tendon (wrist). If you discover that your opponent's arm suddenly tenses up to resist your control, simply use your right hand to punch his nose first, then lock him down.

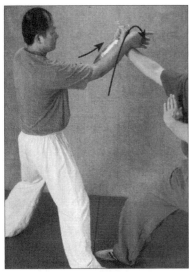 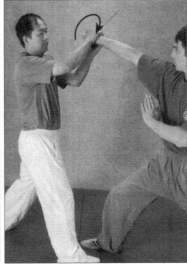 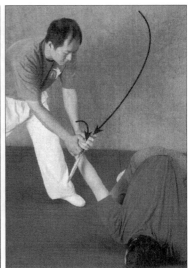

Figure 5–77   Figure 5–78   Figure 5–79

Technique #2: Wild Chicken Spreads Its Wings

(Ye Ji Zhan Chi) 野雞展翅

This is similar in theory to the last technique. Cover the attack with your right hand while clamping upward with your left hand (Figure 5-77). Twist his wrist clockwise (Figure 5-78) and finally step your right leg backward and press his hand downward until his face touches the floor (Figure 5-79).

Theory:

Dividing the Muscle/Tendon (wrist). To make the control effective, keep your opponent's arm as straight as possible. In addition, when you control his wrist, use the entire body's momentum for your turning and pressing instead of just using arms.

Technique #3: White Tiger Turns Its Head or Upward Elbow Wrap

(Bai Hu Fan Shou or Shang Chan Zhou) 白虎返首 ，上纏肘

If your opponent stabs at your chest, step your right leg backward and cover the attack with your left hand while clamping upward with your right hand (Figure 5-80). Move his forearm counterclockwise while locking his wrist with your left hand (Figure 5-81). Then push his elbow upward with your right hand and lock him in position (Figures 5-82 and 5-83). When you have him controlled, the knife should be pointing at his neck so that you can cut or stab him with it.

Theory:

Misplacing the Bone (elbow) and Dividing the Muscle/Tendon (wrist). The key to control is generated from the wrist twisting. With the wrist's twisting and right hand's pulling, you can generate great pain in his wrist.

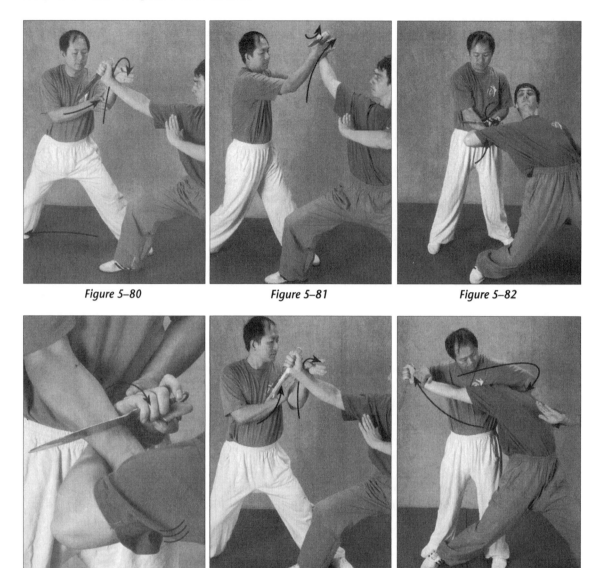

Figure 5–80   Figure 5–81   Figure 5–82

Figure 5–83   Figure 5–84   Figure 5–85

Technique #4: Arm Wraps Around the Dragon's Neck

(Bi Chan Long Jing) 臂 纏 龍 頸

When your opponent stabs at your chest, step your right leg backward and cover his wrist with your left hand while moving your right hand upward (Figure 5-84). Then grab his wrist with your right hand while circling your left arm around his neck (Figure 5-85). Of course, you may instead use your left arm to attack his face or throat (Figure 5-86).

Theory:

Sealing the Artery (neck) and Sealing the Breathing (throat). To prevent your opponent from struggling, lock his neck tightly until his heels are off the ground. You can kill your opponent if you use too much of the power.

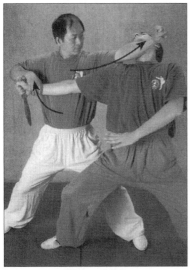

Figure 5–86

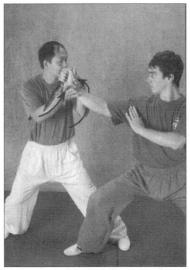

Figure 5–87

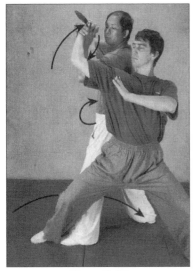

Figure 5–88

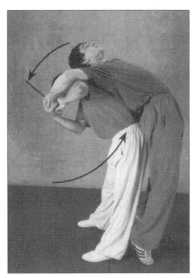

Figure 5–89

Technique #5: The Old Man Carries the Fish on His Back

(Lao Han Bei Yu) 老漢背魚

When your opponent stabs at your chest, step your right leg backward and cover his wrist with your left hand while clamping upward with your right hand (Figure 5-87). Turn your body to your right while pushing upward with your elbow (Figure 5-88). Finally, bow your body forward while pulling his arm with both of your hands (Figure 5-89).

Theory:

Misplacing the Bone (shoulder and elbow). The angle set up at his elbow is very important; too straight or too bent will make the technique ineffective. If necessary, use your right elbow to strike his left kidney.

You can see that there are fewer Qin Na techniques which can be used when the knife is held point-in or point-down than when it is held point-out. However, there are also only a limited number of ways in which your opponent can attack you when he is holding the knife this way. In addition, when he holds the knife this way, his range is more limited. It is therefore safer and more effective for you to use kicks.

The Chinese martial arts have many more Qin Na techniques for use against knife attacks. Remember, however, that it is better to master a few techniques than to learn many techniques poorly. In fact, if you master all of the techniques we have shown, you will find that you can discover or create many other techniques by yourself.

▪ Chapter **6** ▪

QIN NA AGAINST GRABBING

6-1. Introduction

I t is well known that Qin Na specializes against grabbing. When you are grabbed somewhere on your body, other than punching and kicking, Qin Na is probably the most useful and effective tool for dealing with the situation. This is especially true if you want to control your opponent and do not intend to seriously injure him.

Because Qin Na is so effective against grabbing, it has become one of the best methods of dealing with wrestling or Judo, in which grabbing is essential to applying techniques. Not only that, Qin Na can also be the most effective skill against the sticking and adhering in which soft Chinese martial styles specialize. In fact, it is widely known that Japanese Aikido and Jujitsu styles originated from the theories of Taijiquan and Qin Na.

Due to the above reasons, there are abundant Qin Na techniques that have developed in the past which specialize in defense against grabbing. This is because there are so many available techniques which can be used against grabbing, such as wrist grabbing. Therefore, we will only introduce those which are the most representative and effective. After you have mastered all of these techniques, you will be able to comprehend the essence of the art and become proficient in further development.

In this chapter, we will introduce techniques which can be used against the wrist, arm, shoulder, and chest grabs in Sections 6-2, 6-3, 6-4, and 6-5 respectively. Next, some techniques against neck grabbing from both the front and rear will be discussed in Section 6-6. Finally, Qin Na techniques which can be used against special situations, such as grabbing the belt, embracing, and hair pulling will be covered in Sections 6-7, 6-8, and 6-9.

6-2. Qin Na Against Wrist Grabbing

In this section, we will summarize some of the most effective Qin Na techniques against wrist grabbing. We will divide the subject into two categories: opposite side grabbing and same side grabbing.

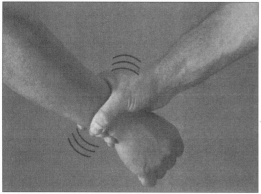

Figure 6–1

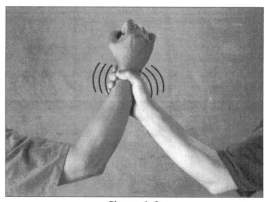

Figure 6–2

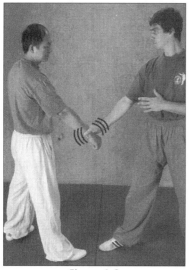

Figure 6–3

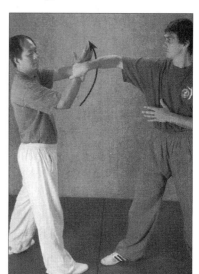

Figure 6–4

I. OPPOSITE SIDE GRABBING

Again, there are two common methods of grabbing for both opposite and same side grabbing. The first way is your opponent grabs from the upper side of the wrist (Figure 6-1) and the second is he grabs from the lower side of the wrist (Figure 6-2). In order to make things clear, we will again divide opposite side grabbing and same side grabbing into two categories: grabbing above the wrist and grabbing under the wrist.

A. GRABBING ABOVE THE WRIST

Technique #1: Small Wrap Finger

(Xiao Chan Zhi) 小纏指

When your opponent's right hand grabs your right wrist (Figure 6-3), immediately use your left hand to cover and push his pinkie toward his wrist to lock it in place while raising up your right hand with the palm facing toward you (Figure 6-4). Finally, step your right leg backward and circle your right hand forward and downward to lock his pinkie and wrist (Figure 6-5). You should continue your circular downward pressing until your opponent's right elbow touches the ground (Figure 6-6).

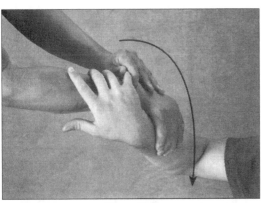

Figure 6–5

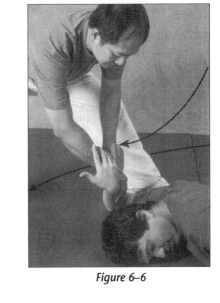

Figure 6–6

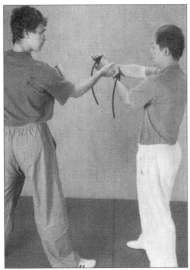

Figure 6–7

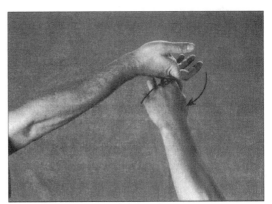

Figure 6–8

Theory:

Dividing the Muscle/Tendon (wrist and pinkie). When you lock your opponent's pinkie with your left hand, the position of locking is important. If the control is too near to the finger tip, your opponent may escape, and if you lock too close to the base of the pinkie joint, it is not as effective. You should try and experience it yourself to get the feeling.

Technique #2: Hand Bend the Index Finger

(Shou Ban Shi Zhi) 手扳食指

When your opponent grabs your right wrist with his right hand, first rotate your right hand counterclockwise while also placing your left hand on his second finger (Figure 6-7). Next, free your right wrist from the gap between his thumb and second finger and let his second finger drop into your left hand, step your right leg backward, and use your thumb and second finger to bend his second finger to lock him up (Figure 6-8). You should increase your locking pressure until his heels are off the ground (Figure 6-9).

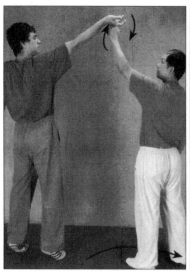
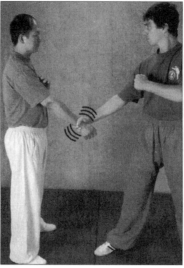
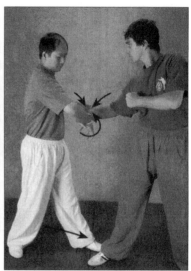

Figure 6–9   *Figure 6–10*   *Figure 6–11*

Theory:

Misplacing the Bone (index finger). The key to locking your opponent upward efficiently is not from raising up your left hand. Instead, it is through the rotation and leverage generated from your left thumb and index finger.

Technique #3: Hand Bends the Thumb

(Shou Ban Mo Zhi) 手扳姆指

When your opponent grabs your right wrist with his right hand (Figure 6-10), immediately rotate your right hand to your left under his wrist while stepping your left leg to the side of his right leg (Figure 6-11). While you are rotating your right forearm, also use your left hand to lock his thumb and forearm, and use your right hand to press his pinkie backward (Figure 6-12). You should increase your pressure until he is in an awkward position to resist or attack you with his left hand (Figure 6-13).

Theory:

Misplacing the Bone (thumb and pinkie) and Dividing the Muscle/Tendon (wrist). This technique can be executed easily for those who have bigger hands. If you have small hands, it will not be easy for you to execute this technique. Therefore, you should use your judgement before you apply this technique.

Technique #4: Hand Bend the Pinkie

(Shou Ban Xiao Zhi) 手扳小指

When your opponent grabs your right wrist with his right hand (Figure 6-14), immediately step your left leg forward to the side of his right leg and swing your right arm to your right, while placing your left hand on his pinkie area (Figure 6-15). Next, free your right arm from the gap between this thumb and index finger and push his thumb backward, while grabbing his pinkie with your left hand and bending it backward (Figure 6-16). You should increase your pressure until his heels are off the ground (Figure 6-17).

Theory:

Misplacing the Bone (thumb and pinkie). The leverage generated from your right hand and left shoulder is very important. Only with this lock can your pinkie lock be effective.

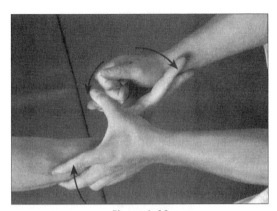

Figure 6–12

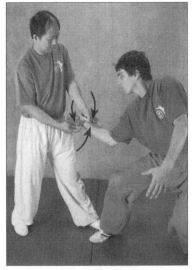

Figure 6–13

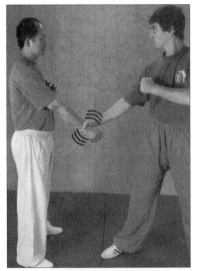

Figure 6–14

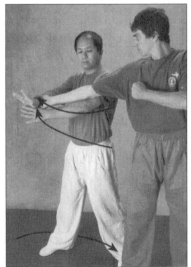

Figure 6–15

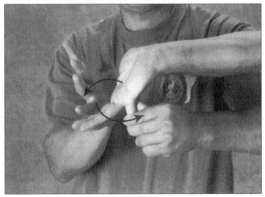

Figure 6–16

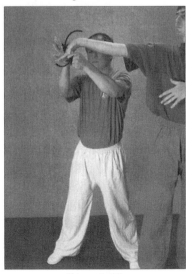

Figure 6–17

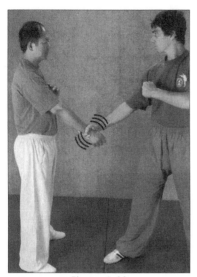

Figure 6–18

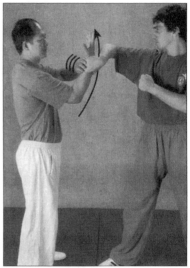

Figure 6–19

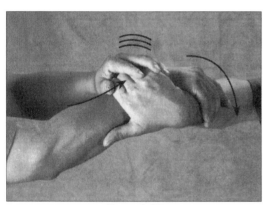

Figure 6–20

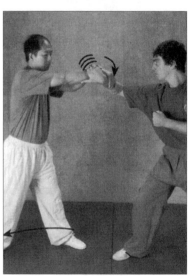

Figure 6–21

Technique #5: Small Wrap Hand

(Xiao Chan Shou) 小纏手

When someone grabs your right wrist with his right hand (Figure 6-18), immediately cover his right hand with your left hand and use your left thumb to push his index finger toward your right wrist, while raising up your right hand with the palm facing you (Figure 6-19). This will prevent him from opening his hand and escaping, and set up a good angle for further locking. Then turn your hand forward and wrap it over his wrist while stepping your right leg backward (Figures 6-20 and 6-21) and finally press him downward with your fingers pointing downward (Figure 6-22). This is a form of crane wing dropping as trained by the crane style. You should press him down until his face touches the ground. If necessary, you may use your right leg to kick his chest or face to injure him.

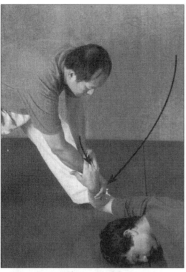

Figure 6–22

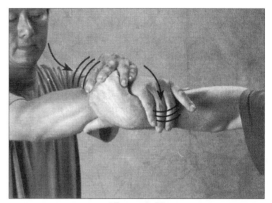

Figure 6–23

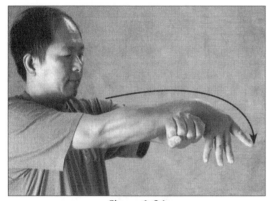

Figure 6–24

Theory:

Dividing the Muscle/Tendon (wrist). When you lock your opponent's right hand with your left hand, you should use your thumb to push the last section of his index finger toward your right wrist while covering your entire hand above his hand. When you lock him down, you should not push to the side. Instead, you should press straight downward. The leverage generated from your right hand and left thumb is the key to locking. When you lock his wrist, his elbow should be lower than his wrist and bent. To accomplish this goal, you must learn how to use your middle, ring, and small fingers to direct your opponent's forearm (Figure 6-23). Furthermore, when you press him down, your should prevent your right arm from bending by extending it until it is straight and your fingers are pointing downward. To train this by yourself, simply place your left forearm right in front of you and file your right wrist forward and then downward against your left wrist area (Figure 6-24).

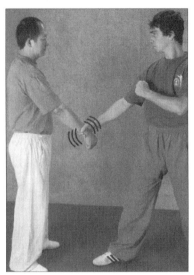

Figure 6–25

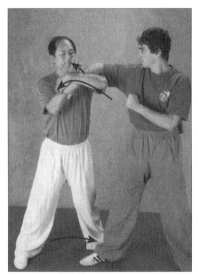

Figure 6–26

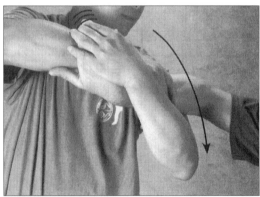

Figure 6–27

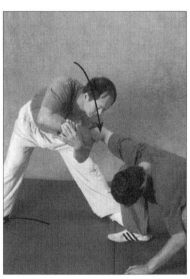

Figure 6–28

Technique #6: Large Wrap Hand

(Da Chan Shou) 大纏手

When someone grabs your right wrist with his right hand (Figure 6-25), step your left leg forward as you raise your right hand up in front of you, and at the same time move your left hand under his forearm to cover and wrap his right hand (Figure 6-26). Lock his right elbow with your left elbow to prevent him from elbowing you. As your left hand is wrapping his hand, raise the fingers of your right hand and then press down on his right wrist (Figures 6-27 and 6-28). You should bow toward him and press him down until his left hand touches the floor, otherwise he can still punch your face with it.

Another option of the Large Wrap Hand is, when your opponent grabs your right wrist with his right hand, again step your left leg behind his right leg and at the same time raise

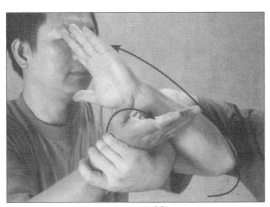

Figure 6–29

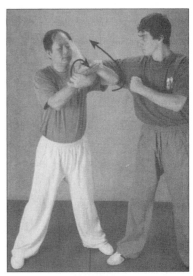

Figure 6–30

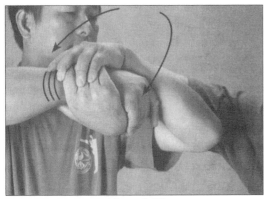

Figure 6–31

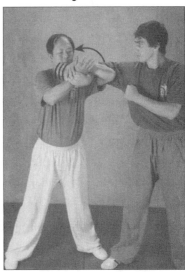

Figure 6–32

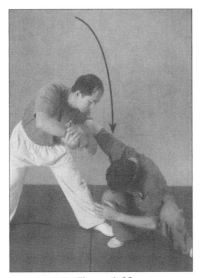

Figure 6–33

your right arm up, while moving your left arm under his right elbow (Figures 6-29 and 6-30). However, this time keep your right palm open. Next, cross your left hand over your right palm and use your left hand to wrap his right fingers (Figures 6-31 and 6-32). Finally, bow toward your opponent while pressing the edge of your right hand to his wrist (Figure 6-33).

Theory:

Dividing the Muscle/ Tendon (wrist). When you lock his wrist, make sure to use the correct angle on his wrist, or he can turn and use his left elbow to strike you. If you find you have failed to control him, you can kick him with your right leg.

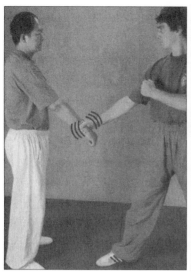

Figure 6–34

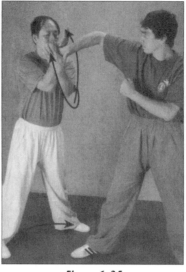

Figure 6–35

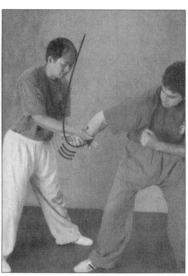

Figure 6–36

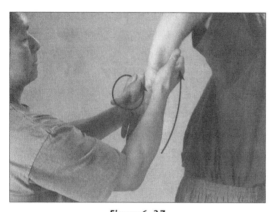

Figure 6–37

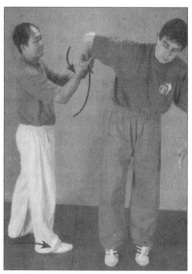

Figure 6–38

Technique #7: Back Wrap Hand

(Fan Chan Shou) 反纏手

When your opponent grabs your right wrist with his right hand (Figure 6-34), step your left leg to his right hand side as you circle your right arm clockwise to weaken his grip (Figure 6-35). Keep circling his arm down while using your left hand to grab his hand (Figure 6-36). Next, use your left hand to twist his hand clockwise and bend it away from you while using your right hand to push upward (Figure 6-37). Finally, step your right leg behind him and lock him up (Figure 6-38). You should lift him up until his heels leave the floor, otherwise he is not completely controlled and can kick you.

Theory:

Dividing the Muscle/Tendon (wrist). The key to control is to twist his wrist as far as possible and then bend. If you use your right hand which is on the wrist to generate good leverage, you may generate great pain in his wrist.

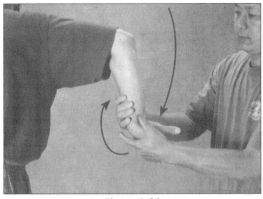

Figure 6–39

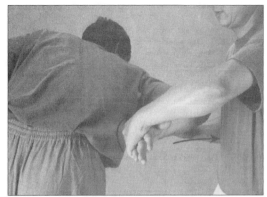

Figure 6–40

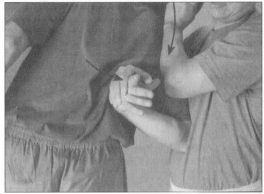

Figure 6–41

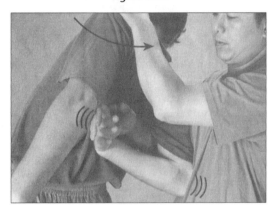

Figure 6–42

Technique #8: Hands Hold Panda

(Shou Bao Wan Xiong) 手抱浣熊

In the last technique, once you have circled his arm down (Figure 6-39) and moved your opponent's hand behind his back, you may use your right hand to pull his elbow in to your right stomach area (Figure 6-40). Immediately use your right hand to grab his hand, and press it toward your stomach to lock his right arm behind him (Figure 6-41). To increase the effectiveness of the locking, use your left hand to grab his hair and pull it down, or simply use your left hand to pull back his left shoulder to cause pain (Figure 6-42).

Theory:

Dividing the Muscle/Tendon (wrist). This technique may not work on those who have double joints. In order to make the control more effective, you may use your left hand to push back any of his fingers.

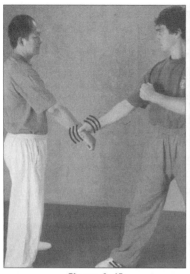

Figure 6–43

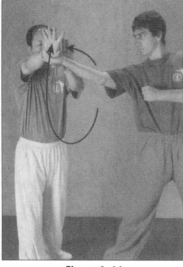

Figure 6–44

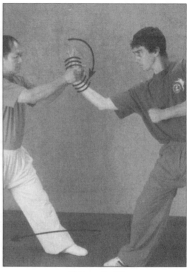

Figure 6–45

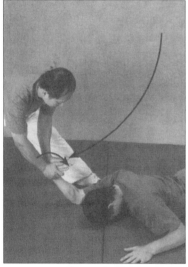

Figure 6–46

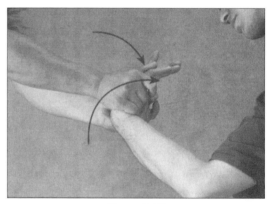

Figure 6–47

Technique #9: White Ape Worships the Buddha or Reverse Wrist Press

(Bai Yuan Bai Fo or Fan Ya Wan) 白猿拜佛 ， 反壓腕

When your opponent has grabbed your right wrist with his right hand (Figure 6-43), simply rotate your right arm and circle your hand counterclockwise and grab his wrist with your left hand, with your thumb pressing the base of his pinkie (Figure 6-44). Press your thumb forward and free your right hand through the gap between his thumb and index finger, then grab his hand with both of your hands and push forward and downward while your right leg steps backward (Figure 6-45). You should press him down until his elbow touches the ground (Figure 6-46). When you press him down, you may twist his hand to the side slightly and therefore generate more pressure on his pinkie tendon (Figure 6-47). This can generate more pain.

Theory:

Dividing the Muscle/Tendon (wrist and pinkie). To make the control effective, you must generate good leverage between your thumbs and pinkie. Once you have locked the hand, press downward with both of your entire hands instead of just the thumbs.

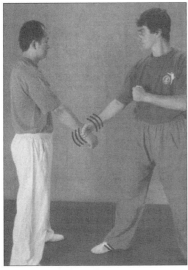

Figure 6–48

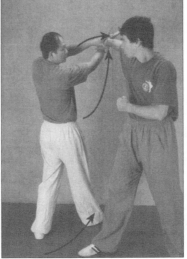

Figure 6–49

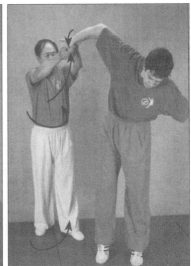

Figure 6–50

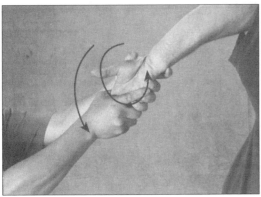

Figure 6–51

Technique #10: Send the Devil to Heaven

(Song Mo Shang Tian) 送魔上天

When your opponent grabs your right wrist with his right hand (Figure 6-48), cover and grab his right hand with your left hand, and swing his arm up as you step your right leg to his right hand side (Figure 6-49). Then, turn to your left and step your left leg beside your right leg while twisting and bending his wrist upward to force his heels off the floor (Figure 6-50).

Theory:

Dividing the Muscle/Tendon (wrist). The important point for executing this technique successfully is, when you have locked your opponent in the final position, you should emphasize the pinkie twisting, which makes the technique more effective. In order to increase the pain, you may use your left hand to twist his hand while using your right hand to grab his fingers and bend them downward (Figure 6-51).

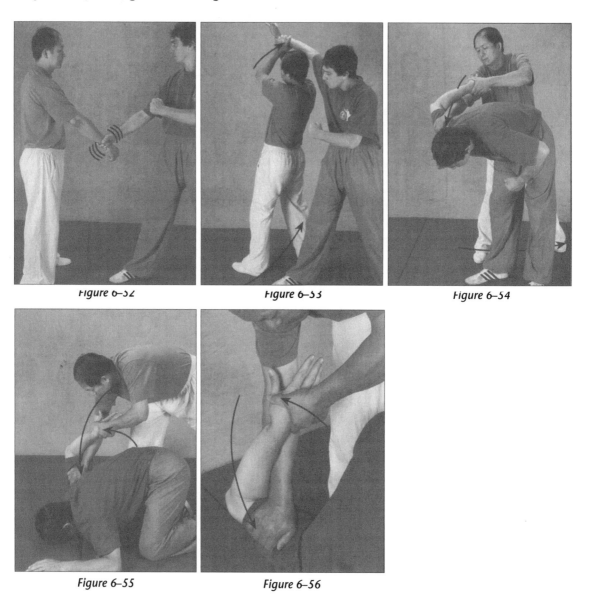

Figure 6–52

Figure 6–53

Figure 6–54

Figure 6–55

Figure 6–56

Technique #11: Lion Worships the Buddha or Large Elbow Wrap

(Shi Zi Bai Fo or Da Chan Zhou) 獅子拜佛 ， 大纏肘

When your opponent has grabbed your right wrist with his right hand (Figure 6-52), immediately step your right leg beside his right leg and raise his right arm up, while using your left hand to grab his right wrist (Figure 6-53). Again, step your left leg behind him while freeing your right hand and coiling it around his arm until it reaches his right elbow (Figure 6-54). Finally, push him downward until his face touches the ground (Figure 6-55).

Theory:

Misplacing the Bone (shoulder) and Dividing the Muscle/Tendon (wrist). When you rotate your body, and twist and bend your opponent's arm, you should use the entire body's power instead of just the arm. In addition, in order to lock him efficiently, you should place your hand on his upper-arm near the elbow area instead of his shoulder (Figure 6-56).

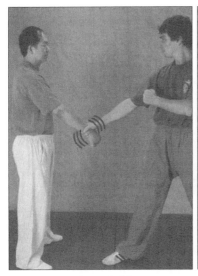
Figure 6–57

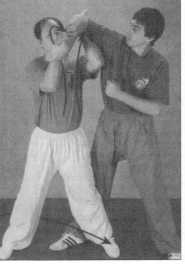
Figure 6–58

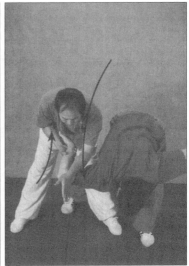
Figure 6–59

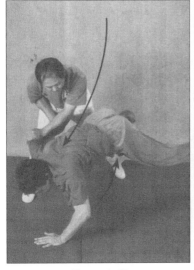
Figure 6–60

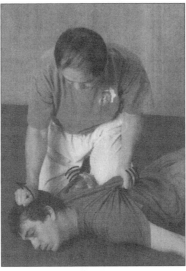
Figure 6–61

Technique #12: Luo Han Bows or Small Elbow Wrap

(Luo Han Xing Li or Xiao Chan Zhou) 羅漢行禮，小纏肘

When your opponent grabs your wrist with his right hand (Figure 6-57), step your left leg to the front of his right leg and use your right hand to grab his wrist, while using your left forearm to press his elbow up (Figure 6-58). Then bend forward, and push his elbow forward and downward (Figure 6-59). If you want to make him fall, simply pull his right arm toward the front of your body to destroy his stability, while bowing your body forward and sweeping your left leg backward (Figure 6-60). When your opponent is on the ground, lock his arm behind his back with your two legs (Figure 6-61). You may also use your right hand to pull his hair toward you to prevent him from escaping.

Theory:

Misplacing the Bone (elbow and shoulder). In order to make your opponent fall, after you have locked him, you should pull him to your front to destroy his balance while sweeping your left leg backward. Once your opponent is on the ground, if necessary you may rotate his arm toward his head and pop his shoulder out of joint.

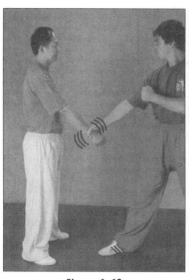
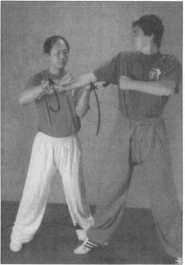
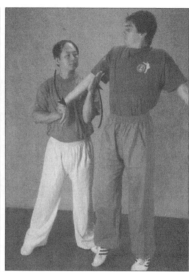

| Figure 6–62 | Figure 6–63 | Figure 6–64 |

Technique #13: Heaven King Supports the Pagoda or Upward Elbow Press

(Tian Wang Tuo Ta or Shang Ya Zhou) 天王托塔，上壓肘

When your opponent grabs your right wrist with his right hand (Figure 6-62), immediately step your left leg beside his right leg, coil your right hand counterclockwise and grab his right wrist while placing your left hand under his elbow (Figure 6-63). Finally, press down on his wrist with your right hand while pressing upward on his elbow with your left hand (Figure 6-64). You should increase your power until his heels are off the ground. You should keep yourself on the right hand side of your opponent. This will prevent him from attacking you with his left hand.

Theory:

Misplacing the Bone (elbow). The leverage generated from both of your hands is the key to the control.

Technique #14: Hands Prop a Large Beam or Prop Up Elbow

(Shou Ban Da Liang or Shang Jia Zhou) 手扳大樑，上架肘

This technique is very similar to the last technique. When your opponent grabs your right wrist with his right hand (Figure 6-65), immediately step your left leg beside his right leg, coil your right hand counterclockwise and grab his wrist and press your left arm upward on his elbow (Figure 6-66). Finally bend your left hand to reach his wrist and use the leverage of both of your hands and your left elbow lock his arm up (Figure 6-67). You should continue your locking pressure until your opponent's heels are off the ground (Figure 6-68).

If you are short, it will be hard for you to use your elbow to control his elbow. In this case, you may simply place his elbow on your left shoulder and lock him up from there.

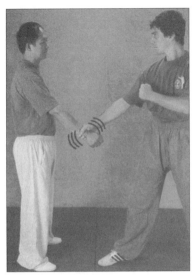

Figure 6–65

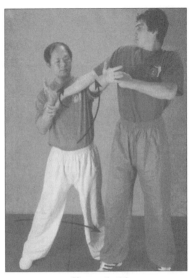

Figure 6–66

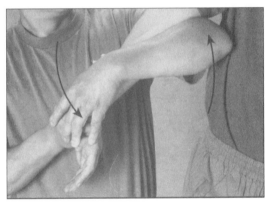

Figure 6–67

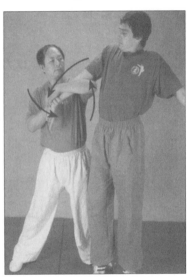

Figure 6–68

Theory:

Misplacing the Bone (elbow). The key to control is from the leverage generated from both of your hands and your left elbow. The position where you stand is very important. You should be in a position from which his left hand cannot reach you.

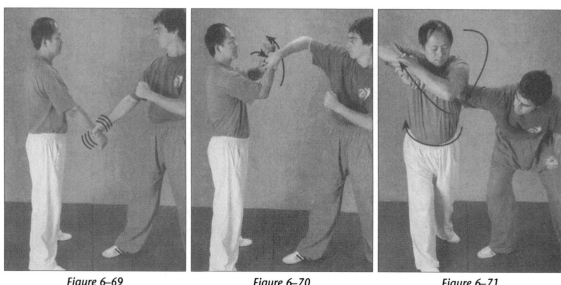

Figure 6–69   Figure 6–70   Figure 6–71

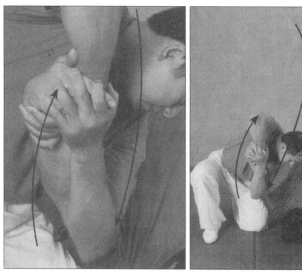

Figure 6–72   Figure 6–73

Technique #15: Old Man Promoted to General

(Lao Han Bai Jiang) 老漢拜將

If your opponent grabs your right wrist with his right hand (Figure 6-69), cover his right hand with your left hand while lifting your right arm upward (Figure 6-70). Next, turn your body to your right and pull his arm straight while placing your left armpit over his elbow (Figure 6-71). Finally, raise your hands while lowering your elbow as you kneel down on your left knee in your stance (Figures 6-72 and 6-73). You must hold his hand at the correct angle so that you will be able to keep his elbow straight and lock his arm; otherwise, he will be able to escape. Remember to press him down until his face touches the floor.

Theory:

Misplacing the Bone (elbow). When you press your opponent down, you should keep his arm straight, and the pressing should be straight on the rear side of his elbow. If you jerk your power, you may break his elbow easily.

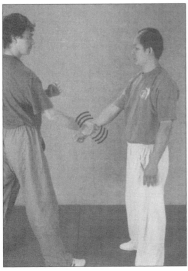

Figure 6–74

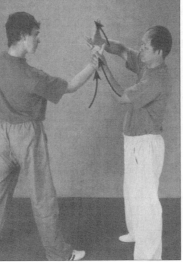

Figure 6–75

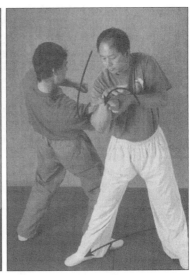

Figure 6–76

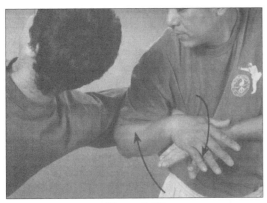

Figure 6–77

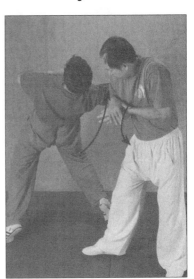

Figure 6–78

Technique #16: Sparrow Hawk Shakes Its Wing or Backward Upward Turning

(Yao Zi Dou Chi or Hou Shang Fan) 鷂子抖翅，後上翻

When your opponent grabs your right wrist with his right hand (Figure 6-74), circle your right arm upward while using your left hand to grab his hand (Figure 6-75). Next, step your right leg behind his right leg and twist your left hand counterclockwise, while circling your right elbow and pressing it against his right elbow (Figure 6-76). Finally, use the leverage of your hands and right elbow to press his elbow upward (Figures 6-77 and 6-78). Alternatively, you may step your left leg behind him, coil your right arm around his right arm and reach his chest to lock his right arm in front of your chest, while using your left hand to push his neck to generate pain in his arm (Figure 6-79).

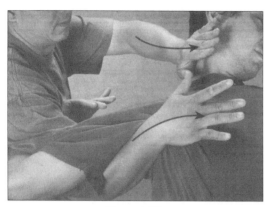

Figure 6–79

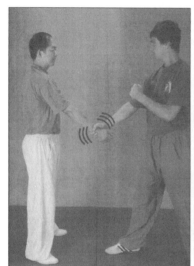

Figure 6–80

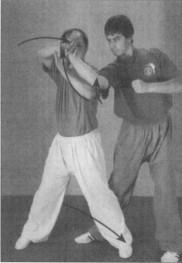

Figure 6–81

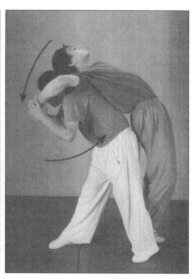

Figure 6–82

Theory.

Dividing the Muscle/Tendon (wrist) and Misplacing the Bones (elbow). Misplacing the Bone (elbow and shoulder) in the optional technique. In order to prevent your opponent from striking you with his left hand, you should step your right leg behind his right leg. This stepping will also offer you an additional option, which allows you to sweep his leg and make him fall.

Technique #17: The Old Man Carries the Fish on His Back

(Lao Han Bei Yu) 老漢背魚

When your opponent grabs your right wrist with his right hand (Figure 6-80), step your left leg to the front of his right leg and grab his right wrist with both of your hands, while using your left elbow to push his right elbow to keep it bent (Figure 6-81). Finally, turn your body to the right and bend forward to lock his arm in place (Figure 6-82).

Theory:

Misplacing the Bone (shoulder and elbow). The angle at which you control your opponent's arm is very important. If you opponent's arm is either too straight or too bent, the control will not be effective. With an accurate angle, you may generate great pain in your opponent's shoulder.

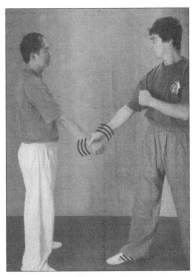

Figure 6–83

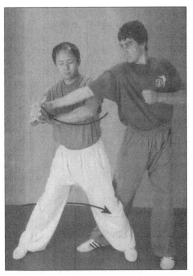

Figure 6–84

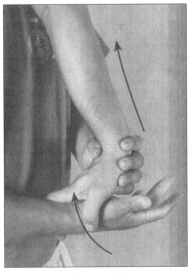

Figure 6–85

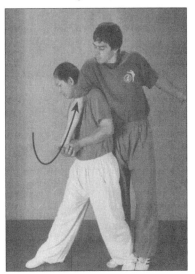

Figure 6–86

Technique #18: One Post to Support the Heavens

(Yi Zhu Ding Tian) 一柱頂天

When your right wrist has been grabbed by your opponent's right hand (Figure 6-83), immediately step your left leg to the front of his right leg and grab his wrist with your left hand, while placing your left shoulder under his right armpit area (Figure 6-84). You should use both hands to control your opponent's wrist and hand, and keep your opponent's entire arm straight (Figure 6-85). Finally, bend his fingers backward while lifting his entire arm upward to increase the pressure on his shoulder joint (Figure 6-86). You should continue lifting until his heels are off the ground.

Theory:

Misplacing the Bone (base of fingers, elbow, and shoulder). In this technique, you control the elbow to lock your opponent's arm in position and lift the arm upward to tear off the ligaments in the shoulder. When you lock your opponent in the final position, you may also place the back side of his upper-arm on your shoulder; this will generate great pain in his upper-arm tendons.

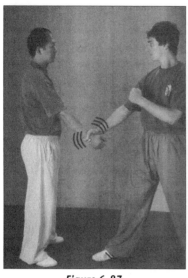
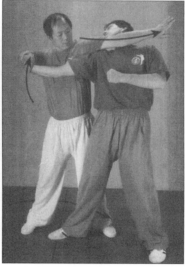
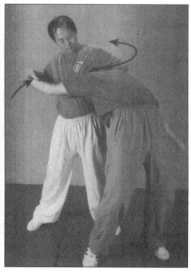

| Figure 6–87 | Figure 6–88 | Figure 6–89 |

Technique #19: Arm Wraps Around the Dragon's Neck

(Bi Chan Long Jing) 臂纏龍頸

When your opponent grabs your right wrist (Figure 6-87), step your left leg behind his right leg, use your right hand to grab his right wrist, and press his arm against your chest while placing your left arm on his neck (Figure 6-88). Finally, circle your left arm around his neck to lock him up (Figure 6-89). If you increase the squeezing pressure, you may seal his arteries on the sides of the neck and stop the oxygen supply to his head, thereby making him pass out. However, you should not do this unless it is absolutely necessary, since this can kill your opponent.

Theory:

Sealing the Artery/Vein (neck) and Misplacing the Bone (elbow). On the sides of the neck are two big blood vessels which supply blood to the brain. When you increase the pressure on the sides of the neck, you seal these vessels. To prevent your opponent from struggling, you must lock his right arm on your chest to put him in an awkward position.

B. GRABBING UNDER THE WRIST

Occasionally, your wrist will be grabbed from underneath. When this happens, normally your arm was already raised for some reason (Figure 6-90). In this sub-section, we will offer you some of the available Qin Na techniques against this grabbing.

Technique #1: Send the Devil to Heaven

(Song Mo Shang Tian) 送魔上天

When your opponent grabs your right wrist with his right hand (Figure 6-91), first step your right leg beside his right leg, rotating your right hand down to loosen his grabbing while using your left hand to grab his right hand (Figure 6-92). Next, continue turning your body to your left, swinging his arm upward while freeing your right hand and grabbing his

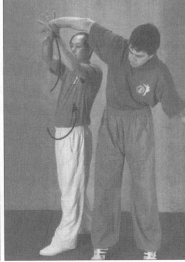

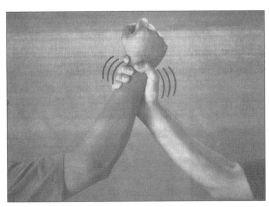

Figure 6–90

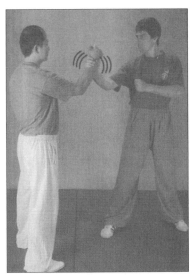

Figure 6–91

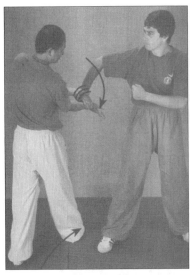

Figure 6–92

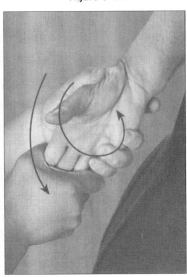

Figure 6–93

Figure 6–94

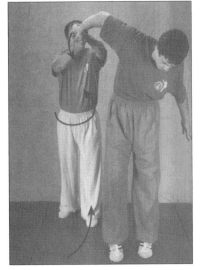

Figure 6–95

vrist (Figure 6-93). Finally, use your left hand to twist his
ιand and lock his pinkie, while using your right hand to
grab his fingers and bend them downward to lock him up
Figure 6-94). You should increase your twisting and bend-
ng pressure until your opponent's heels are off the ground
Figure 6-95).

Theory:

Dividing the Muscle/Tendon (wrist and pinkie) and
Misplacing the Bone (shoulder). An important
point to execute this technique successfully is,
when you have locked your opponent in the final
position, you should emphasize the pinkie twisting
and his fingers' bending, which makes this technique more effective.

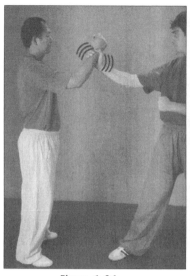
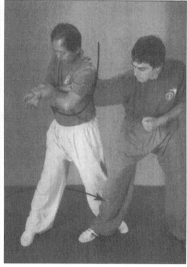
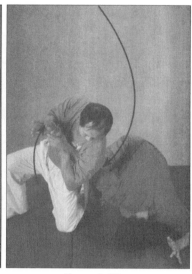

Figure 6–96   Figure 6–97   Figure 6–98

Technique #2: Old Man Promoted to General

(Lao Han Bai Jiang) 老漢拜將

If your opponent grabs your right wrist with his right hand (Figure 6-96), step your left leg behind his right leg and use your left hand to grab his right wrist while swinging his arm to your right and placing your left armpit over his right elbow (Figure 6-97). Finally, use the leverage generated from your hands and left elbow to press him down to the ground (Figure 6-98).

Theory:

Misplacing the Bone (elbow). When you press your opponent down, you should keep his arm straight, and the pressing should be straight on the rear side of his elbow. If you jerk your power, you may break his elbow easily.

Technique #3: Sparrow Hawk Shakes Its Wing or Backward Upward Turning

(Yao Zi Dou Chi or Hou Shang Fan) 鷂子抖翅，後上翻

When your opponent grabs your right wrist with his right hand (Figure 6-99), step your right leg behind his right leg and grab his wrist with your left hand, while circling your right elbow above his elbow (Figure 6-100). Then, swing your right elbow upward against his elbow while twisting his right wrist with your left hand (Figure 6-101). Alternatively, you may again step your left leg behind him, using your right arm to lock his arm in front of you while using your left hand to push his neck (Figure 6-102). This will generate great pain in his arm.

Theory

Dividing the Muscle/Tendon (wrist) and Misplacing the Bones (elbow). In order to prevent your opponent from striking you with his left hand, your stepping to his right is very important. In addition, this stepping will offer you an additional option which allows you to sweep his leg and make him fall.

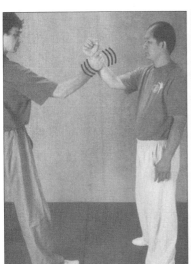

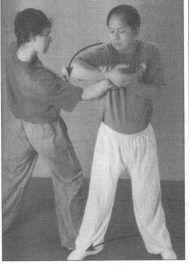

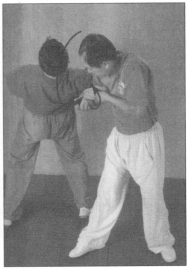

| Figure 6–99 | Figure 6–100 | Figure 6–101 |

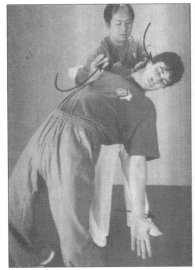

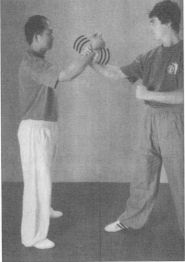

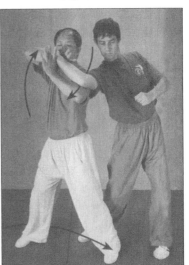

| Figure 6–102 | Figure 6–103 | Figure 6–104 |

Technique #4: The Old Man Carries the Fish on His Back

(Lao Han Bei Yu) 老漢背魚

When your opponent grabs your right wrist with his right hand (Figure 6-103), step your left leg in front of his right leg, grab his right wrist with your left hand and use your left elbow to push his elbow to keep it bent, while also clamping down and grabbing his wrist with your right hand (Figure 6-104). Then, continue turning your body to your right and bow forward while pulling his arm down (Figure 6-105).

Theory:

Misplacing the Bone (shoulder and elbow). The angle at which you control your opponent's arm is very important. If your opponent's arm is either too straight or too bent, the control will not be effective. With an accurate angle, you may generate great pain in your opponent's shoulder.

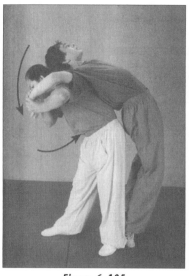
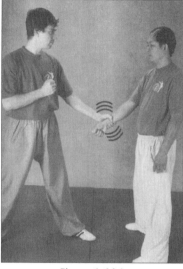
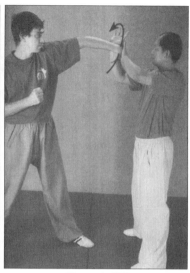

| *Figure 6–105* | *Figure 6–106* | *Figure 6–107* |

II. SAME SIDE GRABBING

A. GRABBING ABOVE THE WRIST

Technique #1: Small Wrap Hand

(Xiao Chan Shou) 小纏手

When your opponent has grabbed your right wrist with his left hand (Figure 6-106), immediately circle your right hand upward, while using your left hand to cover his fingers and thumb to lock his index finger (Figure 6-107). Then, wrap your right hand around his wrist from the outside of his wrist and press down (Figure 6-108). Make sure you bring him down until his elbow touches the floor, and step your left leg back so you will be able to kick him if necessary.

Theory:

Dividing the Muscle/Tendon (wrist). When you lock your opponent's wrist, you must have a good angle for locking. In order to do this, you must extend your right arm while also dropping your right fingers downward. Your opponent's elbow should be bent and lower than his wrist, otherwise he will be able to turn his body and escape from your locking.

Technique #2: Green Snake Turns Its Body

(Qing She Fan Shen) 青蛇翻身

When your opponent grabs your right wrist with his left hand (Figure 6-109), immediately rotate your right hand clockwise while also using the left hand to grab his left hand (Figure 6-110). Finally, use your right hand to press his pinkie backward (Figures 6-111 and 6-112). This will cause great pain in his wrist and pinkie.

Alternatively, once your left hand has twisted and locked your opponent's left hand, use your right hand to push against his left neck (Figure 6-113).

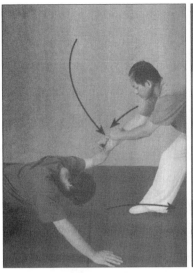

Figure 6–108

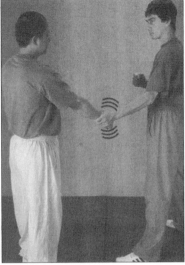

Figure 6–109

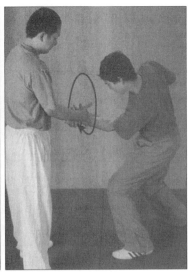

Figure 6–110

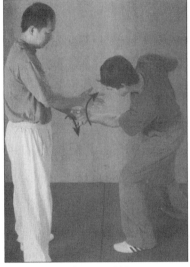

Figure 6–111

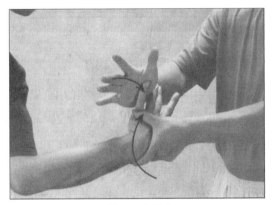

Figure 6–112

Theory:

Dividing the Muscle/Tendon (wrist) and Misplacing the Bones (shoulder, elbow, and pinkie). The position where you stand is very important. Where you stand should be beyond his right hand's reach.

Technique #3: Push the Boat to Follow the Stream

(Shun Shui Tui Zhou) 順水推舟

When your opponent grabs your right wrist with his left hand (Figure 6-114), immediately circle your right arm clockwise while also using your left hand to grab his wrist (Figure 6-115). Coil your right hand around his wrist and grab his forearm near the wrist area, while using your left hand to twist his left hand (Figure 6-116). Next, use the entire body's power

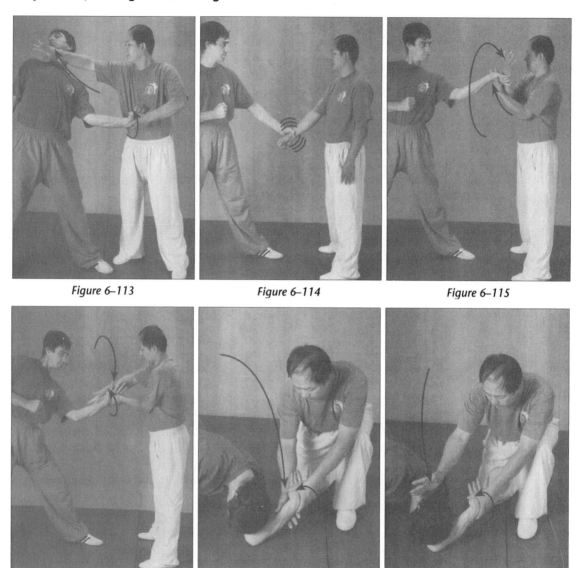

Figure 6–113　　　　　Figure 6–114　　　　　Figure 6–115

Figure 6–116　　　　　Figure 6–117　　　　　Figure 6–118

to turn your body to your left and squat downward to lock your opponent on the ground (Figure 6-117). If you wish to knock him out, continue using your left hand to twist his left wrist while using your right hand to chop the back muscle of his neck (Figure 6-118).

If you wish to take him down, right after you have controlled his wrist with your left hand (Figure 6-119), you may use your right hand to push against his neck area while sweeping your right leg forward (Figure 6-120).

Theory:
Dividing the Muscle/Tendon (wrist). When you swing your opponent down to the ground, you should use your entire body's momentum instead of just using arms. Remember, good Qin Na techniques always use the body to generate power.

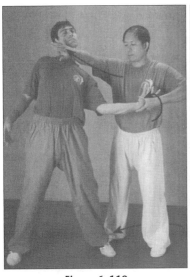

Figure 6–119

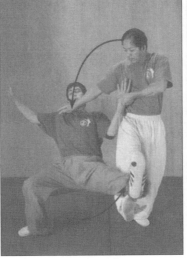

Figure 6–120

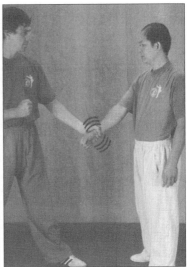

Figure 6–121

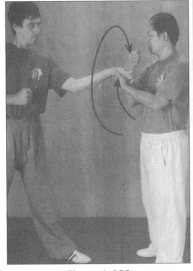

Figure 6–122

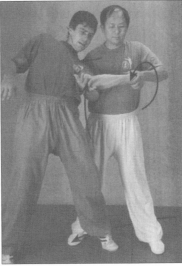

Figure 6–123

Technique #4: Lion Shakes Its Head

(Shi Zi Yao Tou) 獅子搖頭

This technique is very similar to the last one. Again, when your opponent grabs your right wrist with his left hand (Figure 6-121), immediately circle your right arm upward while using your left hand to grab his left wrist (Figure 6-122). Then, step your right leg behind his left leg, twisting his left wrist with your left hand while moving your right hand to his left elbow, and lock his arm up (Figure 6-123).

Theory:

Dividing the Muscle/Tendon (wrist) and Misplacing the Bone (elbow). In order to set up a good angle for locking, his arm should be neither too straight nor too bent (Figure 6-124). The trick to keeping the correct distance for this angle is to use your right shoulder to push his left shoulder to prevent him from changing the locking angle.

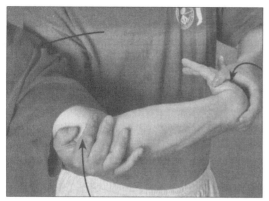

Figure 6–124

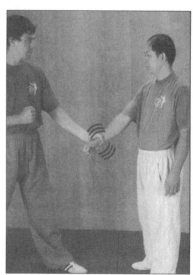

Figure 6–125

Technique #5: Heaven King Supports the Pagoda or Upward Elbow Press

(Tian Wang Tuo Ta or Shang Ya Zhou) 天王托塔，上壓肘

When your opponent uses his left hand to grab your right wrist (Figure 6-125), again use your left hand to grab his left wrist, while circling your right arm to free your right wrist from the grab (Figure 6-126). Then, step your right leg behind his left leg while sliding your right hand along his forearm to reach his elbow. Finally, use the leverage generated from both of your hands to lock his arm up (Figure 6-127).

Theory:

Misplacing the Bone (elbow). The leverage generated from your left and right hands is very important. If necessary, you may jerk your right hand to break his elbow joint.

Technique #6: Old Man Promoted to General

(Lao Han Bai Jiang) 老漢拜將

When your opponent grabs your right wrist with his left hand (Figure 6-128), immediately use your left hand to grab his left hand, while moving your right armpit over his left elbow (Figure 6-129). Next, place his elbow under your armpit while keeping his arm straight (Figure 6-130). Finally, use the leverage generated from both of your hands and right shoulder to press him down until his face touches the ground (Figure 6-131). As you do this, you should also kneel down on your right leg; this will provide a better position for your control. The option to this control is to use your right arm to strike his face (Figure 6-132).

Theory:

Misplacing the Bone (elbow). When you press your opponent down, you should keep his arm straight, and the pressing should be straight on the rear side of his elbow. If you jerk your power, you may break his elbow easily.

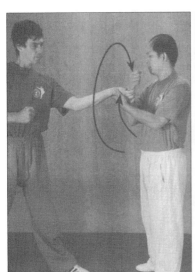

Figure 6–126

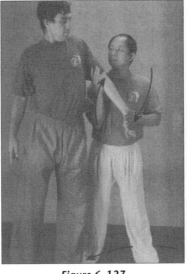

Figure 6–127

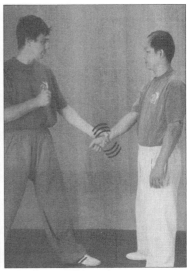

Figure 6–128

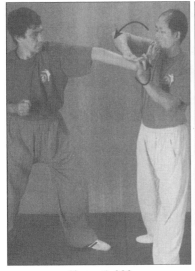

Figure 6–129

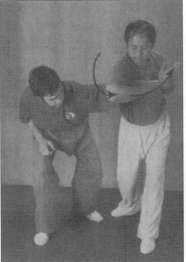

Figure 6–130

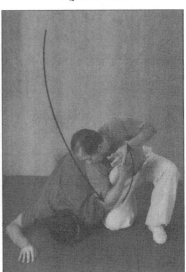

Figure 6–131

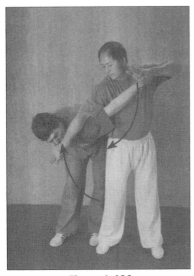

Figure 6–132

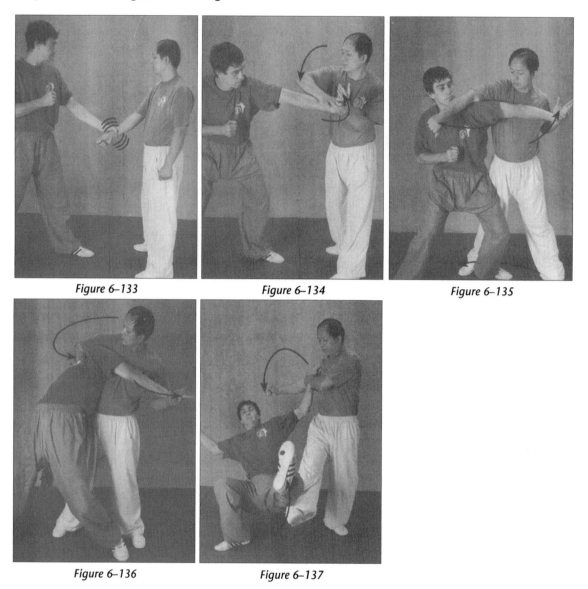

Figure 6–133

Figure 6–134

Figure 6–135

Figure 6–136

Figure 6–137

Technique #7: Arm Wraps Around the Dragon's Neck

(Bi Chan Long Jing) 臂纏龍頸

When your opponent uses his left hand to grab your right wrist (Figure 6-133), again use your left hand to grab his left wrist and twist it counterclockwise, while circling your right elbow above his left arm (Figure 6-134). Next, step your right leg behind his left leg, and lock his left arm in front of your chest while placing your right arm on his throat (Figure 6-135). Finally, circle your right arm around his neck and press his upper body backward (Figure 6-136).

If you wish to take him down, you may push your right arm backward while sweeping your right leg forward (Figure 6-137).

Theory:

Sealing the Artery/Vein (neck). In order to keep your opponent from struggling strongly, you should push your right arm until his upper body bends backward. This will destroy his balance and prevent him from resisting or counterattacking you.

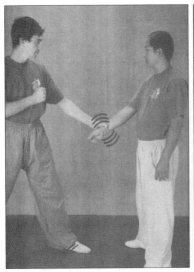

Figure 6–138

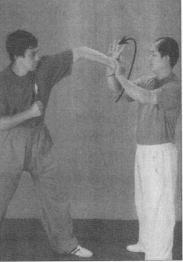

Figure 6–139

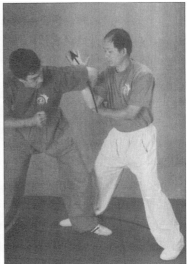

Figure 6–140

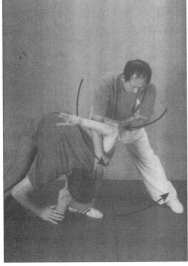

Figure 6–141

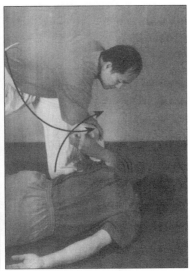

Figure 6–142

Technique #8: Spiritual Dragon Waves Its Tail or Reverse Elbow Wrap

(Shen Long Bai Wei or Fan Chan Zhou) 神龍擺尾，反纏肘

When your opponent grabs your right wrist with his left hand (Figure 6-138), immediately use your left hand to grab his left wrist, while circling your right hand upward to escape from his grabbing (Figure 6-139). Immediately step your right leg behind his left leg, while coiling your right arm around his left arm until your right hand is on his upper-arm near the elbow (Figure 6-140). Next, use the leverage generated from your right hand and elbow to lock his arm behind him while using your left hand to keep his arm bent (Figure 6-141). Finally, circle him down by pressing his elbow until his face touches the ground (Figure 6-142).

Theory:

Misplacing the Bone (shoulder and elbow). When apply this technique, you should keep your opponent's arm bent all the time. If he is able to straighten his arm, he will be able to get out. The trick to keeping his arm bent is through the help of your left hand and right upper-arm. Once your opponent is on the ground, if you continue your pressure forward, you may pop his shoulder joint out of its socket easily.

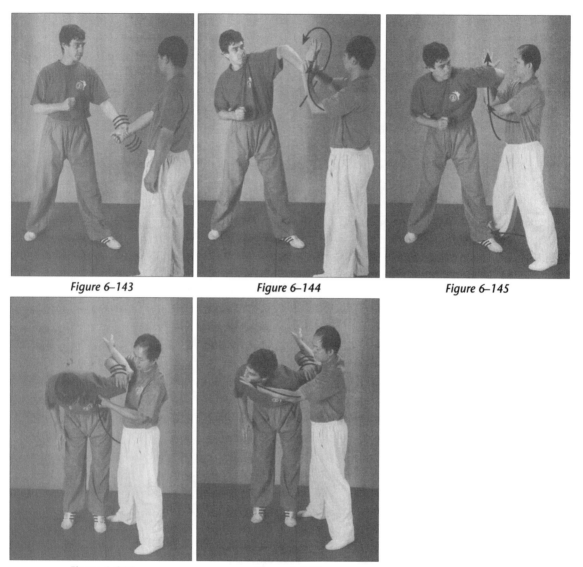

Figure 6–143   Figure 6–144   Figure 6–145

Figure 6–146   Figure 6–147

Technique #9: Pressing Shoulder with Single Finger and Extending the Neck for Water

(Yi Zhi Ding Jiang and Yin Jing Qiu Shui) 一指頂肩， 引頸求水

This technique is very similar to the last technique. When your opponent grabs your right wrist with his left hand (Figure 6-143), immediately use your left hand to grab his left wrist, while circling your right hand upward to escape from his grabbing (Figure 6-144). Immediately step your right leg behind his left leg, while coiling your right arm around his left arm until your right hand is on his upper-arm near the elbow (Figure 6-145). Next, lift his left arm upward to lock all of his tendons and ligaments in his shoulder while pressing your index finger on his *Jianneiling* cavity (M-UE-48) to generate great pain in his shoulder area (Figure 6-146). You should increase the pressure on your index finger until your opponent's heels leave the floor. Alternatively, you may use your left hand to push his chin upward (Figure 6-147). This will also produce great pain.

Theory:

Misplacing the Bone (shoulder) and Cavity Press (*Jianneiling* cavity). When you use your right arm to lock your opponent's left arm and lift it upward, you generate

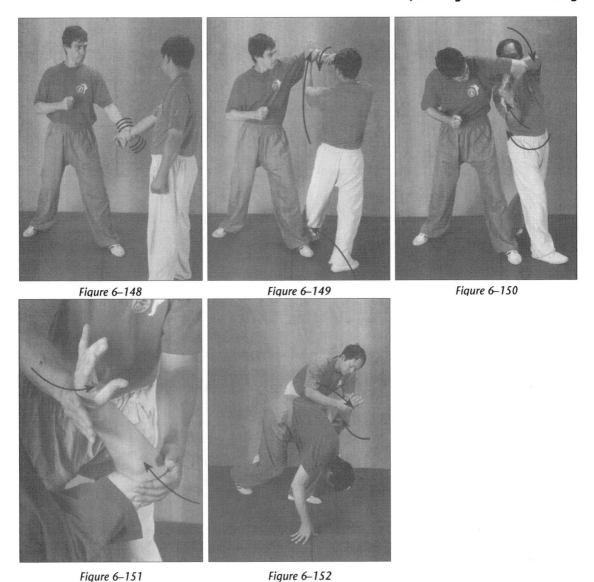

Figure 6–148

Figure 6–149

Figure 6–150

Figure 6–151

Figure 6–152

a strain on his left shoulder's tendons and ligaments. This action also exposes his *Jianneiling* cavity for your cavity press attack. Without an accurate locking position of the shoulder, the cavity press will not be effective.

Technique #10: Large Python Turns Its Body
(Da Mang Fan Shen) 大蟒翻身

When your opponent grabs your right wrist with his left hand (Figure 6-148), immediately step your left leg beside his left leg and coil your right hand around his left wrist, while placing your left hand on his elbow (Figure 6-149). Next, rotate your body to your right and under his left arm, while twisting his left arm (Figure 6-150). Finally use the leverage of the left and right hands (Figure 6-151) to press him down to the ground (Figure 6-152).

Theory:
Misplacing the Bone (shoulder and elbow); Taking down in the final action. In order to make your opponent fall, his controlled arm should be neither too straight nor too bent. A good angle will put him into an undefensible position.

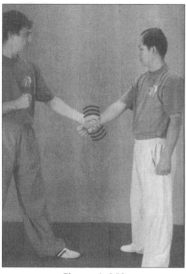
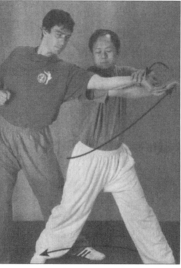
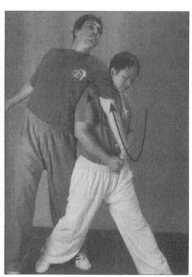

| Figure 6–153 | Figure 6–154 | Figure 6–155 |

Technique #11: One Post to Support the Heavens

(Yi Zhu Ding Tian) 一柱頂天

When your opponent uses his left hand to grab your right wrist (Figure 6-153), immediately step your right leg to the front of his left leg, while swinging your right arm to your left and grabbing his wrist with your left hand (Figure 6-154). Next, place your right shoulder under his left armpit, while pulling his arm downward to keep it straight and then lift his arm straight upward toward his shoulder to lock him up (Figure 6-155). You should continue your lifting until his heels are off the ground. In addition, you should stand at a position where it is hard for your opponent's left hand to attack.

Theory:

Misplacing the Bone (elbow and shoulder). In this technique, you control the elbow to lock your opponent's arm in position and lift the arm upward to tear off the ligaments of the shoulder. Alternatively, you may place your right shoulder under his upper-arm area to press the tendons there. This can also cause significant pain.

Technique #12: The Hand Twists Snake's Head

(Shou Niu She Tou) 手扭蛇頭

When your opponent grabs your right wrist with his left hand (Figure 6-156), immediately circle your right arm upward counterclockwise, while using your left hand to grab his left hand (Figure 6-157). Next, step your right leg behind his left leg, while twisting his left wrist with your left hand and holding his left elbow in with your right hand (Figure 6-158). Finally, use the leverage of both of your hands to lock him downward (Figure 6-159).

Theory:

Dividing the Muscle/Tendon (wrist). In this technique, you should beware of your opponent's possible attack to your groin with his right hand. To prevent him from so doing, you should twist and bend his wrist until his right elbow touches the ground.

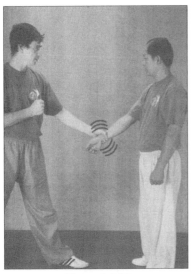

Figure 6-156

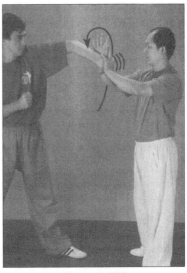

Figure 6-157

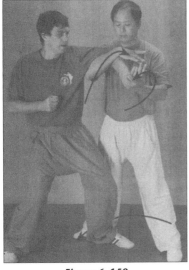

Figure 6-158

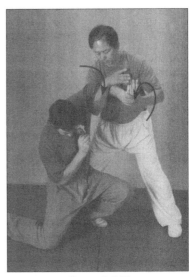

Figure 6-159

Technique #13: The Hand Bends the Pine Branch

(Shou Ban Shong Zhi) 手扳松枝

When your opponent grabs your right wrist with his left hand (Figure 6-160), immediately circle your right arm upward clockwise while using your left hand to grab his left pinkie (Figure 6-161). Next, step your right leg backward, while using your left thumb and index finger to bend his pinkie backward to lock him up (Figures 6-162 and 6-163). You should continue your locking pressure until his heels are off the ground.

Theory:

Misplacing the Bone (pinkie). The leverage generated from your left thumb and index finger is the key to locking.

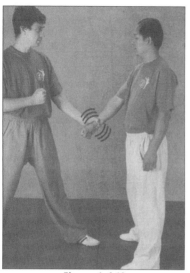

Figure 6–160

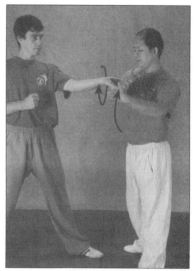

Figure 6–161

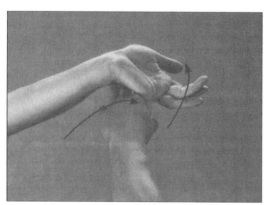

Figure 6–162

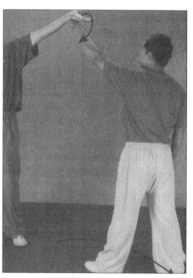

Figure 6–163

B. GRABBING UNDER THE WRIST

Technique #1: Forgive Me for not Going with You

(Shu Bu Tong Xing) 恕不同行

When your opponent grabs your right wrist with his left hand (Figure 6-164), immediately lower your right wrist and use your left hand to grab his left hand, and circle your right elbow above his elbow while also stepping your right leg to his left hand side (Figure 6-165). Next, use your right elbow to push his elbow inward to keep his arm bent (Figure 6-166). Finally, bend your body to your right and lock your opponent in position (Figure 6-167).

Theory:
Dividing the Muscle/Tendon (wrist). In order to lock your opponent effectively, your left hand grabbing must be firm and strong and your right arm should keep his arm bent. Only then, when you bow to your right, will you generate great pain in your opponent's wrist.

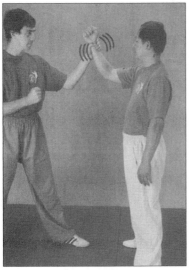

Figure 6–164

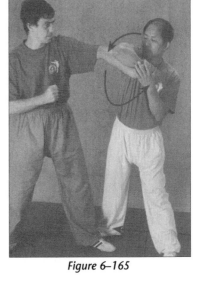

Figure 6–165

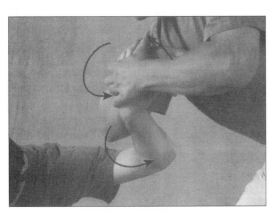

Figure 6–166

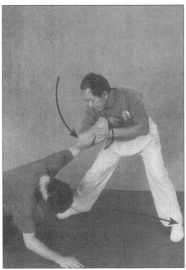

Figure 6–167

Technique #2: Send the Devil to Heaven

(Song Mo Shang Tian) 送魔上天

When your opponent grabs your right wrist with his left hand (Figure 6-168), immediately step your left leg beside his left leg, while lowering your right arm and using your left hand to grab his left hand (Figure 6-169). Continue rotating your body to your right, using your right hand to twist his wrist and using your left hand to grab his fingers and bend them downward (Figure 6-170). You should increase your twisting pressure until your opponent's heels are off the ground.

Theory:

Dividing the Muscle/Tendon (wrist and pinkie). An important point for executing this technique is, when you have locked your opponent in the final position, you should emphasize the pinkie lock and finger bending.

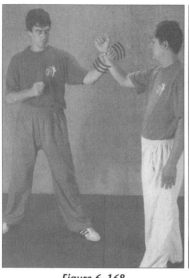

Figure 6–168

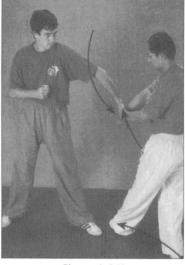

Figure 6–169

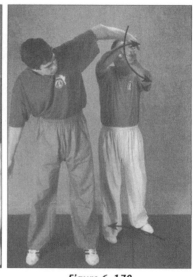

Figure 6–170

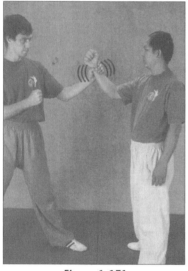

Figure 6–171

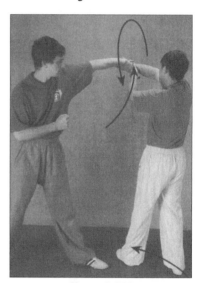

Figure 6–172

Technique #3: Hand Twists the Snake's Neck or Upward Finger Turn

(Shou Niu She Jing or Shang Fen Zhi) 手扭蛇頸，上分指

When your opponent grabs your right wrist with his left hand (Figure 6-171), immediately step your left leg to his left hand side while swinging your right arm upward counterclockwise and using your left hand to grab his pinkie (Figure 6-172). Next, step your right leg next to your left leg while using your thumb and index finger to bend his pinkie backward (Figure 6-173). You should continue your locking pressure until his heels are off the ground (Figure 6-174).

Theory:

Misplacing the Bone (pinkie). The key to locking is not from lifting your opponent's pinkie. It is from the rotation of his pinkie.

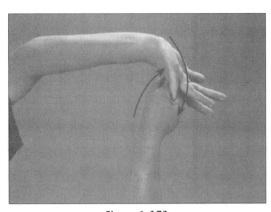

Figure 6–173

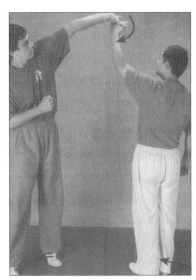

Figure 6–174

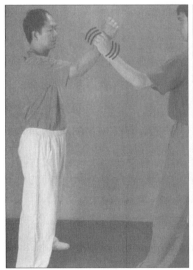

Figure 6–175

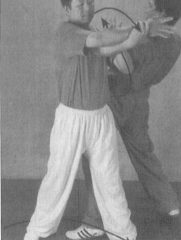

Figure 6–176

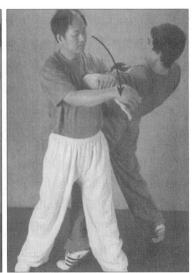

Figure 6–177

Technique #4: Twist the Wing with Both Hands or Forward Upward Turning

(Shuang Shou Ban Chi or Qian Shang Fan) 雙手扳翅，前上翻

When your opponent grabs your right hand with his left hand (Figure 6-175), immediately step your left leg behind his left leg, while pushing his forearm backward and circling your left arm to lock his left arm (Figure 6-176). Finally, use both hands to bend his left arm backward (Figure 6-177). Naturally, you may also sweep your left leg backward to make him fall.

Theory

Misplacing the Bones (elbow and shoulder). In order to prevent your opponent from striking you with his right hand, your stepping to his left is very important. In addition, this stepping will offer you an additional option, which allows your to sweep his leg and make him fall.

6-3. Qin Na Against Arm Grabbing

Very often a wrestler, a Judo expert, or a Taiji martial artist will grab the sleeves of your arms to immobilize you. When you encounter this situation, you may kick your opponent's shin, or even groin before he pulls your arms downward and destroys your centering and balance. Once he has pulled your arms downward, you will be in an awkward position to fight back. Therefore, Qin Na knowledge and skill is vital to dealing with this situation. In this section, we will introduce some effective Qin Na techniques for this scenario.

We will divide the techniques into two categories: opposite side grabbing and same side grabbing. You should understand that, if your opponent grabs you with both his hands to both of your sleeves, you may treat the situation as though you are only grabbed by single arm.

I. OPPOSITE SIDE GRABBING

Technique #1: Small Wrap Hand

(Xiao Chan Shou) 小纏手

When your opponent grabs your right sleeve on the forearm area with his right hand (Figure 6-178), use your left hand to cover and grab his right hand, while raising up your right arm to set up an effective controlling angle (Figure 6-179). Finally, step your right leg backward, while wrapping your right hand around his wrist and pressing downward with your forearm to his wrist (Figure 6-180). When you press him down, you should step your right leg backward. You should press him down until his elbow touches the ground.

Theory:
Dividing the Muscle/Tendon (wrist). When you press your opponent's right wrist down, your right leg stepping is very important. This stepping is to prevent your opponent from attacking you with his left hand. In addition, this will offer you an opportunity to kick him with your right leg when necessary.

Technique #2: Heaven King Supports the Pagoda or Upward Elbow Press

(Tian Wang Tuo Ta or Shang Ya Zhou) 天王托塔，上壓肘

When your opponent grabs your right sleeve on the forearm area with his right hand (Figure 6-181), immediately step your left leg behind his right leg and use your right hand to grab his right wrist, while also placing your left hand on his right elbow. Next, press your right hand down and push his elbow upward with your left hand to lock him up (Figure 6-182). You should increase your controlling power until his heels are off the ground. You should keep yourself on the right hand side of your opponent. This will prevent him from attacking you with his left hand.

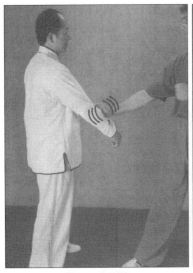

Figure 6–178

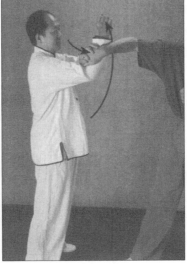

Figure 6–179

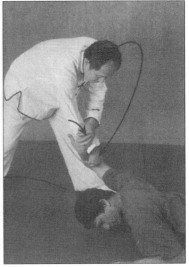

Figure 6–180

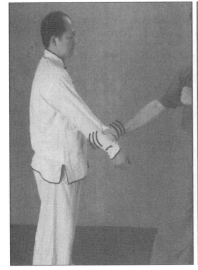

Figure 6–181

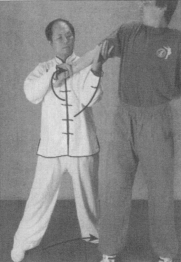

Figure 6–182

Theory:

Misplacing the Bone (elbow). The leverage generated from both of your hands is the key to the control. From the beginning, you should keep your opponent's elbow as straight as possible. If he keeps it bent, it will be difficult to lock him with this technique. However, if he bends his elbow before you have locked him in place, you should immediately push his elbow to your right and pull his wrist toward you. In this case, you will still be able to lock him.

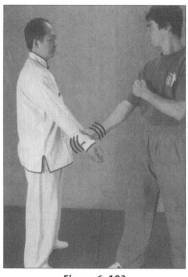
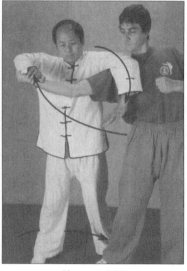
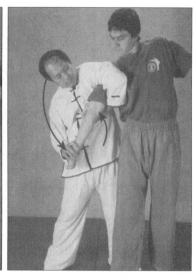

Figure 6–183   Figure 6–184   Figure 6–185

Technique #3: Hands Holding a Large Beam

(Shou Wo Da Liang) 手握大樑

In the same situation, if your opponent grabs your right sleeve with his right hand (Figure 6-183), immediately step your left leg behind his right leg and pull his arm to your right to keep it straight, while placing your left arm around his upper-arm (Figure 6-184). Finally, pull his wrist downward while raising your forearm against the tendons in his upper-arm to generate pain (Figure 6-185).

Theory:

Misplacing the Bone (elbow) and Pressing the Tendons (upper-arm). In this technique, you should beware of your opponent's left hand attack. In addition, if you are shorter than your opponent, it will be harder for your to lock his upper-arm tendon.

Technique #4: The Old Man Carries the Fish on His Back

(Lao Han Bei Yu) 老漢背魚

Again, if your opponent grabs your right sleeve with his right hand (Figure 6-186), immediately step your left leg to the front of his right leg, while grabbing his wrist with both of your hands (Figure 6-187). As you do this, you should also use your left elbow to push his elbow to keep it bent. Next, turn your body and bow forward, while pulling his arm downward to generate pressure on his elbow and shoulder joints (Figure 6-188). If you increase your controlling pressure or jerk your locking arms, you may pull his shoulder out of its socket.

Theory:

Misplacing the Bone (shoulder and elbow). The angle at which you control your opponent's arm is very important. If his arm is either too straight or too bent, the control will not be effective. With an accurate angle, you may generate great pain in your opponent's shoulder.

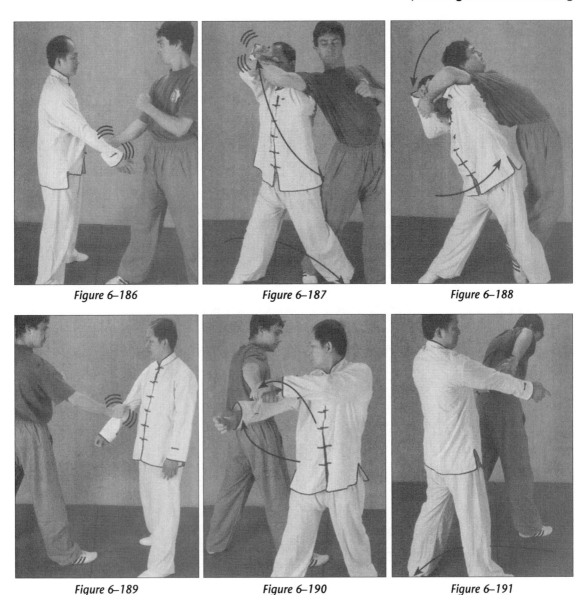

Figure 6–186   Figure 6–187   Figure 6–188

Figure 6–189   Figure 6–190   Figure 6–191

Technique #5: Send the Devil to Heaven

(Song Mo Shang Tian) 送魔上天

When your opponent grabs your right sleeve with his right hand (Figure 6-189), immediately step your right leg beside his right leg and grab his hand with your left hand, while raising up your right arm (Figure 6-190). Next, step your left leg behind your opponent while twisting his right hand with your left hand (Figure 6-191). Finally, continue to twist his right hand hard with your left hand, free your right hand and grab his right fingers and bend them downward (Figure 6-192). You should increase your twisting and bending pressure until your opponent's heels are off the ground.

Theory:

Dividing the Muscle/Tendon (wrist) and Misplacing the Bone (shoulder). The key point of making this technique effective is, when you have locked your opponent in the final position, you should emphasize the pinkie lock and fingers' bending. When you twist your opponent's arm, you should use your entire body's rotation momentum instead of just using your arms.

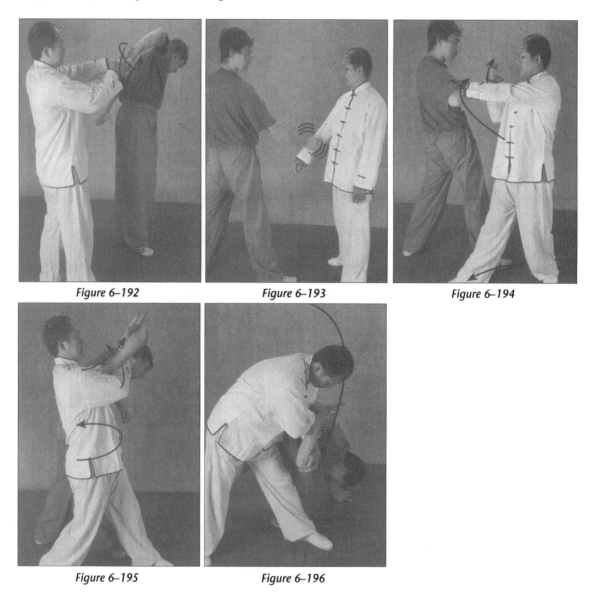

Figure 6–192   Figure 6–193   Figure 6–194

Figure 6–195   Figure 6–196

Technique #6: Large Python Turns Its Body

(Da Mang Fan Shen) 大蟒翻身

When your opponent grabs your right sleeve with his right hand (Figure 6-193), immediately step your right leg to his right hand side and raise up your right hand, while placing your left forearm on his elbow (Figure 6-194). Next, move your body under his right arm while rotating his right arm with both of your hands (Figure 6-195). Finally, bow forward while pressing his arm forward to lock him (Figure 6-196). Alternatively, you may continue to push his arm forward to dislocate his shoulder joint.

Theory:

Misplacing the Bone (elbow and shoulder). The angle you set up for your opponent's arm is very important. If its either too straight or too bent, the control will not be effective. Since this is a large circle Qin Na, it is easier for your opponent to sense what you intend to do, therefore speed becomes critical.

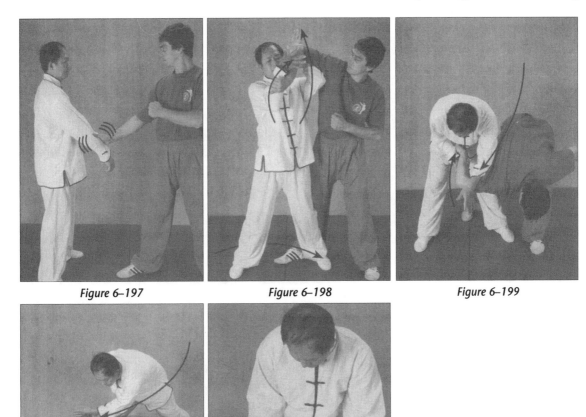

Figure 6–197   Figure 6–198   Figure 6–199

Figure 6–200   Figure 6–201

Technique #7: Luo Han Bows or Small Elbow Wrap

(Luo Han Xing Li or Xiao Chan Zhou) 羅漢行禮，小纏肘

If your opponent grabs your right sleeve with his right hand (Figure 6-197), immediately step your left leg to the front of his right leg, while circling your right hand upward around his forearm to grab his wrist and pressing your left forearm upward to his elbow to keep his arm bent (Figure 6-198). Next, bow your body forward and pull his arm to your front to destroy his balance (Figure 6-199). Once he has lost his balance, immediately sweep his right leg backward with your left leg while continuing your pulling of his arm to make him fall (Figure 6-200). When your opponent is on the ground, lock his arm behind his back with both of your legs while pulling his hair toward you to prevent further resistance (Figure 6-201).

Theory:

Misplacing the Bone (elbow and shoulder). In order to make your opponent fall, after you have locked him, you should pull him to your front to destroy his balance while sweeping your left leg backward. Once your opponent is on the ground, if necessary you may rotate his arm toward his head and pop his shoulder out of joint.

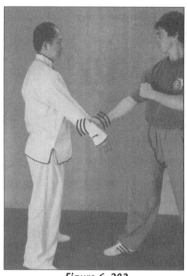
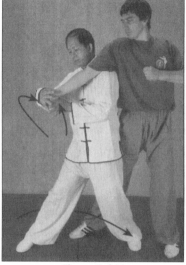
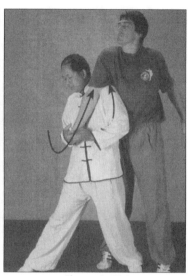

| Figure 6–202 | Figure 6–203 | Figure 6–204 |

Technique #8: One Post to Support the Heavens

(Yi Zhu Ding Tian) 一柱頂天

Again, when your opponent grabs your right forearm area with his right hand (Figure 6-202), immediately step your left leg to the front of his right leg, grab his right wrist with both of your hands, and place your left shoulder under his right armpit (Figure 6-203). You should pull your hands to keep his arm straight. Finally, lift his entire arm upward to increase the pressure on his shoulder (Figure 6-204). You should continue your lifting until his heels are off the ground. In addition, you should stand at the position from which is harder for your opponent's left hand to attack. You may also place his upper-arm on your shoulder. In this case, the tendons in his upper-arm will be pressed and pain will be generated.

Theory:

Misplacing the Bone (elbow and shoulder). In this technique, you control the elbow to lock your opponent's arm in position and lift the arm upward to tear off the ligaments in the shoulder. Alternatively, you may place your right shoulder under his upper-arm area to press the tendons there. This can also cause significant pain.

Technique #9: Arm Wraps Around the Dragon's Neck

(Bi Chan Long Jing) 臂纏龍頸

When your opponent grabs your right sleeve with his right hand (Figure 6-205), immediately step your left leg behind his right leg, grab his right wrist with your right hand and pull to keep his arm straight, and lock it in front of your chest while placing your left arm on his neck area (Figure 6-206). Finally, circle your left arm around his neck and press his body backward (Figure 6-207). In this case, you have locked your opponent's neck.

If you want to take your opponent down, simply sweep his right leg forward with your left leg while pushing his upper body down with your left arm. If necessary, you may increase the locking power of your left arm, and this will cut off the oxygen supply to his brain, sealing his breath. However, you should not do so unless it is a life and death situation.

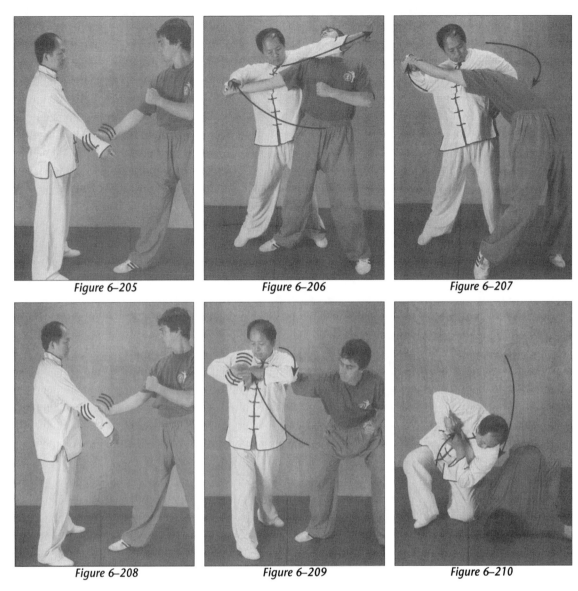

Figure 6–205   Figure 6–206   Figure 6–207

Figure 6–208   Figure 6–209   Figure 6–210

Theory:

Sealing the Breath (neck). To prevent your opponent from struggling strongly, simply push his body backward with your left arm. This will destroy his balance and his capability of resisting.

Technique #10: Old Man Promoted to General

(Lao Han Bai Jiang) 老漢拜將

When your opponent grabs your right sleeve with his right hand (Figure 6-208), again use both of your hands to grab his right wrist while placing your left armpit over his elbow (Figure 6-209). Next, kneel down on your left leg and use the leverage of your hands and left armpit to lock him down to the ground (Figure 6-210).

Theory:

Misplacing the Bone (elbow). When you press your opponent down, you should keep his arm straight, and the pressing should be directly on the rear side of his elbow. If you jerk your power, you may break his elbow easily. In addition, in order to provide a good angle for your locking, you should kneel down on your left leg.

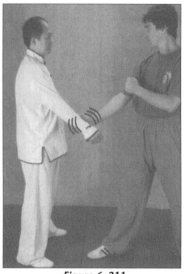

Figure 6–211

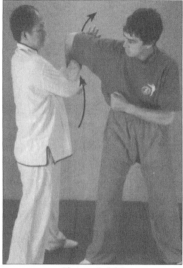

Figure 6–212

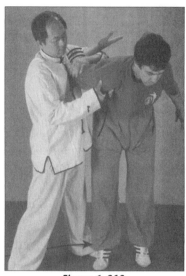

Figure 6–213

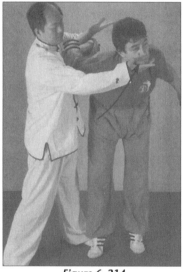

Figure 6–214

Technique #11: Pressing Shoulder with Single Finger and Extending the Neck for Water

(Yi Zhi Ding Jiang and Yin Jing Qiu Shui)
一指頂肩， 引頸求水

When your opponent grabs your right sleeve with his right hand (Figure 6-211), immediately grab his right wrist with your right hand, while inserting your left arm under his right elbow area (Figure 6-212). Then, lift his arm up behind him to increase the pain in his shoulder while using your index finger to press the *Jianneiling* cavity (M-UE-48)(Figure 6-213). This will cause significant pain in the shoulder area. You should increase the pressure on your index finger until your opponent's heels are off the ground. Alternatively, you may use your right hand to push his chin upward to lock him up (Figure 6-214). This will also produce great pain.

Theory:
Misplacing the Bone (shoulder), and Cavity Press (*Jianneiling* cavity). When you use your left arm to lock your opponent's right arm and lift it upward, you generate strain on his right shoulder's tendons and ligaments. This action exposes his *Jianneiling* cavity for your cavity press. Without an accurate locking position for the shoulder, the cavity press will not be effective.

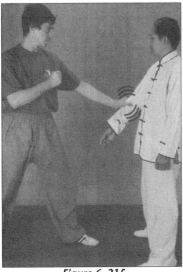

Figure 6–215

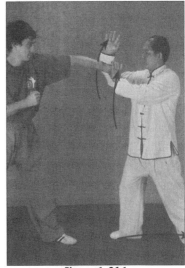

Figure 6–216

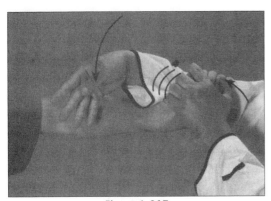

Figure 6–217

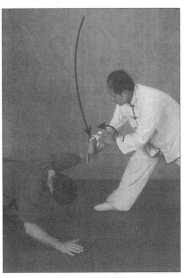

Figure 6–218

II. SAME SIDE GRABBING

Technique #1: Small Wrap Hand

(Xiao Chan Shou) 小纏手

When your opponent has grabbed your right forearm or sleeve with his left hand (Figure 6-215), immediately grab his left hand with your left hand and raise up your right arm while stepping backward with your left leg (Figure 6-216). In your left hand grabbing, you should use your thumb to push his index finger toward his wrist, while covering all other fingers with your left hand (Figure 6-217). Once your right arm has reached the top of his left arm, press it down and keep his left elbow bent (Figure 6-218). You should press him down until his right hand touches the ground.

Theory:

Dividing the Muscle/Tendon on the wrist. To make the control effective, your opponent's elbow must be bent and also be lower than the wrist. This will offer you a proper locking angle.

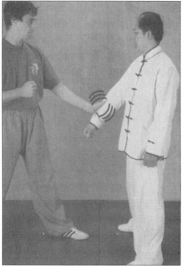

Figure 6–219

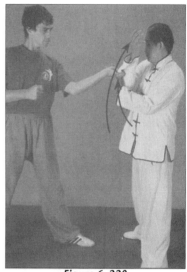

Figure 6–220

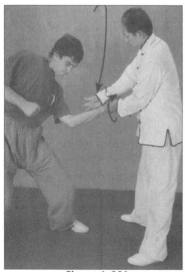

Figure 6–221

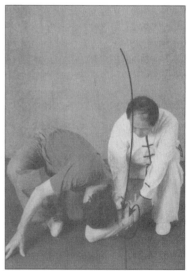

Figure 6–222

Technique #2: Push the Boat to Follow the Stream

(Shun Shui Tui Zhou) 順水推舟

When your opponent grabs your right sleeve with his left hand (Figure 6-219), first circle your right arm upward, and at the same time use your left hand to grab his left hand (Figure 6-220). Next, twist his left wrist with your left hand while coiling your right hand to his forearm area (Figure 6-221). Use your entire body's power to turn to your left and squat downward, while twisting his wrist continuously until he is locked to the ground (Figure 6-222).

Theory:

Dividing the Muscle/Tendon (wrist). When you swing your opponent down to the ground, you should use your entire body's momentum instead of just using arms. Remember, good Qin Na techniques always use the body to generate power.

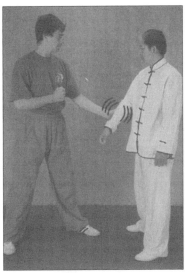
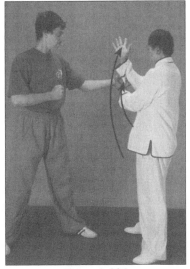
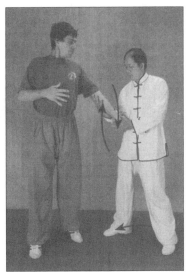

| *Figure 6–223* | *Figure 6–224* | *Figure 6–225* |

Technique #3: Heaven King Supports the Pagoda or Upward Elbow Press

(Tian Wang Tuo Ta or Shang Ya Zhou) 天王托塔，上壓肘

When your opponent grabs your right sleeve with his left hand (Figure 6-223), again raise up your right arm while grabbing his left wrist with your left hand (Figure 6-224). Next, coil your right hand around his left arm until it reaches his elbow, and use the leverage of your left and right hands to lock his arm upward (Figure 6-225). You should increase your controlling power until his heels are off the ground. You should also keep yourself on the left side of your opponent. This will prevent him from attacking you with his left hand.

Theory:

Misplacing the Bone (elbow). The leverage generated from both of your hands is the key to the control. From the beginning, you should keep your opponent's arm as straight as possible. If he keeps it bent, it will be difficult to lock him with this technique. However, if he bends his elbow before you have locked him in place, you should immediately push his elbow to your left and pull his wrist toward you. In this case, you will still be able to lock him.

Technique #4: Send the Devil to Heaven

(Song Mo Shang Tian) 送魔上天

When your opponent grabs your right forearm or sleeve with his left hand (Figure 6-226), immediately step your left leg beside his left leg and grab his wrist with your left hand, while circling your right arm upward (Figure 6-227). Next, step your right leg behind him while using your body's turning momentum to twist his arm (Figure 6-228). Finally, use your right hand to twist his wrist while bending his fingers downward with your left hand (Figure 6-229). You should increase your twisting pressure until your opponent's heels are off the ground.

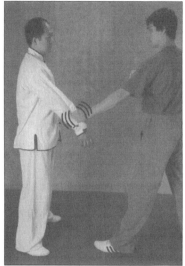

Figure 6–226

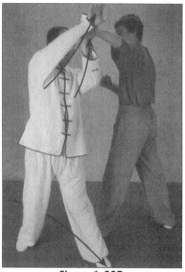

Figure 6–227

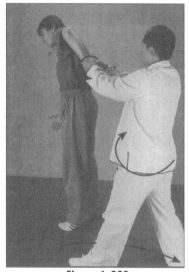

Figure 6–228

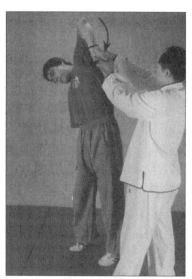

Figure 6–229

Theory:

Dividing the Muscle/Tendon (wrist) and Misplacing the Bone (shoulder). The trick to making this technique effective is when you have locked your opponent in the final position, you should emphasize the pinkie's twisting and fingers' bending.

Technique #5: Large Python Turns Its Body

(Da Mang Fan Shen) 大蟒翻身

When your opponent grabs your right sleeve or forearm with his left hand (Figure 6-230), immediately step your left leg beside his left leg and raise up your right arm while placing your left forearm on his elbow (Figure 6-231). Next, step your right leg behind him and use the body's turning momentum to twist his arm behind him (Figure 6-232). Then,

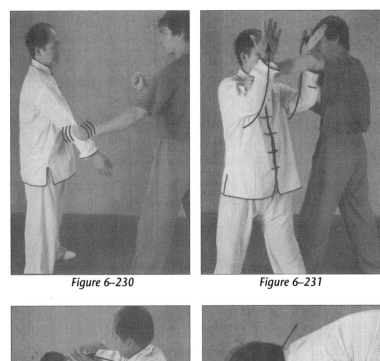

| Figure 6–230 | Figure 6–231 | Figure 6–232 |

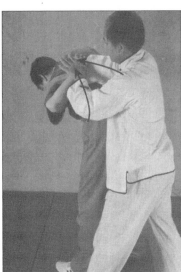
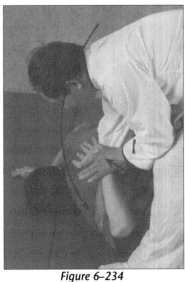

| Figure 6–233 | Figure 6–234 |

place your right hand on his upper-arm near the elbow area while using your left hand to lock his arm to prevent it from straightening out (Figure 6-233). Finally, use the leverage generated from both of your hands to rotate his arm forward and downward to lock him on the ground (Figure 6-234).

Theory:

Misplacing the Bone (elbow and shoulder). When you rotate your body, you should be on your opponent's left hand side instead of in front of him. Otherwise, you are in a position which allows your opponent to strike you or pull you down.

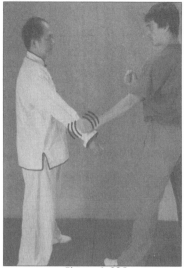

Figure 6–235

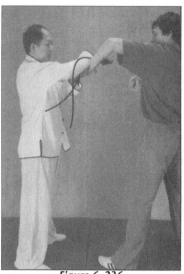

Figure 6–236

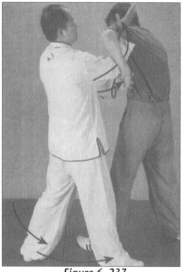

Figure 6–237

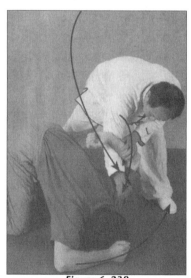

Figure 6–238

Technique #6: Spiritual Dragon Waves Its Tail or Reverse Elbow Wrap

(Shen Long Bai Wei or Fan Chan Zhou) 神龍擺尾，反纏肘

When your right forearm or sleeve is grabbed by your opponent's left hand (Figure 6-235), immediately coil your right arm upward while grabbing his left wrist with your left hand (Figure 6-236). Next. reposition yourself to his left, while coiling your right arm around his left arm until your hand reaches his upper-arm near the elbow area (Figure 6-237). Finally, step your left leg backward and use the body's turning momentum to press him downward until his face reaches the ground (Figure 6-238).

Theory:

Misplacing the Bone (shoulder and elbow). When applying this technique, you should keep your opponent's arm bent at all times. If he is able to straighten his arm, he will be able to get out. The trick to keeping his arm bent is through the help of your left hand and right upper-arm. Once your opponent is on the ground, if you continue your forward pressure, you may pop his shoulder joint out of its socket easily.

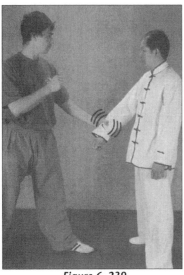

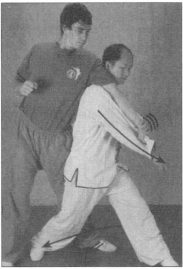

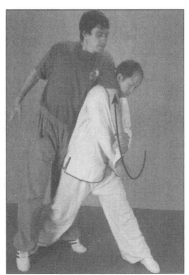

| Figure 6–239 | Figure 6–240 | Figure 6–241 |

Technique #7: One Post to Support the Heavens

(Yi Zhu Ding Tian) 一柱頂天

When your opponent grabs your right forearm with his left hand (Figure 6-239), immediately step your right leg to the front of his left leg and grab his left wrist with your left hand, while placing your right shoulder under his left armpit (Figure 6-240). At this time, you should also pull his arm down to keep it straight. Finally, lift his entire arm upward to increase the pressure on his shoulder (Figure 6-241). You should continue your lifting until his heels are off the ground. In addition, you should stand at a position from which it is harder for your opponent's left hand to attack.

Theory:

Misplacing the Bone (elbow and shoulder). In this technique, you control the elbow to lock your opponent's arm in position, and lift the arm upward to tear off the ligaments in the shoulder. Alternatively, you may place your right shoulder under his upper-arm area to press the tendons there. This can also cause significant pain.

Technique #8: Old Man Promoted to General

(Lao Han Bai Jiang) 老漢拜將

When your opponent grabs your right forearm or sleeve with his left hand (Figure 6-242), immediately circle your right hand upward and grab his wrist while placing your right armpit over his left elbow (Figure 6-243). As you do this, you should also use your left hand to grab and bend his wrist. Finally, use the leverage of your left hand and right shoulder to press him down (Figure 6-244). You should also kneel on your right leg; this will provide a better position for your control.

Theory:

Misplacing the Bone (elbow). When you press your opponent down, you should keep his arm straight, and the pressing should be directly on the rear side of his elbow. If you jerk your power, you may break his elbow easily.

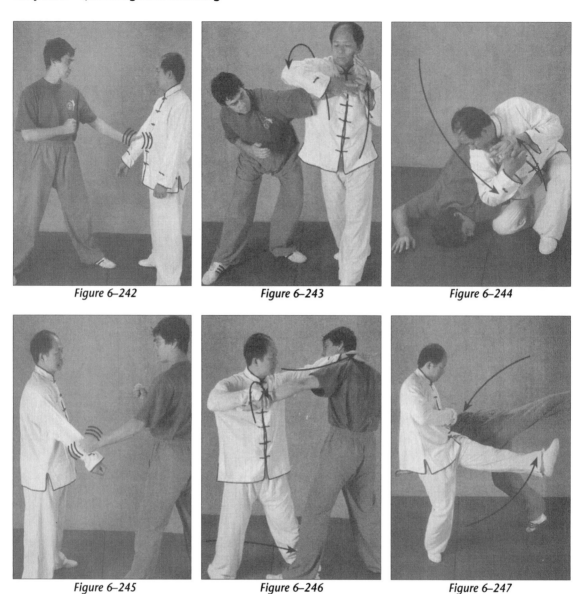

| Figure 6–242 | Figure 6–243 | Figure 6–244 |

| Figure 6–245 | Figure 6–246 | Figure 6–247 |

Technique #9: The Leg Trips the Lo Han

(Tui Ban Luo Han) 腿絆羅漢

When your opponent grabs your right forearm or sleeve with his left hand (Figure 6-245), immediately step your left leg to the front of his left leg, circle your right hand around his forearm and grab his wrist, while placing your left arm on the back of his neck (Figure 6-246). Finally, use the leverage of your left arm and left leg to sweep him down (Figure 6-247).

Theory:

Taking down. In order to make the take down technique more effective, you may also use your right hand to push his left arm backward. This will prevent him from struggling.

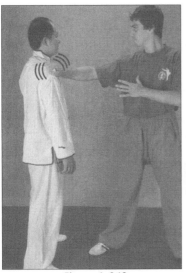

Figure 6–248

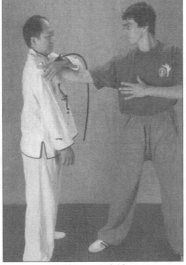

Figure 6–249

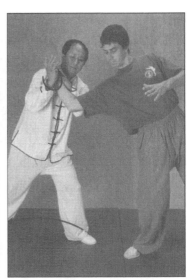

Figure 6–250

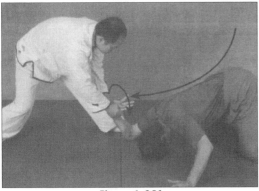

Figure 6–251

6-4. Qin Na Against Shoulder Grabbing

I. FROM THE FRONT

A. OPPOSITE SIDE GRABBING

Technique #1: White Ape Worships the Buddha or Reverse Wrist Press

(Bai Yuan Bai Fo or Fan Ya Wan) 白猿拜佛 ， 反壓腕

When your opponent's right hand is on your right shoulder (Figure 6-248), first use your left hand to cover and grab his left hand (Figure 6-249). Immediately step your right leg backward while twisting his right wrist until his palm faces upward (Figure 6-250). This will enable you to free your right arm. Finally, use both of your hands to bend his hand inward until his elbow touches the ground (Figure 6-251). When you press him down, you may twist his hand to the side slightly, and thereby generate more pressure on his pinkie's tendon. This will generate more pain.

Theory:

Dividing the Muscle/Tendon (wrist and pinkie). To make the control efficient, you must generate good leverage between your thumbs and pinkie. Once you have locked the hand, press downward with the entirety of both of your hands instead of just the thumbs.

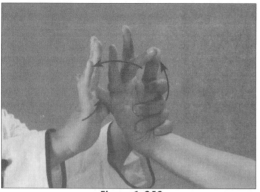

Figure 6–252

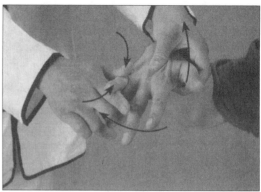

Figure 6–253

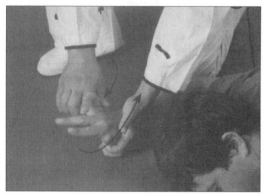

Figure 6–254

Technique #2: Fingers Lock the Dragon's Tail or Turning Finger Dividing

(Zhi Suo Long Wei or Zhuan Fen Zhi) 指鎖龍尾 ，轉分指

In the last technique, after you have turned your opponent's right hand until his palm faces upward, immediately sandwich his pinkie between your right thumb and index finger and bend his pinkie backward (Figure 6-252). Next, use the thumb to push the base of his pinkie, while using your index finger to push his pinkie backward and the other three fingers to lock his ring finger (Figure 6-253). As you do this, you should also use your left hand to push the base of his thumb backward   Finally, lead him down to the ground before you release your left hand control (Figure 6-254).

Theory:

Dividing the Muscle/Tendon and Misplacing the Bone (ring finger and pinkie). In this technique, before your opponent is completely controlled to the ground, you should not release your left hand control on his thumb.

Technique #3: Butterfly Bores Through the Flowers or Back Turning

(Hu Die Chuan Hua or Fan Bei Zhuan) 蝴蝶穿花 ，反背轉

When your opponent's right hand is on your right shoulder (Figure 6-255), immediately use your left hand to cover and grab his right fingers (Figure 6-256). Next, rotate his right

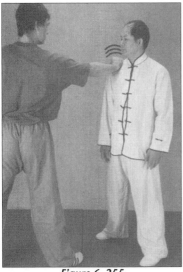

Figure 6–255

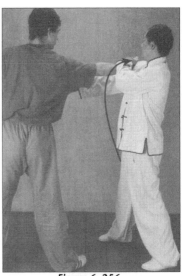

Figure 6–256

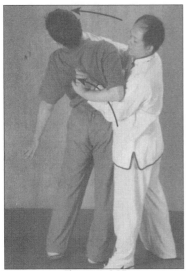

Figure 6–257

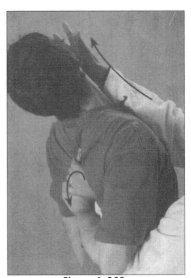

Figure 6–258

arm to lock his arm behind him, while repositioning yourself to his right hand side and pushing his chin upward with your right hand (Figure 6-257).

Theory:
Misplacing the Bone (base of fingers). In order to lock him effectively, you should twist your left hand and bend his fingers backward while also using your right hand to push his chin (Figure 6-258).

Technique #4: Heaven King Supports the Pagoda or Upward Elbow Press

(Tian Wang Tuo Ta or Shang Ya Zhou) 天王托塔，上壓肘

When your opponent's right hand is on your right shoulder (Figure 6-259), first relocate yourself to his right and use your right hand to grab his right forearm near the wrist area, while also placing your left hand on his right elbow area (Figure 6-260). Finally, rotate his right arm until his palm is facing upward, and then use the leverage of your right

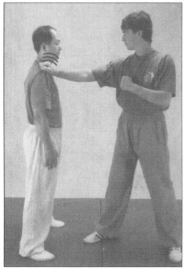

Figure 6–259

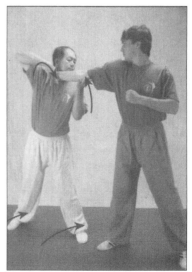

Figure 6–260

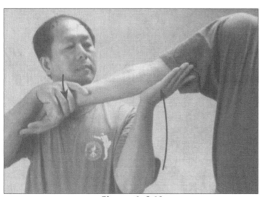

Figure 6–261

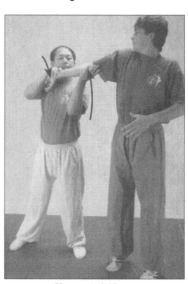

Figure 6–262

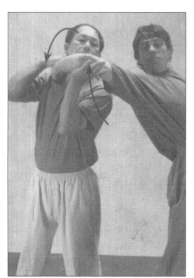

Figure 6–263

hand and left hand to press his elbow up (Figure 6-261). You should increase your power until his heels are off the ground (Figure 6-262).

Theory:

Misplacing the Bone (elbow). The leverage generated from both of your hands is the key to the control. If your opponent bends his elbow before you have locked him in place, you should immediately push his elbow forward while pulling his wrist toward you (Figure 6-263). In this case, you will still be able to lock him. Remember, you should keep yourself on the right hand side of your opponent. This will prevent him from attacking you with his left hand.

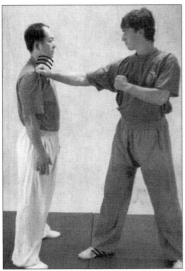

Figure 6–264

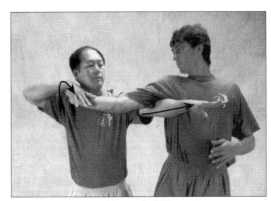

Figure 6–265

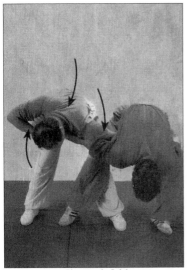

Figure 6–266

Technique #5: Two Children Worship the Buddha

(Shuang Tong Bai Fo) 雙童拜佛

When your opponent's right hand is on your right shoulder (Figure 6-264), step your left leg behind his right leg while using your right hand to grab his right wrist, and extending your left arm under his right arm to reach his left chest (Figure 6-265). Finally, bow forward while pulling his right wrist backward and pushing your left shoulder forward against his upper-arm to lock him (Figure 6-266).

Theory:

Pressing the Tendon (upper-arm) and Misplacing the Bone (elbow). In order to control your opponent more efficiently, you should press your left shoulder forward and pull your right hand backward. The controlling leverage is generated from your left shoulder and your right hand. This technique can only control your opponent temporarily. It is very difficult to dislocate your opponent's elbow. Therefore, this technique serves only to lock temporarily in order to set up further striking.

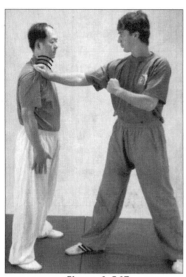

Figure 6–267

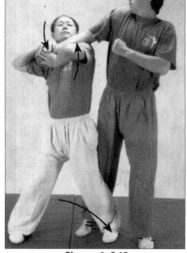

Figure 6–268

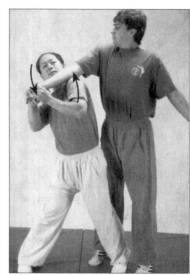

Figure 6–269

Technique #6: Carry a Pole on the Shoulder

(Jian Tiao Bian Dan) 肩挑扁擔

When your opponent grabs your right shoulder with his right hand (Figure 6-267), step your left leg to the front of his right leg and grab his right wrist with your right hand, while placing your left arm under his right arm and locking him upward (Figure 6-268). The leverage generated from both the hands and the left upper-arm is the key to locking.

You may also place his right elbow on your left shoulder to lock him up (Figure 6-269). Through the leverage of both of your hands and your left shoulder, you may lock him up until his heels are off the ground.

Theory:

Misplacing the Bone (elbow). In this technique, if you jerk your right arm downward, you may break his elbow joint.

Technique #7: The Old Man Carries the Fish on His Back

(Lao Han Bei Yu) 老漢背魚

If your opponent grabs your right shoulder area with his right hand (Figure 6-270), immediately use both of your hands to grab his right wrist while using your left elbow to push his right elbow to bend it (Figure 6-271), Finally, step your left leg to the front of his right leg and bow forward to lock his right arm (Figure 6-272). If you keep pulling both of your hands downward, you may pull his shoulder out of its socket.

Theory:

Misplacing the Bone (shoulder and elbow). The angle at which you control your opponent's arm is very important. If your opponent's arm is either to straight or too bent, the control will not be effective. With an accurate angle, you may generate great pain in your opponent's shoulder.

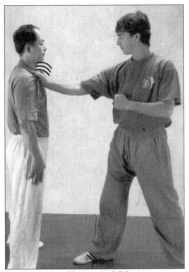

Figure 6–270

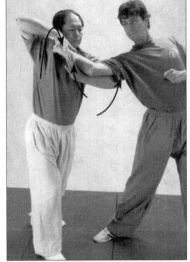

Figure 6–271

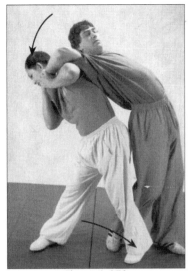

Figure 6–272

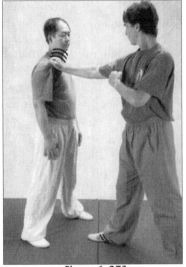

Figure 6–273

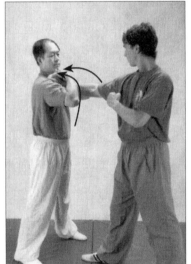

Figure 6–274

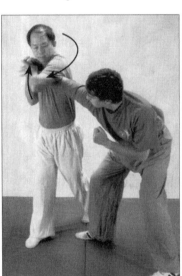

Figure 6–275

Technique #8: Old Man Promoted to General

(Lao Han Bai Jiang) 老漢拜將

When your opponent's right hand is on your right shoulder (Figure 6-273), again grab his right wrist with both of your hands (Figure 6-274). Next, place your left armpit over his right elbow while turning your body to your right (Figure 6-275). Finally, use the leverage of both of your hands and your left shoulder to press him down (Figure 6-276). As you do this, you should also kneel down on your left leg; this will provide you a better position for your control.

Theory:

Misplacing the Bone (elbow and shoulder). When you press your opponent down, you should keep his arm straight and the pressing should be straight on the rear side of his elbow. If you jerk your power, you may break his elbow easily.

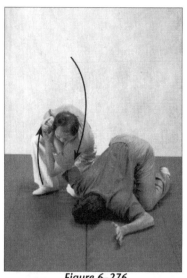

Figure 6–276

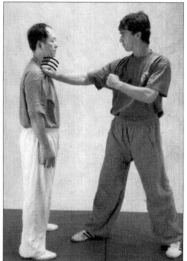

Figure 6–277

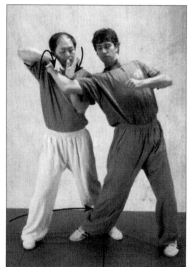

Figure 6–278

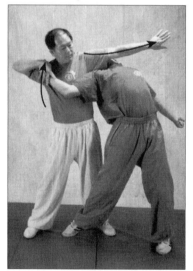

Figure 6–279

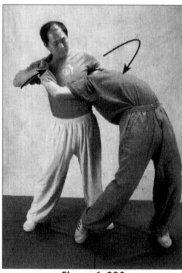

Figure 6–280

Technique #9: Arm Wraps Around the Dragon's Neck

(Bi Chan Long Jing) 臂纏龍頸

When your opponent grabs your right shoulder with his right hand (Figure 6-277), step your left leg behind his right leg and grab his right wrist with your right hand, while pushing his elbow with your left forearm (Figure 6-278). Next, extend your left arm to his neck area while locking his right arm on your chest (Figure 6-279). Finally, circle your left arm around his neck while pulling his right wrist backward (Figure 6-280).

Theory:

Sealing the Breath or Artery (neck). When you control your opponent, in order to prevent him from struggling or counterattacking, you should push his neck backward so his balance is destroyed.

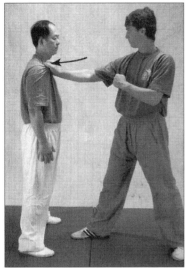

Figure 6-281

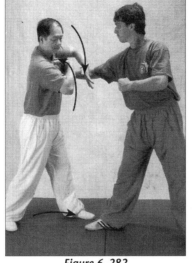

Figure 6-282

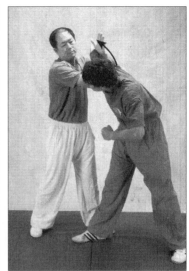

Figure 6-283

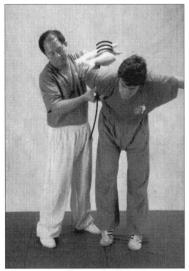

Figure 6-284

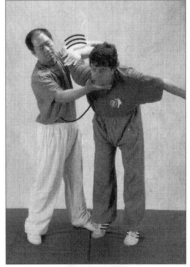

Figure 6-285

Technique #10: Pressing Shoulder with Single Finger and Extending the Neck for Water

(Yi Zhi Ding Jiang and Yin Jing Qiu Shui) 一指頂肩 ， 引頸求水

When your opponent's right hand is on your right shoulder (Figure 6-281), step your left leg to his right hand side and grab his right wrist with your right hand, while placing your left hand on his elbow (Figure 6-282), Next, coil your left arm around his right arm (Figure 6-283) and lock his arm behind his back, while using your index finger to press his *Jianneiling* cavity (M-UE-48)(Figure 6-284). You should increase the pressure on your index finger until your opponent's heels leave the floor. Alternatively, you may use your right hand to push his chin upward (Figure 6-285). This will also produce great pain.

Theory:

Misplacing the Bone (shoulder) and Cavity Press (*Jianneiling* cavity). When you use your left arm to lock your opponent's right arm and lift it upward, you generate a strain on his right shoulder's tendons and ligaments. This action also exposes his *Jianneiling* cavity for your cavity press attack. Without an accurate locking position for the shoulder, the cavity press will not be effective.

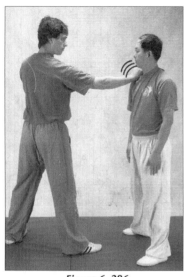

Figure 6–286

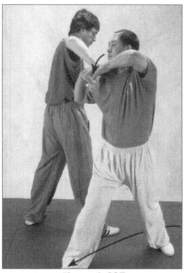

Figure 6–287

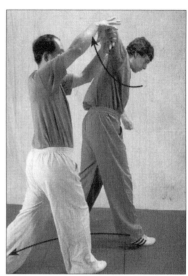

Figure 6–288

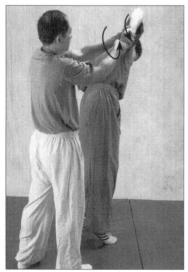

Figure 6–289

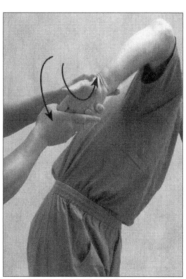

Figure 6–290

Technique #11: Send the Devil to Heaven

(Song Mo Shang Tian) 送魔上天

When your opponent's right hand is on your right shoulder (Figure 6-286), use both of your hands to grab his right hand while stepping your right leg to his right hand side (Figure 6-287). Next, step your left leg to his back while twisting his right arm with both of your hands (Figure 6-288). Finally, lock his right arm upward until his heels are off the ground (Figure 6-289).

Theory:

Dividing the Muscle/Tendon (wrist) and Misplacing the Bone (shoulder). An important point for executing this technique is, when you have locked your opponent in the final position, you should use your left hand to twist his hand while using your right hand to grab his fingers and bend them downward (Figure 6-290).

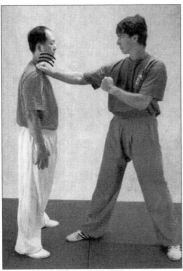

Figure 6-291

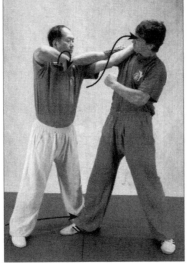

Figure 6-292

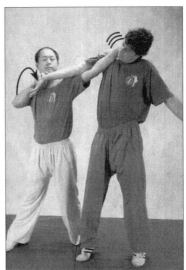

Figure 6-293

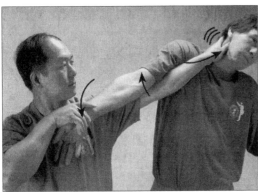

Figure 6-294

Technique #12: Roast Peking Duck

(Bei Ping Kao Ya) 北平烤鴨

When your opponent's right hand is on your right shoulder (Figure 6-291), again step your left leg behind his right leg and grab his right wrist with your right hand, while inserting your left hand under his right arm and reaching his right neck area (Figure 6-292). Next, turn his right arm until his palm is facing upward and then press his arm downward to lock his arm (Figure 6-293). When you do this, you should also straighten your left arm to increase the pressure on his upper-arm tendon (Figure 6-294).

In this technique, you may use your left thumb to press the main artery on the right side of his neck. This will seal the oxygen supply to his brain and make him lose consciousness.

Theory:

Misplacing the Bone (elbow and shoulder) and Sealing Artery (neck for optional technique). Once you have locked your opponent's arm in place, if you push your left hand down against his right shoulder and push your left forearm upward, you may produce significant pain in his shoulder.

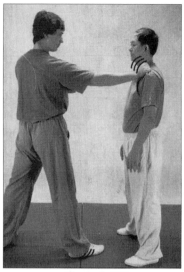

Figure 6–295

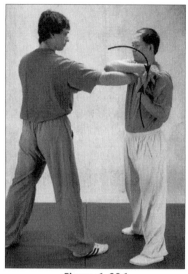

Figure 6–296

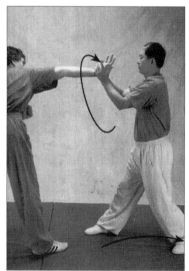

Figure 6–297

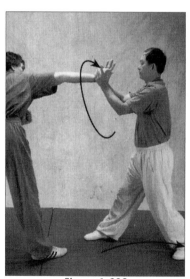

Figure 6–298

B. SAME SIDE GRABBING

Technique #1: Wild Chicken Spreads Its Wings

(Ye Ji Zhan Chi) 野雞展翅

When your opponent's right hand is on your left shoulder (Figure 6-295), first use both hands to grab his right hand (Figure 6-296). Next, step your left leg backward while twisting his right wrist clockwise until his palm faces upward (Figure 6-297). Finally, use both of your hands to press his wrist down until he is on the ground (Figure 6-298).

Theory:

Dividing the Muscle/Tendon (wrist). When you press your opponent down, the power is generated from the leverage of your pinkie and thumb area. Keep trying until the most effective angle and leverage are found.

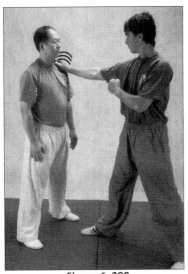
Figure 6–299

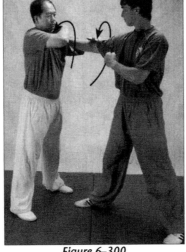
Figure 6–300

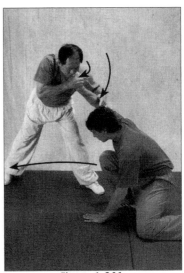
Figure 6–301

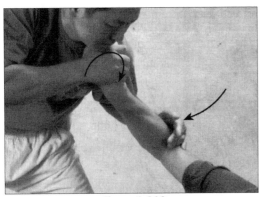
Figure 6–302

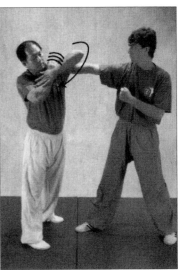
Figure 6–303

Technique #2: Wild Chicken Breaks Its Wings

(Ye Ji Ao Chi) 野雞拗翅

When your opponent's right hand is on your left shoulder (Figure 6-299), first use your right hand to cover and grab his right hand while placing your left hand on his right elbow (Figure 6-300). Next, step your right leg back and bow toward him to lock him down (Figure 6-301). When you do this, your right hand must grab his hand tightly while using your left hand to keep his elbow bent (Figure 6-302).

Alternatively, after using your right hand to grab his right hand, your may place your left elbow on his right elbow (Figure 6-303). Then bend your body toward him to lock his wrist (Figure 6-304). Again, your right hand grabbing must be strong while you use your left elbow to keep his right arm bent (Figure 6-305).

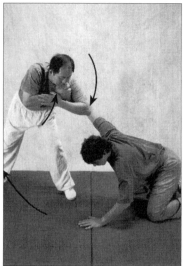

Figure 6–304

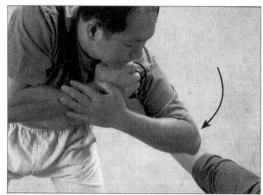

Figure 6–305

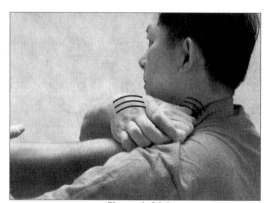

Figure 6–306

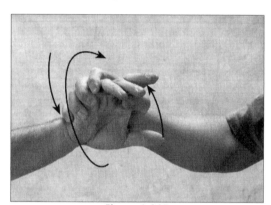

Figure 6–307

Theory:

Dividing the Muscle/Tendon (wrist). When you lock your opponent, right after you have grabbed his right hand (Figure 6-306), turn his hand clockwise and then bend it down (Figure 6-307). The power for locking is generated from the leverage of your pinkie and the thumb area. Keep trying until the most effective angle and leverage are found.

Technique #3: Luo Han Bows or Small Elbow Wrap

(Luo Han Xing Li or Xiao Chan Zhou) 羅漢行禮，小纏肘

When your opponent's right hand is on your left shoulder (Figure 6-308), first step your right leg backward, while using your right hand to grab your opponent's right wrist and using your left forearm to press his right arm upward (Figure 6-309). Next, bow your body forward, while pulling your opponent to the front of you and pressing downward

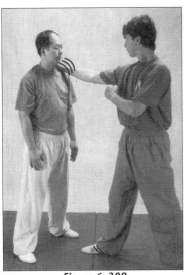

Figure 6–308

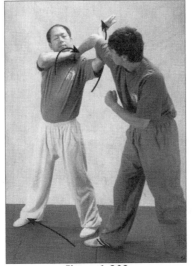

Figure 6–309

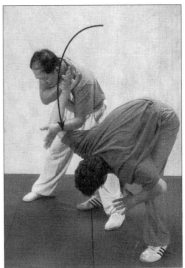

Figure 6–310

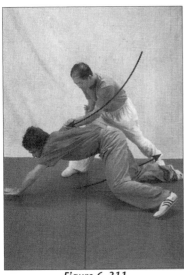

Figure 6–311

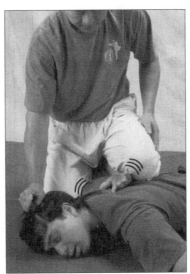

Figure 6–312

with your left hand (Figure 6-310). Finally, sweep your left leg backward to make him fall (Figure 6-311). When your opponent is on the ground, lock his arm behind his back. With the help of both of your legs, you will be able to lock him there firmly (Figure 6-312).

Theory:

Misplacing the Bone (elbow and shoulder). In order to make your opponent fall, after you have locked him, you should pull him to your front to destroy his balance while sweeping your left leg backward. Once your opponent is on the ground, if necessary you may rotate his arm toward his head and pop his shoulder out of joint.

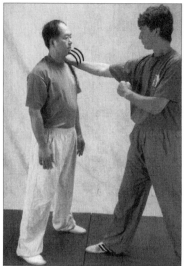

Figure 6–313

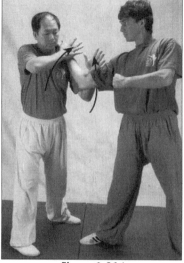

Figure 6–314

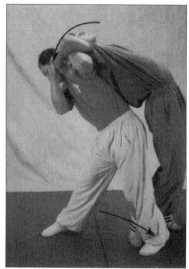

Figure 6–315

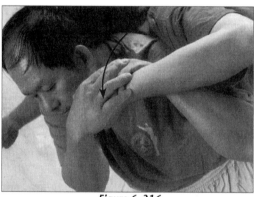

Figure 6–316

Technique #4: The Old Man Carries the Fish on His Back

(Lao Han Bei Yu) 老漢背魚

When your opponent's right hand is on your left shoulder (Figure 6-313), first use your right hand to cover his right hand while using your left forearm to push and bend his right elbow (Figure 6-314). Finally, step your left leg to the front of his right leg while turning your body and bowing forward to generate pressure on his elbow and shoulder joints (Figure 6-315). If you increase your control pressure or jerk your locking arms, you may pull his shoulder out of its socket.

Theory:

Misplacing the Bone (shoulder and elbow). The angle at which you control your opponent's arm is very important. If you opponent's arm is either too straight or too bent, the control will not be effective. With an accurate angle, you may generate great pain in your opponent's shoulder (Figure 6-316).

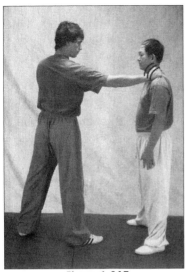

Figure 6–317

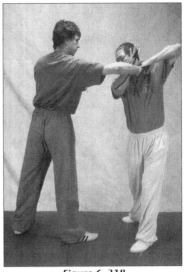

Figure 6–318

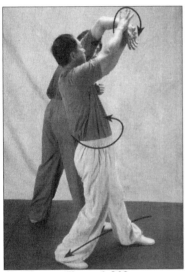

Figure 6–319

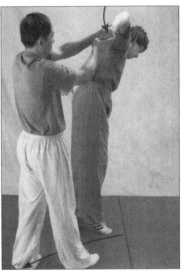

Figure 6–320

Technique #5: Send the Devil to Heaven

(Song Mo Shang Tian) 送魔上天

When your opponent's right hand is on your left shoulder (Figure 6-317), turn your body to your left and grab his right wrist with your left hand, while clamping upward your right hand toward his wrist (Figure 6-318). Next, step your right leg beside his right leg while turning your body and using both of your hands to twist his right arm (Figure 6-319). Finally, step your left leg backward, while twisting his right hand with your left hand and bending his fingers downward with your right hand to lock him upward (Figure 6-320).

Theory:

Dividing the Muscle/Tendon (wrist) and Misplacing the Bone (shoulder). The trick to making this technique effective is, when you have locked your opponent in the final position, emphasize the pinkie lock through twisting his hand. This can cause great tension in his pinkie's tendon. In this case, if you bend his fingers downward, you may generate great pain.

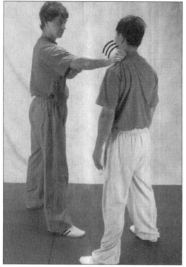

Figure 6–321

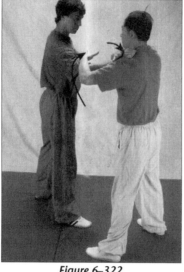

Figure 6–322

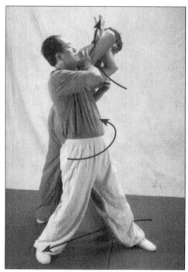

Figure 6–323

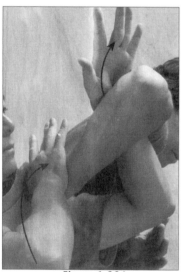

Figure 6–324

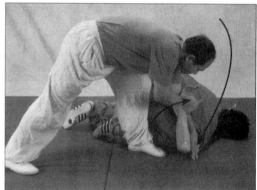

Figure 6–325

Technique #6: Large Python Turns Its Body

(Da Mang Fan Shen) 大蟒翻身

When your opponent's right hand is on your left shoulder (Figure 6-321), use your right hand to grab his right hand while placing your left forearm on his right elbow (Figure 6-322). Next, step your right leg behind his right leg and turn your body to your left while rotating his arm (Figures 6-323 and 6-324). Finally, bow forward and use the leverage of both of your hands to press him down to the ground (Figures 6-325 and 6-326).

Theory:

Misplacing the Bone (elbow and shoulder). The angle to lock your opponent's arm is very important. Too straight or too bent is not effective for locking. Since this technique is a large circle Qin Na, the speed is very important. Taking too much time will allow your opponent to resist you.

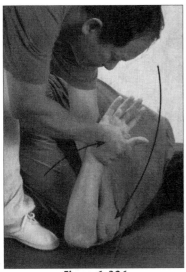

Figure 6–326

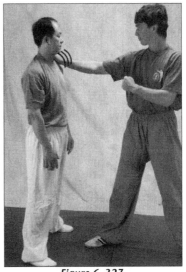

Figure 6–327

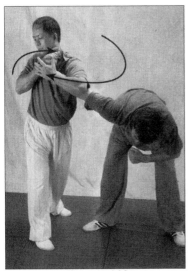

Figure 6–328

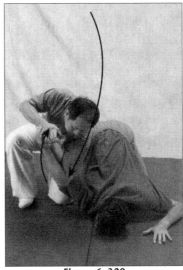

Figure 6–329

Technique #7: Old Man Promoted to General

(Lao Han Bai Jiang) 老漢拜將

When your opponent's right hand is on your left shoulder (Figure 6-327), first turn your body to your right and grab his right hand with your right hand while placing your left armpit on his right elbow (Figure 6-328). Next, bend your left knee down while using the leverage of your left shoulder and both hands to press him down until his face touches the ground (Figure 6-329).

Theory:

Misplacing the Bone (elbow and shoulder). When you press your opponent down, you should keep his arm straight, and the pressing should be straight on the rear side of his elbow. If you jerk your power, you may break his elbow easily.

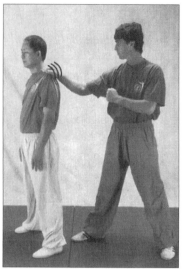
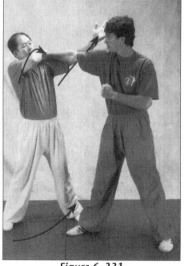
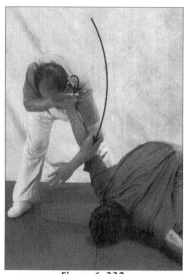

| *Figure 6–330* | *Figure 6–331* | *Figure 6–332* |

II. FROM THE REAR

A. OPPOSITE SIDE GRABBING

When your opponent touches your shoulder from behind you, since you cannot see which hand he is using, it is harder to decide what technique should be used. However, there are some techniques which can effectively be applied for either possibility. Naturally, these techniques are considered better than those which can be used only for special occasions.

Technique #1: Turn the Body and Bow

(Zhuan Shen Ju Gong) 轉身鞠躬

When your opponent is behind you and his right hand is on your left shoulder (Figure 6-330), turn your body to your left, step your left leg behind his right leg, and use your right hand to cover and grab his right hand, while placing your left forearm on his right elbow (Figure 6-331). Finally, use the leverage of your right hand and left forearm to press him down to the ground (Figure 6-332).

Theory:
Dividing the Muscle/Tendon (wrist) and Misplacing the Bone (elbow and shoulder). The keys to making this technique effective are your right hand's twisting and bending on his wrist, and your left forearm's locking and pressing while keeping your opponent's arm straight.

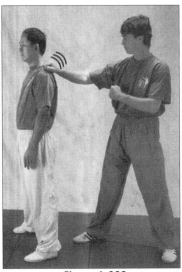

Figure 6-333

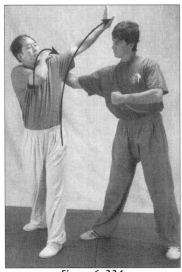

Figure 6-334

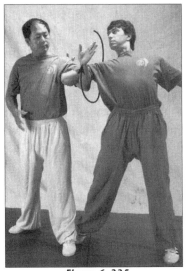

Figure 6-335

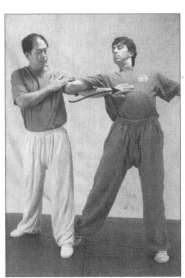

Figure 6-336

Technique #2: Turn Back to Seize the Ape

(Hui Tou Qin Yuan) 回頭擒猿

When your opponent is behind you and uses his right hand to touch your left shoulder (Figure 6-333), first use your right hand to cover his right hand to prevent him from escaping, while turning your body to your left and circling your left arm over his right arm (Figure 6-334). Next, use your left arm to lock up his right elbow while releasing your right hand grab (Figure 6-335). Finally, extend your left arm and push his chest with your left hand (Figure 6-336).

Theory:

Misplacing the Bone (elbow). When you turn your body, you should beware of your opponent's left hand. When you scoop your left arm upward to his elbow, you should release your right hand's grabbing. This will offer you a better angle for his elbow control. If you wish to dislocate your opponent's elbow, simply straighten your left arm.

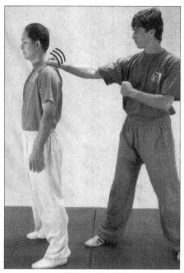
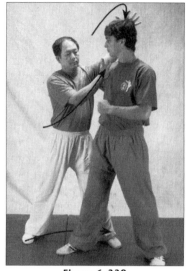
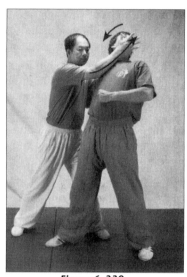

| Figure 6–337 | Figure 6–338 | Figure 6–339 |

Technique #3: Twist the Neck to Kill a Chicken

(Sha Ji Niu Jing) 殺雞扭頸

When your opponent is behind you and his right hand is on your left shoulder (Figure 6-337), turn your body to the left, step your left leg behind his right leg, and place your left hand behind his head and your right hand on his chin (Figure 6-338). Finally, use the leverage of both of your hands to twist his neck to the side and 45 degrees upward (Figure 6-339). If you wish to break his neck, you may simply jerk your power. However, you should not do so unless it is necessary.

Theory:
Misplacing the Bone (neck). This technique can also be used when your opponent is using the other hand to touch your left shoulder.

Technique #4: Send the Devil to Heaven

(Song Mo Shang Tian) 送魔上天

When your opponent's right hand touches your left shoulder from behind (Figure 6-340), first step your left leg back while grabbing his right hand with your right hand (Figure 6-341). Immediately turn your body to your left while also using your right hand to grab his right hand (Figure 6-342). Finally, step your right leg to his back while using your body's rotation momentum to twist his arm and lock it upward (Figure 6-343).

Theory:
Dividing the Muscle/Tendon in the wrist and Misplacing the Bone in the shoulder. The trick to making this technique effective is, when you have locked your opponent in the final position, you should use your left hand to twist his hand while using your right hand to grab his fingers and bend them downward.

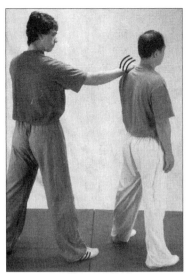

Figure 6–340

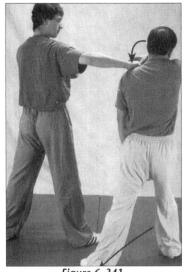

Figure 6–341

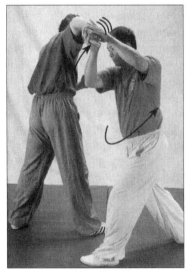

Figure 6–342

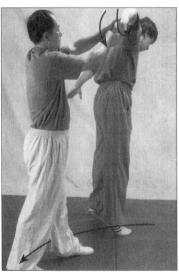

Figure 6–343

Technique #5: Large Python Turns Its Body

(Da Mang Fan Shen) 大蟒翻身

When your opponent's right hand touches your left shoulder from behind (Figure 6-344), step your left leg behind his right leg and grab his right hand with your right hand while placing your left forearm on his elbow area (Figure 6-345). Next, step your right leg behind him while rotating your body to your left (Figure 6-346). Finally, use the leverage of both of your hands to press him down to the ground (Figure 6-347).

Theory:

Misplacing the Bone (elbow and shoulder). The angle for locking his arm is very important. Too straight or too bent can make the technique ineffective.

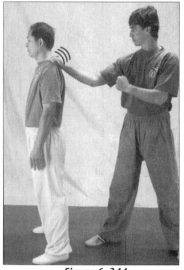

Figure 6-344

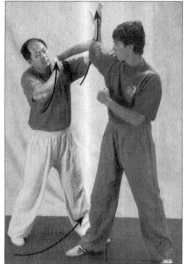

Figure 6-345

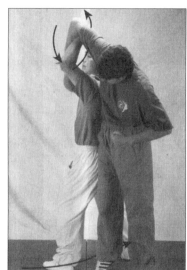

Figure 6-346

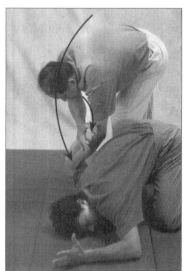

Figure 6-347

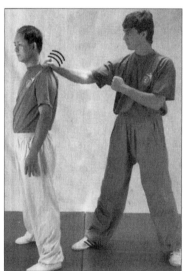

Figure 6-348

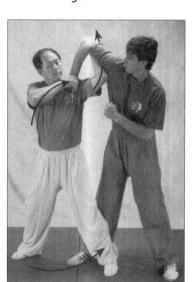

Figure 6-349

Technique #6: Luo Han Bows or Small Elbow Wrap

(Luo Han Xing Li or Xiao Chan Zhou) 羅漢行禮 , 小纏肘

When your opponent's right hand touches your left shoulder (Figure 6-348), step your left leg to the front of his right leg, grab his right hand with your right hand while placing your left forearm on his elbow (Figure 6-349). Finally, bow your body forward and use the leverage of your right hand and left forearm to press him downward (Figure 6-350).

If you wish to take him down, simply sweep your left leg backward while pulling his arm to the front of your body (Figure 6-351).

Theory:

Misplacing the Bone (elbow and shoulder). To make this technique effective, your turning must be fast and the coordination of your right hand and left forearm is very important. You should keep his arm bent all the time.

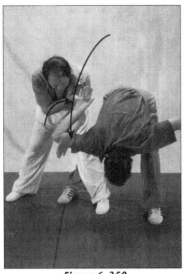

Figure 6–350

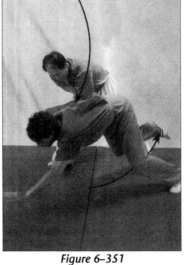

Figure 6–351

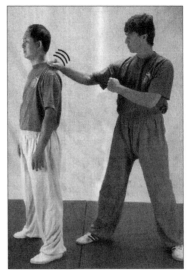

Figure 6–352

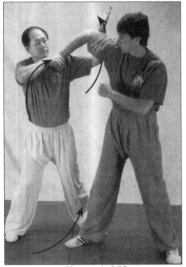

Figure 6–353

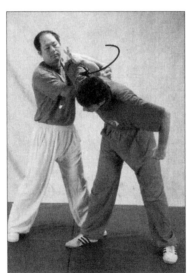

Figure 6–354

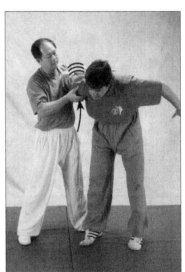

Figure 6–355

Technique #7: Pressing Shoulder with Single Finger and Extending the Neck for Water

(Yi Zhi Ding Jiang and Yin Jing Qiu Shui) 一指頂肩，引頸求水

If your opponent's right hand touches your left shoulder from behind (Figure 6-352), again step your left leg behind his right leg, grab his right hand with your right hand while placing your left forearm on his elbow area (Figure 6-353). Next, coil your left hand around his right arm until it reaches his elbow and lock his arm behind his back (Figure 6-354). At this stage, all of the tendons and ligaments in your opponent's shoulder are very tense. Next, press your index finger on his *Jianneiling* cavity (M-UE-48); you will be able to generate great pain in his shoulder area (Figure 6-355). You should increase the pressure on

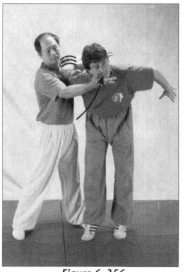

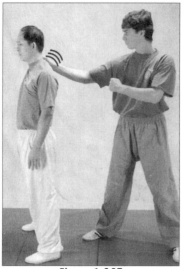

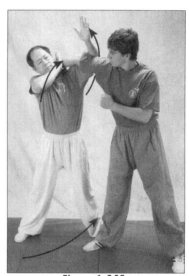

| Figure 6–356 | Figure 6–357 | Figure 6–358 |

your index finger until your opponent's heels leave the floor. Alternatively, you may use your right hand to push his chin upward (Figure 6-356). This will also produce great pain.

Theory:

Misplacing the Bone (shoulder) and Cavity Press (*Jianneiling* cavity). When using your left arm to lock your opponent's right arm and lift it upwards, you generate a strain on his right shoulder's tendons and ligaments. This action also exposes his *Jianneiling* cavity for your cavity press attack. Without an accurate locking position for the shoulder, the cavity press will not be effective.

B. SAME SIDE GRABBING

Technique #1: The Heavens Turn and the Earth Circles

(Tian Xuan Di Zhuan) 天 旋 地 轉

When your opponent's right hand touches your right shoulder (Figure 6-357), step your left leg behind his right leg and grab his right hand with your right hand, while placing your left arm behind his upper-arm (Figure 6-358). Finally, use the leverage of your neck and left forearm to press him down (Figure 6-359).

If you wish to take him down, simply move your left leg to the front of his right leg and sweep backward while circling his arm to your front (Figure 6-360).

Theory:

Misplacing the Bone (elbow and shoulder) and Pressing the Tendons (upper-arm). This technique is also commonly used in the situation when your opponent grabs your middle upper back. When you apply this technique, if you find that your opponent is using his left hand to touch your left shoulder instead of his right hand

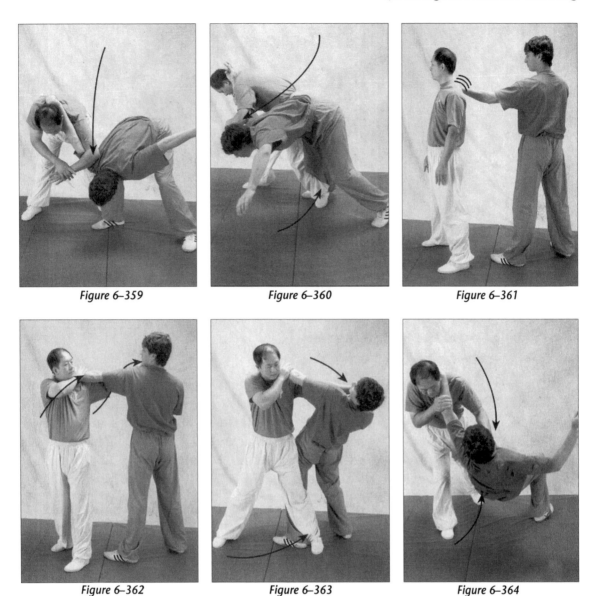

Figure 6–359   Figure 6–360   Figure 6–361

Figure 6–362   Figure 6–363   Figure 6–364

(Figure 6-361), after you have turned your body and raised up both of your arms (Figure 6-362), simply grab his throat with your left hand while stepping your left leg behind his left leg (Figure 6-363). Naturally, you may sweep your left leg backward to take him down (Figure 6-364).

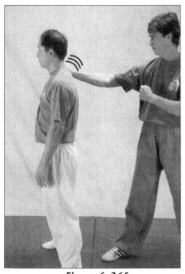
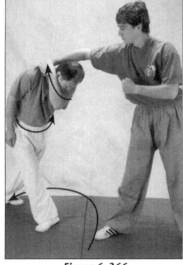
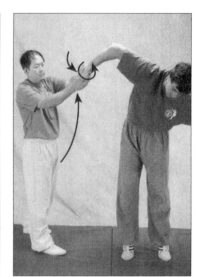

| Figure 6–365 | Figure 6–366 | Figure 6–367 |

Technique #2: Send the Devil to Heaven

(Song Mo Shang Tian) 送魔上天

When your opponent's right hand touches your right shoulder (Figure 6-365), use your left hand to grab his right hand while stepping your left leg backward toward his right hand side (Figure 6-366). Next, use both of your hands to grab his right hand, and twist and bend his hand and wrist to lock him upward (Figure 6-367). You should increase your twisting pressure until your opponent's heels are off the ground.

Theory:
Dividing the Muscle/Tendon (wrist) and Misplacing the Bone (shoulder). To make the control most effective, you should use your left hand to twist his hand while bending his fingers downward with your right hand.

Technique #3: Large Python Turns Its Body

(Da Mang Fan Shen) 大蟒翻身

When your opponent's right hand touches your right shoulder behind you (Figure 6-368), again step your left leg behind his right leg and grab his right hand with your right hand, while placing your left forearm on his elbow (Figure 6-369). Next, step your right leg behind him while rotating your body under his right arm (Figure 6-370). Finally, use the leverage of your right hand and left forearm to press him down to the ground (Figure 6-371).

Theory:
Misplacing the Bone (elbow and shoulder). The angle of your opponent's arm is the key to the control. If his arm is either too straight or too bent, the control will not be effective. When you execute this technique, speed is crucial. Without good speed, your opponent can sense your intention easily.

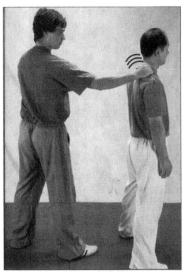

Figure 6–368

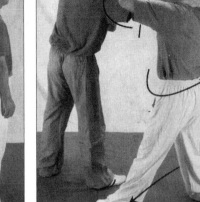

Figure 6–369

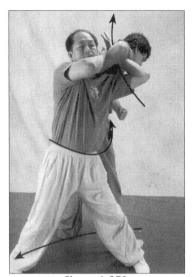

Figure 6–370

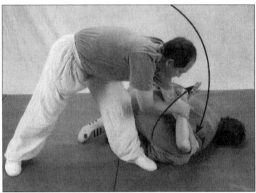

Figure 6–371

Technique #4: Arm Wraps Around the Dragon's Neck

(Bi Chan Long Jing) 臂纏龍頸

When your opponent's right hand touches your right shoulder from behind (Figure 6-372), first turn your body to the right while using your right hand to grab his right wrist and placing your left arm on his neck (Figure 6-373). Next, step your left leg behind his right leg and use your left arm to circle his neck, while locking his arm on your chest (Figure 6-374).

Theory:

Seal the Artery/Vein (neck). In order to prevent your opponent from striking you with his left hand, you should increase your left arm's wrapping and make his body lean backward. This will destroy his balance and center and thus prevent him from attacking you powerfully.

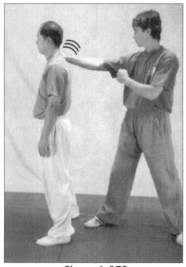

Figure 6–372

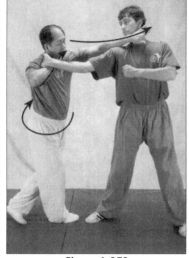

Figure 6–373

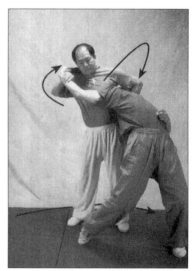

Figure 6–374

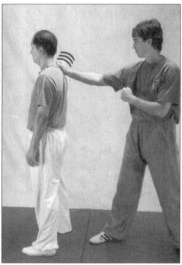

Figure 6–375

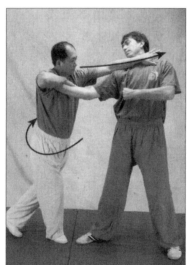

Figure 6–376

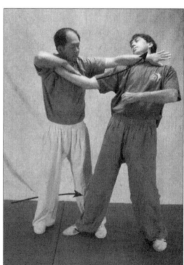

Figure 6–377

Technique #5: Face the Heavens and Fall Down

(Yang Tian Fan Die) 仰天翻跌

When your opponent's right hand touches your right shoulder (Figure 6-375), again turn your body to your right, while using your right hand to grab his right wrist and extending your left arm on his neck area (Figure 6-376). Next, step your left leg behind his right leg while pressing his head backward (Figure 6-377). Finally, use your left arm to press his neck down while using your left leg to sweep his right leg to make him fall (Figure 6-378).

Theory:

Taking Down. The leverage generated from your left leg sweeping and left arm pushing is very important. With practice, you will make your opponent fall easily.

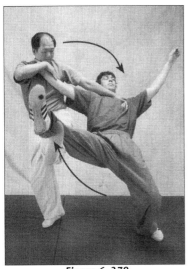

Figure 6–378

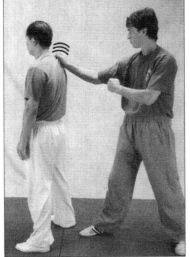

Figure 6–379

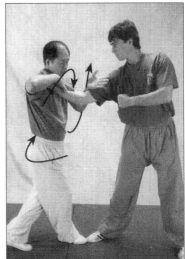

Figure 6–380

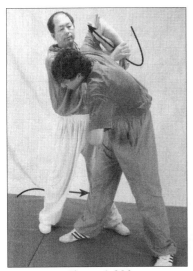

Figure 6–381

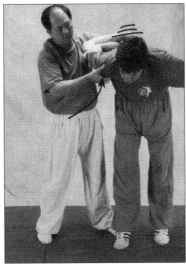

Figure 6–382

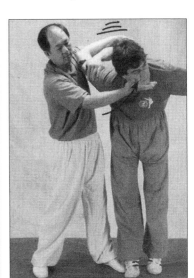

Figure 6–383

Technique #6: Pressing Shoulder with Single Finger and Extending the Neck for Water

(Yi Zhi Ding Jiang and Yin Jing Qiu Shui) 一指頂肩 ， 引頸求水

When your opponent's right hand touches your right shoulder from behind (Figure 6-379), again turn your body to your right, while using your right hand to grab his right wrist and placing your left forearm on his right elbow (Figure 6-380). Next, step your left leg behind his right leg, while coiling your left hand around his right arm and finally reaching his elbow, and lock his arm upward behind his back (Figure 6-381). At this stage, all of the tendons and ligaments in your opponent's shoulder are very tensed. Next, press your index finger into his *Jianneiling* cavity (M-UE-48); you will be able to generate great pain in his shoulder area (Figure 6-382). You should increase the pressure on your index finger until your opponent's heels leave the floor. Alternatively, you may use your right hand to push his chin upward (Figure 6-383). This will also produce great pain.

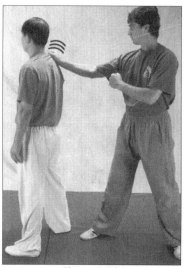

Figure 6–384

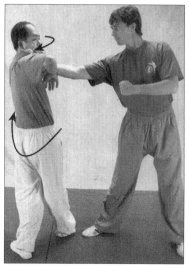

Figure 6–385

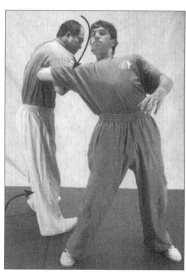

Figure 6–386

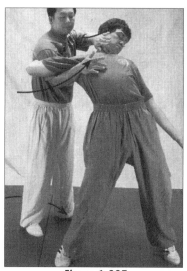

Figure 6–387

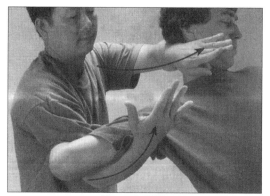

Figure 6–388

Theory:

Misplacing the Bone (shoulder) and Cavity Press (*Jianneiling* cavity). When you use your left arm to lock your opponent's right arm and lift it upward, you generate a strain on his right shoulder's tendons and ligaments. This action also exposes his *Jianneiling* cavity for your cavity press attack. Without an accurate locking position for the shoulder, the cavity press will not be effective.

Technique #7: Sparrow Hawk Shakes Its Wing or Backward Upward Turning

(Yao Zi Dou Chi or Hou Shang Fan) 鷂子抖翅，後上翻

When your opponent's right hand touches your right shoulder from behind (Figure 6-384), turn your body to your right, while lifting your right elbow upward and grabbing his right hand with your left hand (Figure 6-385). Next, reposition yourself to his back, while twisting his hand with your left hand and raising up his elbow with your right elbow (Figure 6-386). Finally, move your right hand to his chest to lock his right arm, while using your left hand to push his neck to his left (Figures 6-387 and 6-388).

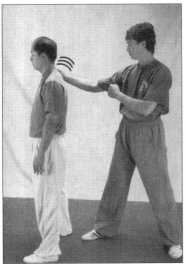

Figure 6–389

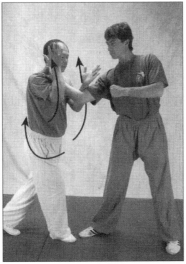

Figure 6–390

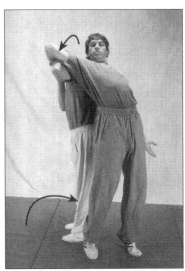

Figure 6–391

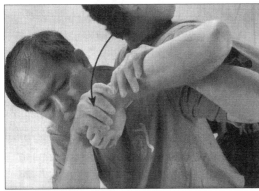

Figure 6–392

Theory.

Dividing the Muscle/Tendon (wrist) and Misplacing the Bones (elbow and shoulder). In order to prevent your opponent from striking you with his left hand, your stepping to his right is very important. In addition, this stepping will offer you an additional option which allows your to sweep his leg and make him fall.

Technique #8: The Old Man Carries the Fish on His Back

(Lao Han Bei Yu) 老漢背魚

When your opponent's right hand is on your right shoulder (Figure 6-389), again turn your body to your right, while raising up your right arm to his wrist and left forearm to his elbow (Figure 6-390). Next, step your left leg to his back while turning your body to your right, and use the leverage of both of your hands and left shoulder to lock him up (Figures 6-391 and 6-392).

Theory:

Misplacing the Bone (shoulder and elbow). The angle you set up at his elbow is very important. Too straight or too bent will make the technique ineffective. If necessary, you may use your right elbow to strike his left kidney.

6-5. Qin Na Against Chest and Rear Back Grabbing

In this section, we will introduce some Qin Na techniques which can be used against chest grabs, and also grabs to the area under the back of your neck. For chest grabs, we will again use two categories: before the grabbing and after the grabbing. If your opponent is grabbing you with both his hands, simply treat it the same as the case of a single hand grab.

I. CHEST GRABBING

A. BEFORE GRABBING

When your opponent grabs your chest, his hand must first be opened before it approaches your chest. Therefore, most of the techniques introduced in Chapter 2 which were used against stationary open hand attacks can be applied here. The only distinction is that the strategy of using Qin Na against a moving open hand attack is different from that of a stationary open hand attack. When your opponent's hand is extended and opened in front you, you must move forward and use your hands to reach his. Also, because your opponent's mind is in a defensive mode, you must act very fast in order to make your techniques effective.

However, when your opponent's hand is approaching your chest very fast, his mind is on attacking. In this situation, if you are able to step back to yield and accurately intercept his hand's forward momentum with the correct timing, your techniques can be executed successfully.

a. RIGHT HAND AGAINST RIGHT HAND

Technique #1: White Crane Nods Its Head

(Bai He Dian Tou) 白 鶴 點 頭

When your opponent's right hand is approaching your chest to grab you, first step your right leg back while using your right hand to grab his right fingers (Figure 6-393). Next, press his fingers backward and force him down with both of your hands (Figures 6-394 and 6-395).

Theory:
Misplacing the Bone (base of fingers). When you grab your opponent's fingers, you may grab all four (except the thumb), three, two, or even one fingers. The whole idea is to bend the base joints of the fingers backward until the ligaments are strained or torn off. When this happens, you may cause significant pain and lock your opponent in place.

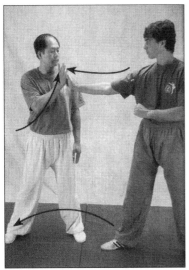

Figure 6–393

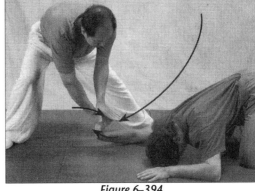

Figure 6–394

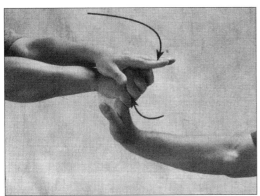

Figure 6–395

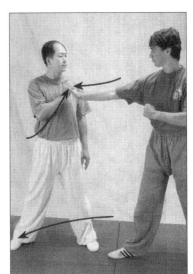

Figure 6–396

Technique #2: White Crane Twists Its Neck

(Bai He Niu Jing) 白鶴扭頸

In action, this technique is very similar to the last one. However, in theory, it is very different. If your opponent intends to grab your chest, again step your right leg back and use your right hand to grab his right finger(s) (Figure 6-396). Next, turn his hand to your right and then bend to lock his pinkie's tendon in position (Figure 6-397). Finally, press him down to the ground (Figure 6-398). When you apply this technique, it is very important that, in order to lock your opponent at a correct angle, his elbow must always be lower than his wrist. To make the technique most effective, you should use both hands to execute the twisting and bending (Figure 6-399).

Theory:

Dividing the Muscle/Tendon (wrist and pinkie). After you grab your opponent's fingers and twist to your right, you have placed his fingers in a correct angle for locking. Right after twisting, if you immediately bend his fingers backward, you have twisted and bent the pinkie's tendon, which could result in serious pain.

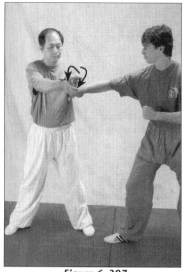

Figure 6–397

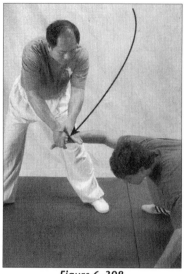

Figure 6–398

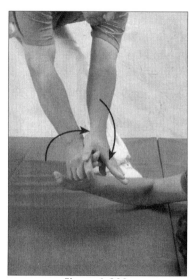

Figure 6–399

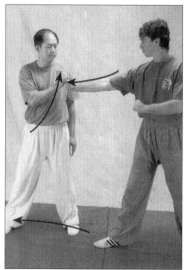

Figure 6–400

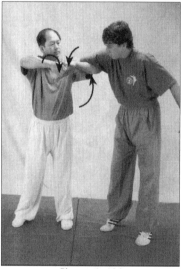

Figure 6–401

Technique #3: White Crane Covers Its Wings

(Bai He Yan Chi) 白鶴掩翅

This is an option for the pinkie's tendon lock. Again, step your right leg backward while using your right hand to grab your opponent's approaching hand (Figure 6-400). After you grab his fingers, turn them to your right and bend them backward while moving your left hand under his right arm, and reach his pinkie to lock his pinkie's tendon (Figure 6-401). Then, use your left hand to press his pinkie down, while using your left elbow to stop him from moving his elbow downward.

Theory:

Dividing the Muscle/Tendon (wrist and pinkie). When you twist and bend your opponent's pinkie downward, his right elbow will automatically move downward in order to release the pressure. At this time, if use your left elbow to stop his right elbow from going down, you may produce great pain in his pinkie tendon.

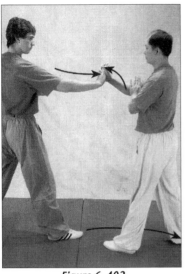

Figure 6-402

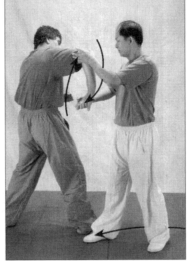

Figure 6-403

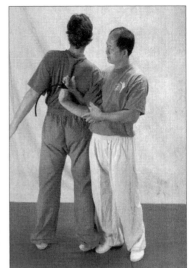

Figure 6-404

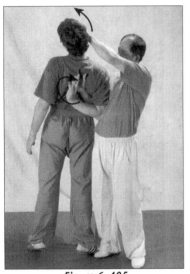

Figure 6-405

Technique #4: White Crane Bores the Bush

(Bai He Chuan Cong) 白鶴穿叢

In this technique, again step your right leg backward and use your right hand to grab your opponent's fingers (Figure 6-402). Next, turn his wrist to your right, and bend and lock his pinkie's tendon while also using your left hand to push his right elbow (Figure 6-403). Then, with the help of your left hand, lock your opponent's entire right arm behind his back by controlling his right hand (Figure 6-404). In order to control your opponent more efficiently, you may also use your left hand to pull either his second, middle, or ring finger backward to increase the pain. Alternatively, you may also use your left hand to push his neck to his left (Figure 6-405).

Theory:

Dividing the Muscle/Tendon (pinkie) and Misplacing the Bone (shoulder). In order to control him more effectively, you should increase the pressure toward the pinkie side. It is very important to know that when you step in to lock his right arm behind him, you should not step in with your left leg, since it will also expose your groin to attack. Once you have locked him in position with the leverage of your chest and right hand, free your left hand for many other options. Once you have locked your opponent's hand behind his back, if you lift his arm upward, you may also cause the ligaments in his shoulder to tear off.

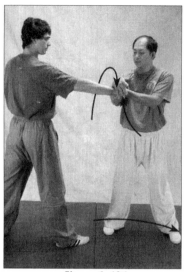

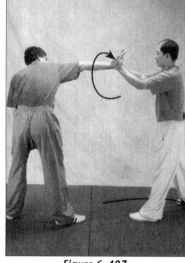

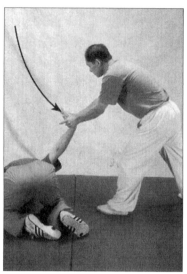

Figure 6–406   Figure 6–407   Figure 6–408

Technique #5: Wild Chicken Spreads Its Wings

(Ye Ji Zhan Chi) 野雞展翅

In this technique, first step your left leg backward while using your right hand to cover your opponent's right hand and clamping your left hand upward to his wrist (Figure 6-406). Next, step your right leg backward while rotating your opponent's wrist clockwise until his palm faces upward (Figure 6-407). Finally, use both of your hands to press him down to the ground (Figure 6-408). Remember, when you press your opponent down, you are not using the fingers but the entire hand with the coordination of the entire body's movement

Theory:

Dividing the Muscle/Tendon (wrist). After you have grabbed your opponent's wrist with both of your hands, you must use the entire hand and body to generate a turning momentum. This technique will not be useful if your opponent is a double jointed person and is able to touch his fingers to his forearm easily. The reason for this is simply because your opponent has the capability of extending his muscle/tendon on his wrist to a level which is beyond your control. This can be done through continued stretching of the wrist joint. If you have discovered this problem when you use this technique, you should either kick his groin or change your strategy by controlling the fingers instead of the wrist immediately.

Technique #6: Hands Prop a Large Beam or Prop Up Elbow

(Shou Ban Da Liang or Shang Jia Zhou) 手扳大樑，上架肘

When your opponent's right hand is approaching your chest (Figure 6-409), step your right leg backward while circling your right hand on to his wrist and grabbing his thumb and using your left hand to grab his ring finger and pinky (Figure 6-410). Finally, place your left elbow or shoulder under his right elbow, pull his thumb back with your right hand and turn his ring finger and pinkie to the side to lock him upward (Figures 6-411 and 6-412).

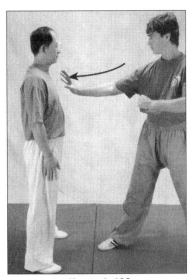

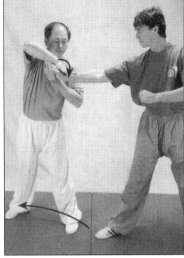

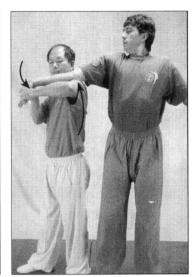

Figure 6–409   Figure 6–410   Figure 6–411

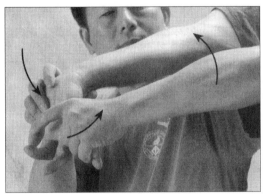

Figure 6–412

Theory:
Misplacing the Bone (elbow) and Dividing the Muscle/Tendon (base of the ring finger). To make the control effective, you should use your right hand to press backward on his thumb while splitting the tendons located between the middle and the ring fingers.

Technique #7: Baby Crane Twists Its Wing or Thumb Press
(You He Niu Chi or Mo Zhi Ya) 幼鶴扭翅 ，拇指壓

In the last technique, once you have locked his arm on your left elbow or shoulder, you may place your right thumb on the base joint and your index finger on the first joint of his right thumb (Figure 6-413). Then, use the leverage of your index finger and thumb to press the base of this thumb and lead him to the ground (Figure 6-414). Once he is locked on the ground, you may use your left hand to pull his hair to his right to prevent him from biting

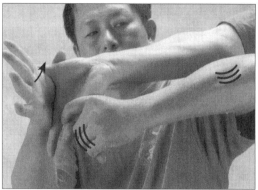

Figure 6–413

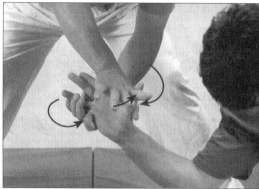

Figure 6–414

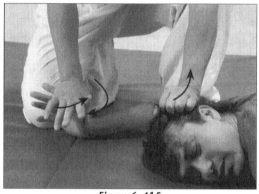

Figure 6–415

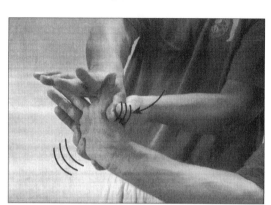

Figure 6–416

you (Figure 6-415). If you find your thumb is too weak to control the base joint of his thumb, you may add your left thumb on your right thumb to increase the pressure (Figure 6-416).

Theory:

Misplacing the Bone (base of thumb). Through the leverage of the thumb and the index finger, you may generate great pressure on the base joint of the thumb and tear the ligaments off.

Technique #8: The Hand Locks the Dragon's Tail or Small Finger Hook

(Shou Kou Long Wei or Xiao Zhi Kou) 手扣龍尾， 小指扣

When your opponent's right hand is approaching your chest to grab you (Figure 6-417), immediately step your right leg backward while covering his hand with your left hand, grab his thumb and turn his hand counterclockwise until his palm faces upward (Figure 6-418). As you do this, also use your right hand to grab his pinkie, while placing your left elbow under his right elbow to lock his arm upward (Figure 6-419). Finally, use your ring finger and pinkie to bend his pinkie, backward until his heels are off the ground (Figure 6-420). Again, if you find your right fingers are too weak to handle the job, you may add your left index finger on his pinkie area to increase the pain (Figure 6-421).

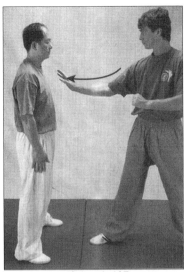

Figure 6–417

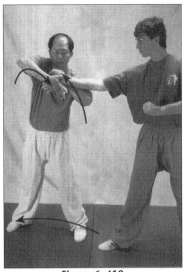

Figure 6–418

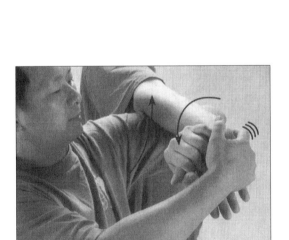

Figure 6–419

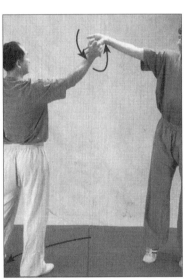

Figure 6–420

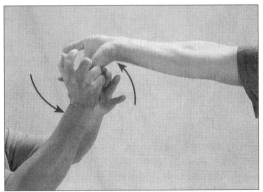

Figure 6–421

Theory:

Misplacing the Bone (elbow and pinkie). The position of your ring finger in locking his pinkie is very important. Your ring finger should be on the base of his pinkie. If you use your left hand to assist your right hand to control, you should place your index finer on the top of your right ring finger, while placing your left thumb on your right thumb area to generate good leverage.

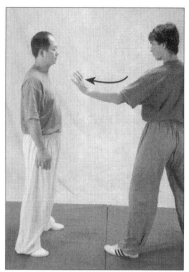

Figure 6–422

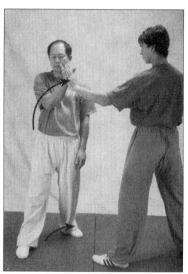

Figure 6–423

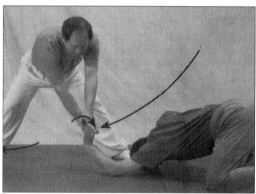

Figure 6–424

b. RIGHT HAND AGAINST LEFT HAND

Technique #1: White Crane Nods Its Head

(Bai He Dian Tou) 白鶴點頭

When your opponent's left hand is approaching your chest (Figure 6-422), immediately step your left leg to his right while using your right hand to grab his left fingers (except the thumb)(Figure 6-423). Finally, bend his fingers backward and lead his body down until his elbow touches the floor (Figure 6-424).

Theory:

Misplacing the Bone (base joint of fingers). In order to set up a good angle for grabbing, you should step your left leg to his right hand side to reposition yourself. This will offer you a good angle for your grabbing. When you grab your opponent's fingers, you may grab all four (except the thumb), three, two, or even one fingers. The whole idea is to bend the base joints of the fingers backward until the ligaments are strained or torn off.

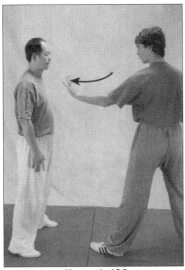

Figure 6–425

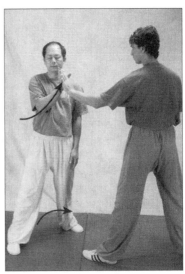

Figure 6–426

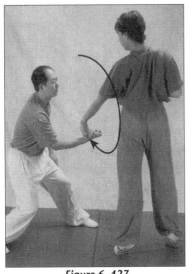

Figure 6–427

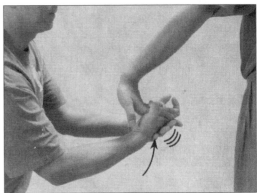

Figure 6–428

Technique #2: Rotating the Sky Post

(Niu Zhuan Tian Zhu) 扭轉天柱

In this technique, when your opponent's left hand is approaching your chest (Figure 6-425), again step your left leg to his right hand side to set up a good angle for grabbing, and use your right hand to grab his fingers (except the thumb)(Figure 6-426). Finally, rotate his arm clockwise and then press his fingers backward to lock him up (Figure 6-427). If you find that your right hand alone is too weak to handle the job, simply add your left hand to help to bend his fingers backward (Figure 6-428). You should continue to increase your pressure until his heels are off the ground.

Theory:

Misplacing the Bone (base joint of fingers). When you grab your opponent's fingers, you may grab all four (except the thumb), three, two, or even one fingers. The whole idea is to bend the base joints of the fingers backward until the ligaments are strained or torn off. When this happens, you may cause significant pain and lock your opponent in place. When you control his arm, you should keep his arm as straight as possible.

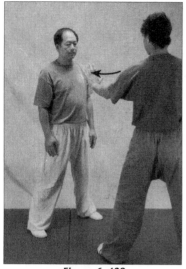

Figure 6–429

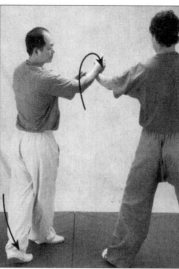

Figure 6–430

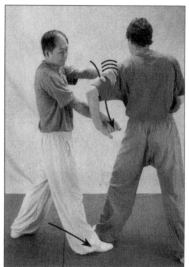

Figure 6–431

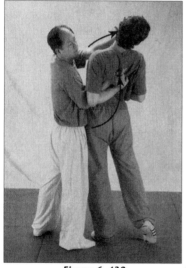

Figure 6–432

Technique #3: Butterfly Bores Through the Flowers or Back Turning

(Hu Die Chuan Hua or Fan Bei Zhuan)

蝴蝶穿花，反背轉

In this technique, when your opponent's left hand is reaching your chest (Figure 6-429), step your left leg behind your right leg while using your right hand to cover and grab his left hand (Figure 6-430). Next, step your right leg behind his left leg while circling your right hand down and toward his back (Figure 6-431). As you do this, you should use your left hand to control his left upper-arm area to generate good leverage for your right hand's circling. Finally, lock his arm behind his back while using your left hand to push his chin backward or to his right (Figure 6-432).

Theory:
Misplacing the Bone (shoulder and the base joint of the left fingers). When you have locked his arm behind him, the key to controlling is in your right hand's twisting. The more you increase your twisting pressure, the more pain you will produce in your opponent's fingers. In addition, the position of his arm should be as high as possible, which can also increase the pain significantly in his shoulder. When you use your left hand to grab your opponent's hair or to push his head upward, you will destroy his centered feeling and put him in a posture from which it is harder for him to resist you.

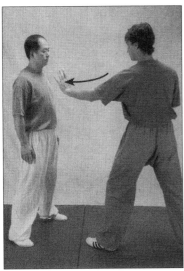
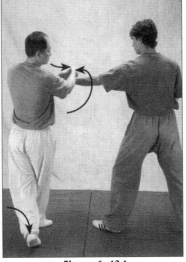
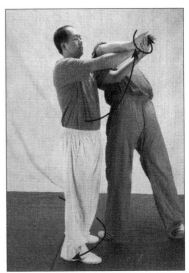

Figure 6–433 *Figure 6–434* *Figure 6–435*

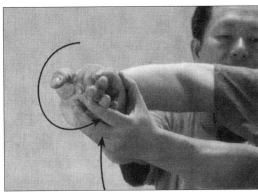

Figure 6–436

Technique #4: White Ape Offers the Fruit

(Bai Yuan Xian Guo) 白猿獻果

Though this technique looks very similar to last one, the theory of the control is different. In this technique, when your opponent's left hand is approaching your chest (Figure 6-433), again step your left leg behind your right leg, use your right hand to cover your opponent's left hand, and clamp your left hand upward (Figure 6-434). Next, step your right leg behind his right leg, swinging his left hand downward and then upward. With the help of your left hand, you may lock your opponent upward (Figure 6-435). When you lock him to the final position, use your right hand to twist his left hand, while using your left hand to support the right hand's lifting (Figure 6-436). In order to prevent your opponent from turning, you should also use your left shoulder to press his left shoulder closely.

Theory:

Misplacing the Bone (shoulder) and Dividing the Muscle/Tendon (wrist). The key to controlling is in your right hand's rotation. The more you increase your rotational pressure, the more pain will increase in your opponent's fingers. In addition, the distance between your opponent's hand and back should be accurate. His arm should be neither too straight nor too bent. A proper distance can make the technique very effective. Furthermore, the position of the control should be high, which can increase the pain significantly in his shoulder. However, if you continue to increase the lifting power, you may pop out your opponent's shoulder joint easily.

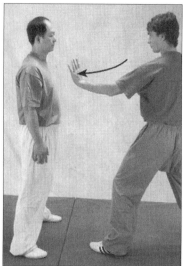

Figure 6–437

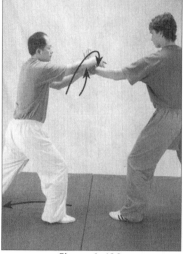

Figure 6–438

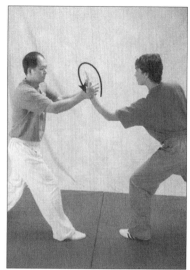

Figure 6–439

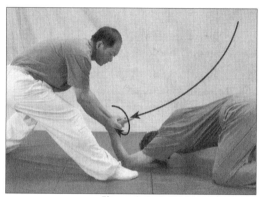

Figure 6–440

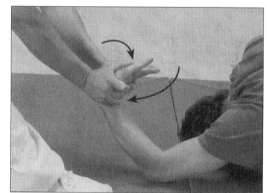

Figure 6–441

Technique #5: White Ape Worships the Buddha or Reverse Wrist Press

(Bai Yuan Bai Fo or Fan Ya Wan) 白猿拜佛，反壓腕

In this technique, when your opponent's left hand is approaching your chest (Figure 6-437), first step your left leg backward and use your right hand to cover your opponent's left hand, while also clamping your left hand upward on his wrist (Figure 6-438). Next, circle his hand clockwise until his palm faces upward (Figure 6-439). Finally, press his wrist down until his left elbow touches the floor (Figure 6-440). When you press him down, you should use the entire hand instead of just the thumbs (Figure 6-441). You may also bend and twist your opponent's hand to his left for your locking (Figure 6-442). In this case, in order to generate good leverage, you may use your right hand to twist his left hand, while using your left hand to push his head to his right (Figure 6-443).

Theory:

Dividing the Muscle/Tendon (wrist through bending and stretching). The key to control is to use the entirety of both of your hands to generate the pressure instead of using just the thumbs.

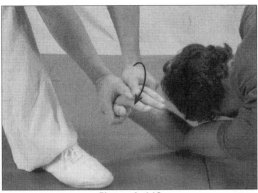

Figure 6–442

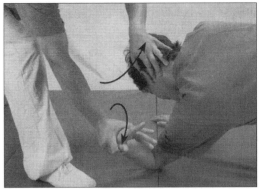

Figure 6–443

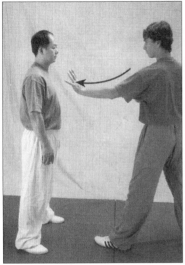

Figure 6–444

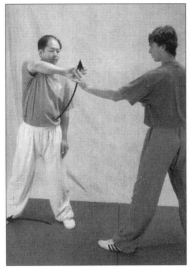

Figure 6–445

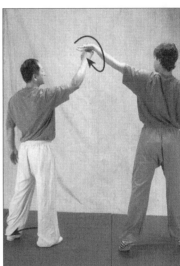

Figure 6–446

Technique #6: Hand Twists the Snake's Neck or Upward Finger Turn

(Shou Niu She Jing or Shang Fen Zhi) 手扭蛇頸，上分指

When your opponent's left hand is approaching your chest (Figure 6-444), immediately step your right leg backward, while moving your right hand upward with your palm facing to the right to reach his hand (Figure 6-445). This will set up an easy angle for you to grab his left index finger. Next, use your right hand to grab your opponent's left index finger and immediately twist them clockwise until the palm faces upward, and use the leverage of your thumb, index and middle fingers to bend down and lift your opponent's body upward until his heels are off the ground (Figure 6-446). To prevent him from escaping and to increase the effectiveness of the control, you may also use your left thumb and index finger to bend his pinkie backward (Figure 6-447).

Theory:

Misplacing the Bone (base of the index finger and pinkie). When you use your right hand to grab your opponent's left hand, the palm of your right hand is facing to the right. This will help you set up a good angle for your grip. In addition, it will also be harder for your opponent to see your hand coming.

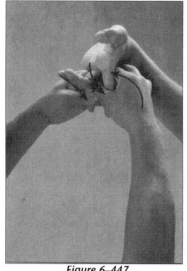

Figure 6–447

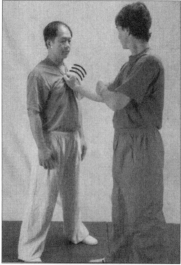

Figure 6–448

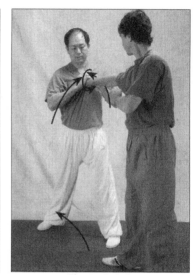

Figure 6–449

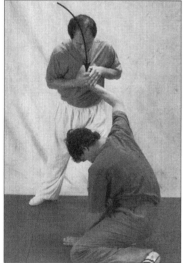

Figure 6–450

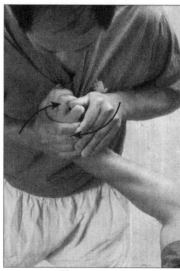

Figure 6–451

B. AFTER GRABBING

a. PALM FACING DOWNWARD

Technique #1: Twisting the Pinkie with the Thumb

(Shou Ya Xiao Zhi) 手壓小指

When your opponent has grabbed your chest with his right hand (palm facing down)(Figure 6-448), first step your right leg backward while using both of your hands to grab his wrist and twist it clockwise (Figure 6-449). Next, bend your body forward to lock his wrist while using your left thumb to push his pinkie apart from the other four fingers (Figure 6-450). When you apply this technique, his elbow should be lower than his wrist (Figure 6-451).

Theory:

Misplacing the Bone (pinkie joints) and Dividing the Muscle/Tendon (wrist). Your right hand grabbing and twisting on his wrist is very important, and can not only

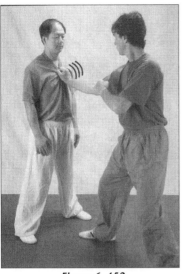

Figure 6–452

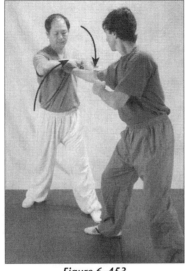

Figure 6–453

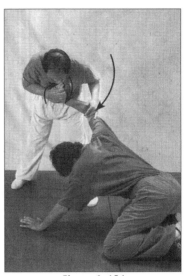

Figure 6–454

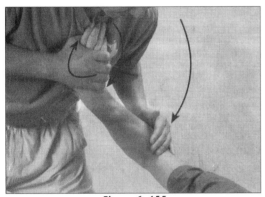

Figure 6–455

prevent him from escaping but can also set up a space for your left hand's pinkie grabbing.

Technique #2: Wild Chicken Breaks Its Wings

(Ye Ji Ao Chi) 野雞拗翅

When your opponent has grabbed your chest with his right hand (Figure 6-452), again use your right hand to grab his hand and then turn it clockwise (Figure 6-453). While you are doing this, also step back your right leg and place your left hand on his right elbow. Finally, bow forward and bend his wrist downward while using your left hand to keep his right elbow bent (Figures 6-454 and 6-455). You should control him until his left hand touches the ground.

Theory:

Dividing the Muscle/Tendon (wrist). When you control your opponent, in order to prevent him from attacking you with his left hand, you must step your right leg backward. The key to control is from the tight locking of his wrist and the bending power of your body.

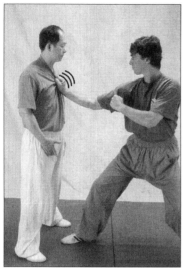
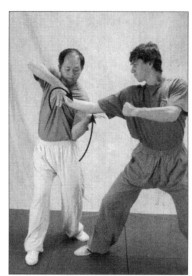
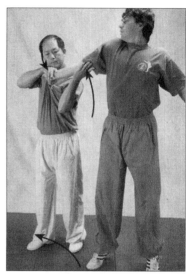

| Figure 6–456 | Figure 6–457 | Figure 6–458 |

Technique #3: Heaven King Supports the Pagoda or Upward Elbow Press

(Tian Wang Tuo Ta or Shang Ya Zhou) 天王托塔，上壓肘

In this technique, when your opponent grabs your chest with his right hand (Figure 6-456), first use your right hand to grab his right wrist and turn it counterclockwise until his palm faces upward, while placing your left hand on his right elbow (Figure 6-457). Finally, step your right leg backward while using the leverage generated from both of your hands to lock him up until his heels are off the ground (Figure 6-458).

Theory:

Misplacing the Bone (elbow). The leverage generated from both of your hands is the key to the control. From the beginning, you should keep your opponent's elbow as straight as possible. If he has kept it bent, it will be difficult to lock him with this technique. However, if he bends his elbow before you have locked him in place, you should immediately change to the technique "Old Man Carries the Fish on His Back," described below.

Technique #4: The Old Man Carries the Fish on His Back

(Lao Han Bei Yu) 老漢背魚

When your opponent has grabbed your chest with your right hand (Figure 6-459), use both of your hands to grab his right wrist, while using your left elbow to push his elbow to keep it bent (Figure 6-460). Finally, turn your body to your right and bow forward to lock his arm on your back (Figure 6-461).

Theory:

Misplacing the Bone (shoulder and elbow). The angle you set up at his elbow is very important. Too straight or too bent will make the technique ineffective.

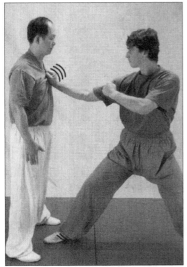

Figure 6-459

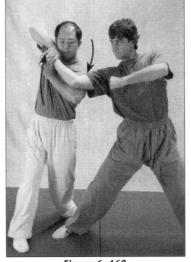

Figure 6-460

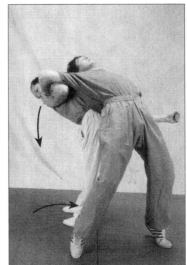

Figure 6-461

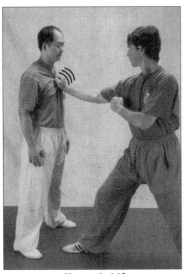

Figure 6-462

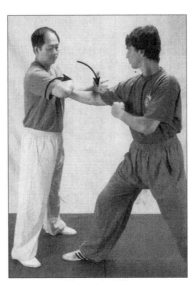

Figure 6-463

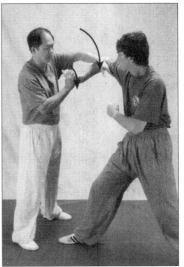

Figure 6-464

Technique #5: Pressing Shoulder with Single Finger and Extending the Neck for Water

(Yi Zhi Ding Jiang and Yin Jing Qiu Shui) 一指頂肩 , 引頸求水

When your opponent's right hand has grabbed your chest (Figure 6-462), again use your right hand to grab his right hand, twist it, and bend it to lock his wrist (Figure 6-463). Next, through the twisting of your right hand, lift his elbow upward while starting to coil his left hand around his right arm (Figure 6-464). Then, use the leverage of your left hand and elbow lock his arm behind him (Figure 6-465). Finally, use your index finger to press the *Jianneiling* cavity (M-UE-48). This will cause significant pain in the shoulder area. You should increase the pressure on your index finger until your opponent's heels leave the floor (Figure 6-466). Alternatively, you may use your right hand to push his chin upward (Figure 6-467). This will also produce great pain.

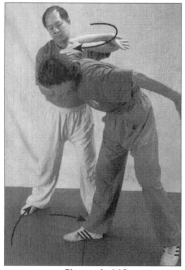
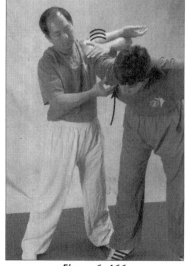
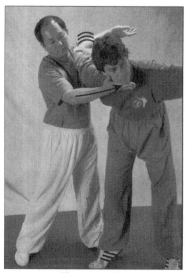

Figure 6–465   *Figure 6–466*   *Figure 6–467*

Theory:

Misplacing the Bone (shoulder), and Cavity Press (*Jianneiling* cavity). When you use your left arm to lock your opponent's right arm and lift it upward, you generate a strain on his right shoulder's tendons and ligaments. This action also exposes his *Jianneiling* cavity for your cavity press attack. Without an accurate locking position for the shoulder, the cavity press will not be effective.

Technique #6: Roast Peking Duck

(Bei Ping Kao Ya) 北平烤鴨

In this technique, when your opponent grabs your chest with his right hand (Figure 6-468), step your left leg behind his right leg, grab his wrist with your right hand and at the same time extend your left arm under his right arm to reach his neck (Figure 6-469). Finally, straighten out your left arm and pull his wrist down to lock his entire arm up (Figure 6-470). Remember, his palm should face upward.

Theory:

Misplacing the Bone (elbow and shoulder). Once you have locked your opponent's arm in place, if you push your left hand down against his right shoulder and push your left wrist upward, you may produce significant pain in his shoulder (Figure 6-471). You may also press your thumb on the path of his artery on the right hand side of his neck, to seal the oxygen supply to his brain. However, you should not do so unless it is absolutely necessary.

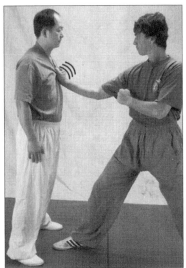

Figure 6-468

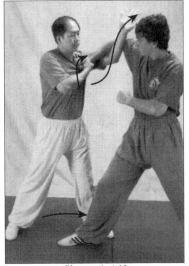

Figure 6-469

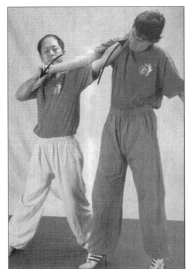

Figure 6-470

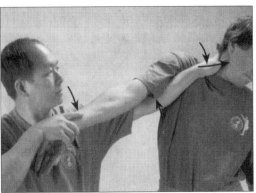

Figure 6-471

Technique #7: Arm Wraps Around the Dragon's Neck

(Bi Chan Long Jing) 臂纏龍頸

When your opponent grabs your chest with his right hand (Figure 6-472), again step your left leg behind his right leg, grab his wrist with your right hand, and at the same time use your left forearm to push his elbow to bend it (Figure 6-473). Then, immediately circle your left arm around his neck to lock it while pulling his right wrist backward to lock his arm on your chest (Figure 6-474). You should press him backward until his face looks upward.

Theory:
Seal the Artery (neck) and Seal the Breathing (throat). To prevent your opponent from struggling or attacking you with his left hand, you should lock his neck tightly until his heels are off the ground. Naturally, you may kill your opponent if you use too much power.

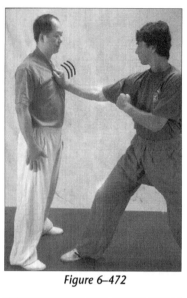

Figure 6–472

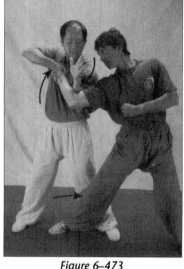

Figure 6–473

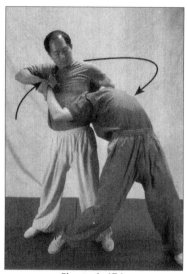

Figure 6–474

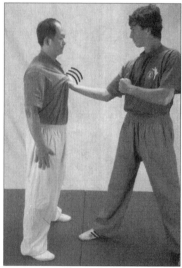

Figure 6–475

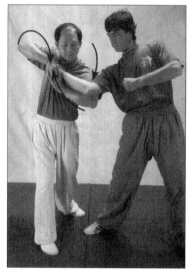

Figure 6–476

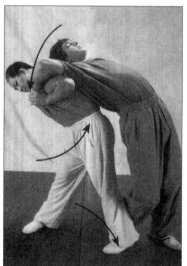

Figure 6–477

b. PALM FACES UPWARD

Technique #1: The Old Man Carries the Fish on His Back

(*Lao Han Bei Yu*) 老漢背魚

If your opponent's right hand has grabbed your chest with his palm facing upward (Figure 6-475), turn your body to your right, while using both of your hands to grab his wrist and left elbow to push his right elbow to keep it bent (Figure 6-476). Finally, step your left leg to the front of his right leg and turn and bend your body forward to lock your opponent's entire arm in position (Figure 6-477).

Theory:

Misplacing the Bone (shoulder and elbow). To make the technique effective, your opponent's arm should not be too straight or too bent. In order to generate strong

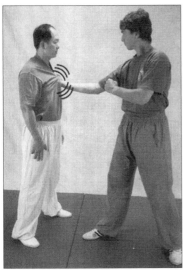
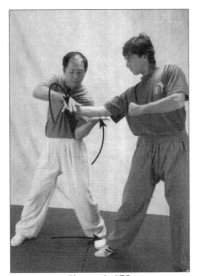
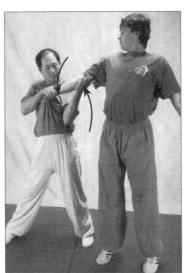

| *Figure 6–478* | *Figure 6–479* | *Figure 6–480* |

power, your locking should be generated from your entire body's bowing. Always look for better leverage to do the job.

Technique #2: Heaven King Supports the Pagoda or Upward Elbow Press

(Tian Wang Tuo Ta or Shang Ya Zhou) 天王托塔，上壓肘

When your opponent has grabbed your chest with his right hand (Figure 6-478), again step your left leg beside his right leg and use your right hand to grab his right wrist, while pressing your left hand upward onto his elbow (Figure 6-479). Finally, use the leverage of both of your hands to lock him upward (Figure 6-480). You should increase your controlling power until his heels are off the ground. You should keep yourself on the right hand side of your opponent. This will prevent him from attacking you with his left hand.

Theory:
Misplacing the Bone (elbow). The leverage generated from both of your hands is the key to the control. From the beginning, you should keep your opponent's elbow as straight as possible. If he has kept it bent, it will be difficult to lock him with this technique.

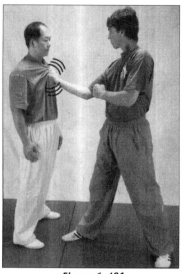

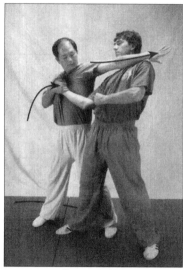

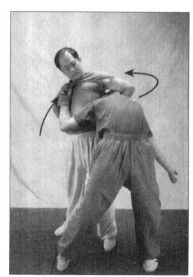

Figure 6–481	Figure 6–482	Figure 6–483

Technique #3: Arm Wraps Around the Dragon's Neck

(Bi Chan Long Jing) 臂纏龍頸

When your opponent grabs your chest with his right hand (Figure 6-481), step your left leg behind his right leg, while using your right hand to grab his right wrist and extending his left arm to his neck area (Figure 6-482). Finally, circle your left arm around his neck while still locking his right arm on your chest (Figure 6-483). You should press him backward until his face looks upward.

Theory:

Seal the Artery (neck) and Seal the Breathing (throat). To prevent your opponent from struggling, you should lock his neck tightly until his heels are off the ground. Naturally, you may kill your opponent if you use too much power.

Technique #4: Eagle Claw to Seal the Throat

(Ying Zhua Suo Hou) 鷹爪鎖喉

When your opponent grabs your chest with his right hand (Figure 6-484), first step your right leg behind his right leg and grab his wrist and twist it counterclockwise with your left hand, while using your right forearm to press in his elbow (Figure 6-485). Then, immediately extend your right hand until it reaches his throat and grab his throat (Figure 6-486) When you grab his throat, you should keep his right arm locked; this will provide you good leverage for your throat grabbing (Figure 6-487). Naturally, if you desire to take him down, simply sweep your right leg backward and push your right hand forward.

Theory:

Dividing the Muscle (wrist) and Sealing the Breath (throat). To make the entire control effective, your left hand control of his wrist is very important.

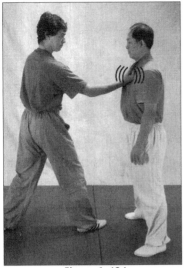

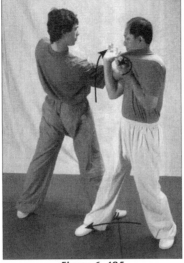

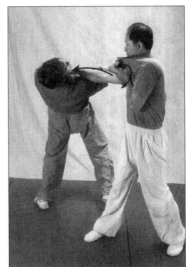

Figure 6–484

Figure 6–485

Figure 6–486

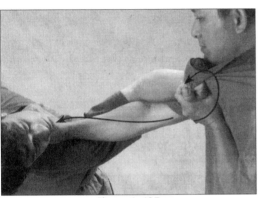

Figure 6–487

II. GRABBING UPPER REAR BACK

When your opponent grabs your upper back area, since you cannot see which hand he has grabbed you with, the best techniques are those which can be used for either hand or those which allow you to have different options right after you discover which hand he has used to grab you.

Technique #1: The Heavens Turn and the Earth Circles-1

(Tian Xuan Di Zhuan -1) 天旋地轉

When your opponent's right hand grabs your shirt from behind (Figure 6-488), turn your body to your right and step your left leg behind his right leg while raising up both of your arms (Figure 6-489). When you do this, your left forearm is on his right upper-arm. Finally, use the leverage generated from your neck and left forearm to press him down (Figure 6-490). Naturally, in order to enhance the pressing power, you may also use right hand to help your left forearm.

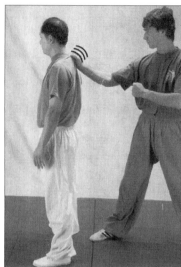

Figure 6–488

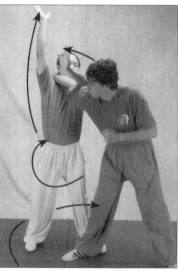

Figure 6–489

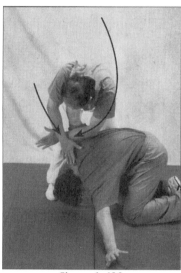

Figure 6–490

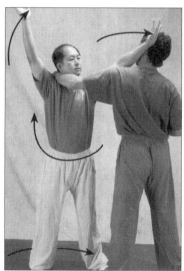

Figure 6–491

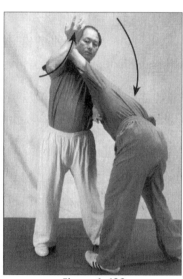

Figure 6–492

Theory:

Misplacing the Bone (elbow and shoulder) and Pressing the Tendons (upper-arm). When you apply this technique, after your turning, if you find that your opponent is using his left hand to touch your left shoulder instead of his right hand (Figure 6-491), simply use your left arm to circle his neck and lock him (Figure 6-492).

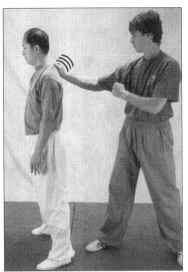 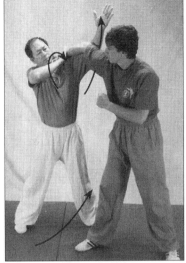 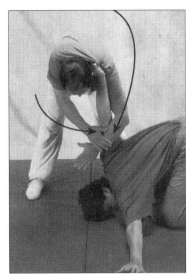

| *Figure 6–493* | *Figure 6–494* | *Figure 6–495* |

Technique #2: The Heavens Turn and the Earth Circles -2

(Tian Xuan Di Zhuan - 2) 天旋地轉

When your opponent's right hand grabs your shirt from behind (Figure 6-493), turn your body to your left and step your left leg behind his right leg, while grabbing his right wrist with your right hand and placing your left arm on his upper-arm (Figure 6-494). Finally, use the leverage of your shoulder and hands to press him down (Figure 6-495).

Theory:

Misplacing the Bone (elbow). When turning your body to your left, you should beware of his left hand. In order to prevent him from attacking you with his left hand, you may reposition yourself to his right hand side when you raise up both of your arms.

Technique #3: Arm Wraps Around the Dragon's Neck

(Bi Chan Long Jing) 臂纏龍頸

When your opponent grabs your shirt with his right hand from behind (Figure 6-496), turn your body to your right and step your left leg behind his right leg, while using your right hand to control his right forearm and placing your left arm on his neck (Figure 6-497). Then, circle your left arm around his neck, while still controlling his right arm with your right hand (Figure 6-498). You should press him backward until his face looks upward.

Theory:

Sealing the Artery (neck) and Sealing the Breath (throat). To prevent your opponent from struggling, you should lock his neck tightly until his heels are off the ground. You can kill your opponent if you use too much power.

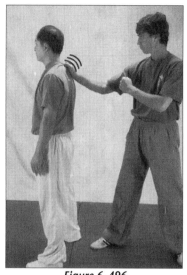

Figure 6–496

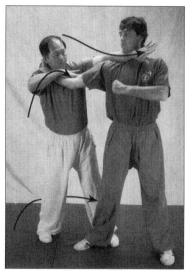

Figure 6–497

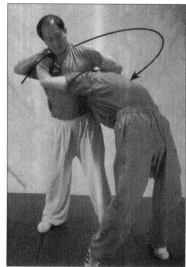

Figure 6–498

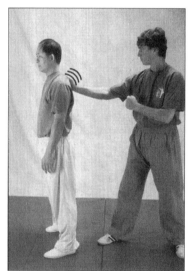

Figure 6–499

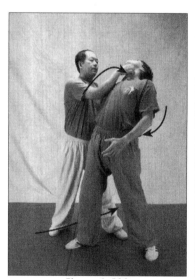

Figure 6–500

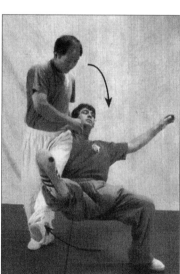

Figure 6–501

Technique #4: Spiritual Dragon Spits the Pearl

(Shen Long Tu Zhu) 神龍吐珠

When your opponent grabs your shirt from behind (Figure 6-499), simply turn your body to your left and step your left leg behind his right leg (Figure 6-500). As you do this, you should also place your left hand on his sacrum, while using your right hand to grab his throat.

If you wish, you may sweep your left leg forward while pushing his head backward to take him down (Figure 6-501).

Theory:

Sealing the Breath (throat). To prevent him from resisting or counterattacking, you must push his head backward and destroy his balance.

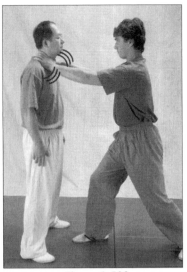
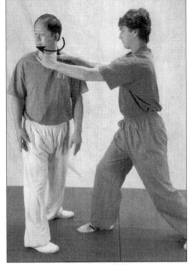
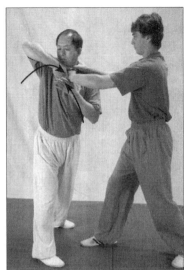

Figure 6–502   *Figure 6–503*   *Figure 6–504*

6-6. Qin Na Against Neck Grabbing

If the opportunity allows, the best way to deal with the problem of someone who is choking your neck is to kick his groin or shin hard. You may also punch his nose with good success. However, there are some neck choking techniques which may put you in the position from which you may not be able to either kick or punch him. Then you must use the following Qin Na techniques to counter his attack.

I. FROM THE FRONT

A. TWO HANDS HOLD THE NECK

Technique #1: Send the Devil to Heaven

(Song Mo Shang Tian) 送魔上天

When your opponent uses both his hands to hold your neck (Figure 6-502), first turn your head to the side to use the neck muscles to protect your throat and loosen up his grabbing (Figure 6-503). Then, immediately use both of your hands to grab his left wrist (Figure 6-504). Next, step your left leg to his left while turning your body to your right under his left arm (Figure 6-505). Finally, use both of your hands to lock him upward until his heels are off the ground (Figure 6-506).

Theory:
Dividing the Muscle/Tendon (wrist) and Misplacing the Bone (shoulder). An important point to making this technique most effective is to use your right hand to twist his hand, while bending his fingers downward with your left hand.

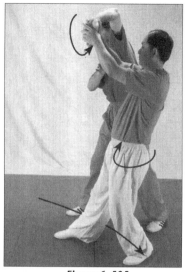

Figure 6–505

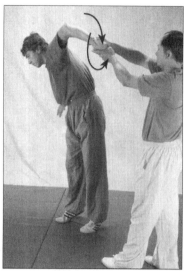

Figure 6–506

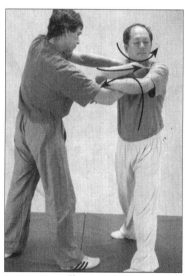

Figure 6–507

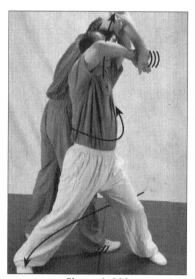

Figure 6–508

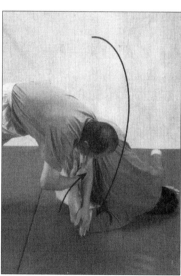

Figure 6–509

Technique #2: Large Python Turns Its Body

(Da Mang Fan Shen) 大蟒翻身

When your opponent uses both his hands to hold your neck, immediately turn your head to your left while grabbing his right hand with your right hand and placing your left forearm on his elbow (Figure 6-507). Next, step your right leg to his right, and turn your body to the left under his right arm while twisting his arm (Figure 6-508). As you do this, also coil your left forearm around his elbow and continue to grab his hand with your right hand. Finally, bow your body forward and lock him down to the ground (Figure 6-509).

Theory:

Misplacing the Bone (elbow and shoulder). In order to make the control effective, you should keep your opponent's arm bent at all times. When you twist his arm, you should use your entire body's turning momentum, instead of just using your arm.

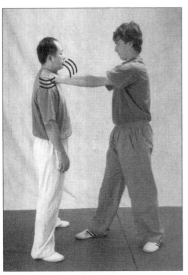
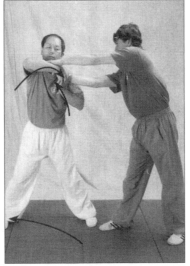
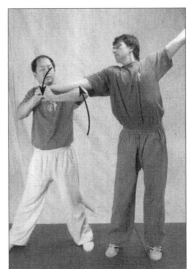

| *Figure 6–510* | *Figure 6–511* | *Figure 6–512* |

Technique #3: Shoulder Carries a Pole

(Jian Tiao Bian Dan) 肩挑扁擔

When your opponent grabs your neck with both his hands (Figure 6-510), immediately step your right leg backward while grabbing his right wrist with both of your hands (Figure 6-511). Finally, use your left upper-arm or shoulder to press his elbow upward, while pushing his right wrist downward to lock him (Figure 6-512). You should control him until his heels are off the ground.

Theory:

Misplacing the Bone (elbow). If you jerk your power, with good leverage, you may break his elbow easily.

Technique #4: The Old Man Carries the Fish on His Back

(Lao Han Bei Yu) 老漢背魚

When your opponent grabs your neck with both his hands (Figure 6-513), immediately turn your body to your right while using both of your hands to grab his right wrist, and using your left elbow to push his right elbow to keep it bent (Figure 6-514). Then, step your left leg to his right hand side while turning your body and bowing forward (Figure 6-515).

Theory:

Misplacing the Bone (shoulder and elbow). The angle at which you control your opponent's arm is very important. If you opponent's arm is either too straight or too bent, the control will not be effective. With an accurate angle, you may generate great pain in your opponent's shoulder.

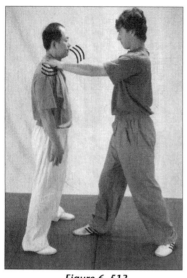

Figure 6–513

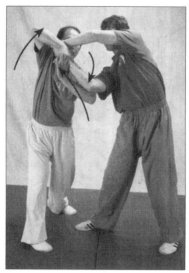

Figure 6–514

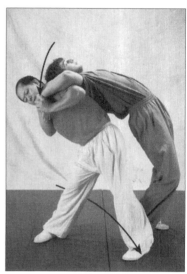

Figure 6–515

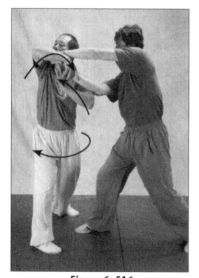

Figure 6–516

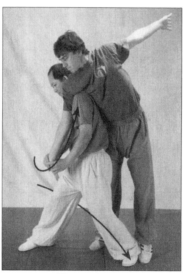

Figure 6–517

Technique #5: One Post to Support the Heavens

(Yi Zhu Ding Tian) 一柱頂天

In the last technique, if your opponent keeps his arm stiff and straight, then after turning your body to your right (Figure 6-516), step your left leg to the front of his right leg while placing your left shoulder under his right upper-arm and then pressing his arm upward (Figure 6-517). This can generate great pain in his upper-arm's tendons and shoulder's ligaments.

Theory:

Misplacing the Bone (elbow and shoulder) and Pressing the Tendons (upper-arm). In this technique, you control the elbow to lock your opponent's arm in position and lift the arm upward to tear off the ligaments of the shoulder.

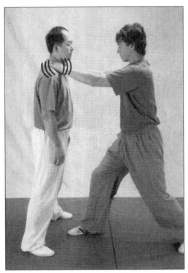

Figure 6–518

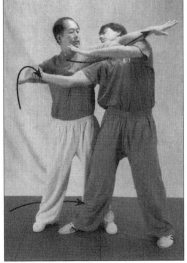

Figure 6–519

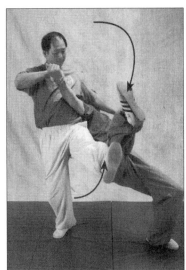

Figure 6–520

Technique #6: Face the Heavens and Fall Down

(Yang Tian Fan Die) 仰天翻跌

When your opponent grabs your neck with his two hands (Figure 6-518), first turn your body to your right and step your left leg behind his right leg (Figure 6-519). As you do this, also use your right hand to grab his right wrist and place your left arm on his neck area. Finally, press his neck down with your left hand while sweeping his right leg with your left leg to make him fall (Figure 6-520).

Theory:
Taking Down. The leverage generated from your left leg sweeping and left arm pushing is very important. With practice, you will make your opponent fall easily.

Technique #7: Fisherman Spreads his Fishing Net

(Yu Fu Sa Wang) 漁夫撒網

In the last technique, right after you have turned your body to your right, stepped your left leg behind his right leg, grabbed his right wrist with your right hand, and placed your left arm on his neck (Figure 6-521), immediately place your right forearm under his right knee (Figure 6-522). Finally, use the leverage of your left hand and right forearm to destroy his root and throw him away (Figure 6-523).

Theory:
Taking Down. When you throw him away, you should use your entire body's rotational power. If you desire to injure him seriously, when you throw him away, also use your right hand to grab his groin. Naturally, you should not do so unless it is absolutely necessary.

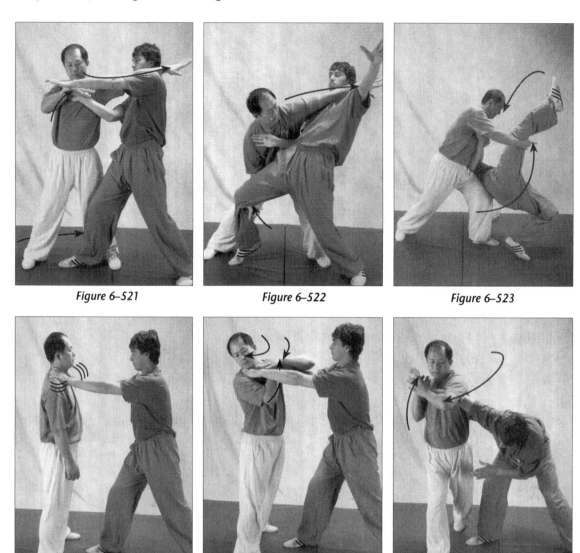

Figure 6–521   Figure 6–522   Figure 6–523

Figure 6–524   Figure 6–525   Figure 6–526

Technique #8: Old Man Promoted to General

(Lao Han Bai Jiang) 老漢拜將

When your opponent grabs your neck with both his hands (Figure 6-524), first turn your head to your right while using both hands to grab his right wrist (Figure 6-525). Then, immediately place your left elbow over his elbow (Figure 6-526) and use the leverage generated from both of your hands and left elbow to press him down to the ground (Figure 6-527).

Theory:

Misplacing the Bone (elbow). When you press your opponent down, you should keep his arm straight and the pressing should be straight on the rear side of his elbow. If you jerk your power, you may break his elbow easily.

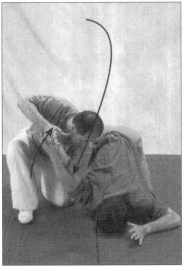

Figure 6–527

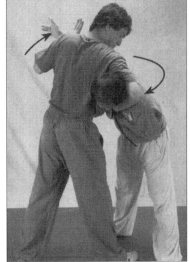

Figure 6–528

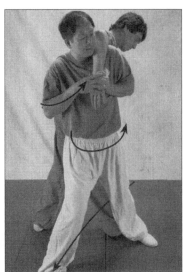

Figure 6–529

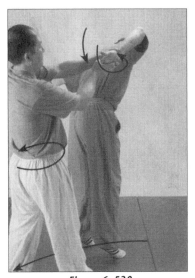

Figure 6–530

B. THE ARM CIRCLES THE NECK

a. FROM THE FRONT

I. RIGHT ARM CIRCLES

Normally, when your opponent uses his right arm to encircle your neck, he is on your right and his left hand has already grabbed your right hand. Here, we will introduce a few techniques for defending in this situation.

Technique #1: Send the Devil to Heaven

(Song Mo Shang Tian) 送魔上天

When your opponent's right arm circles your neck while his left hand grabs your right wrist (Figure 6-528), immediately use your left hand to grab his right wrist and pull it away from wrapping. Next, step your right leg to his right, while freeing your right hand and grabbing his right wrist (Figure 6-529). Finally, step your left leg to his back and at the same time use your body's turning momentum to twist his arm and wrist to lock him up (Figure 6-530).

Theory:

Dividing the Muscle/Tendon (wrist) and Misplacing the Bone (shoulder). An important point is, when you have locked your opponent in the final position, you should use your left hand to twist his hand, while using your right hand to grab his fingers and bend them downward. This can make the control most effective.

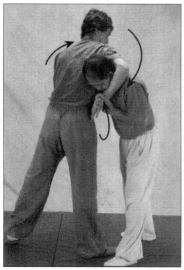

Figure 6–531

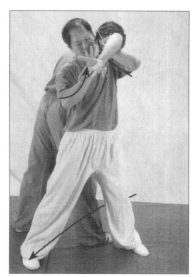

Figure 6–532

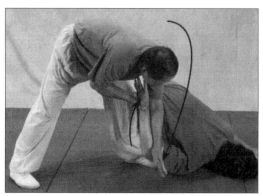

Figure 6–533

Technique #2: Large Python Turns Its Body

(Da Mang Fan Shen) 大蟒翻身

When your opponent's right arm circles your neck, immediately use your left hand to grab his right wrist and pull it away (Figure 6-531). Next, step your right leg to his right hand side and turn your body counterclockwise under his right arm, while freeing your right hand to take over the left hand's wrist grabbing and placing your left forearm on his elbow (Figure 6-532). Finally, use the leverage of your right hand and left forearm to press him down to the ground (Figure 6-533).

Theory:

Misplacing the Bone (elbow and shoulder). In order to make the control effective, your opponent's arm should be straight all the time.

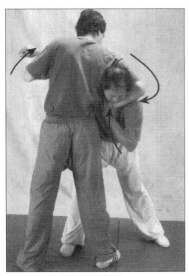

Figure 6–534

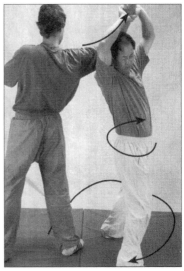

Figure 6–535

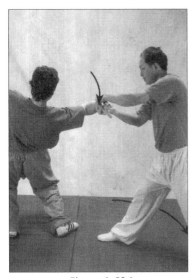

Figure 6–536

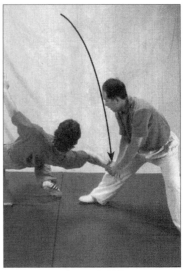

Figure 6–537

Technique #3: Turn the Body and Pull Down

(Zhuan Shen La Dao) 轉身拉倒

When your opponent's right arm circles your neck, immediately use your left hand to grab his right wrist and pull it away (Figure 6-534). Next, free your right hand and grab his right wrist while turning your body clockwise and lifting his right arm upward (Figure 6-535). Then, again step your left leg to your right and at the same time pull your opponent's right arm downward to put his arm in awkward position (Figure 6-536). Finally, pull him down to the floor (Figure 6-537).

Theory:

Misplacing the Bone (elbow and shoulder) and Taking Down. In order to make the control effective, your opponent's arm should be neither too straight nor bent too much. The correct angle will offer you a good set up for your control.

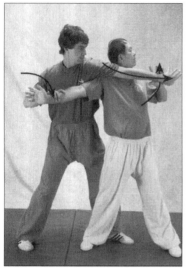

Figure 6–538

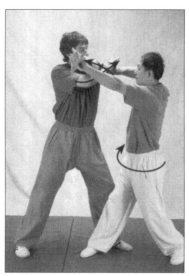

Figure 6–539

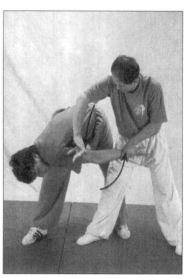

Figure 6–540

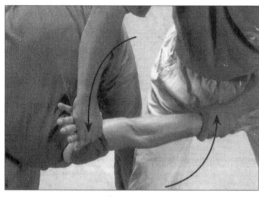

Figure 6–541

II. LEFT ARM CIRCLES

Normally, when your opponent uses his left arm to encircle your neck, he is on your right and his right hand has already grabbed your right hand. Here, we will introduce a few techniques for defending in this situation.

Technique #1: Left Right Cross Elbow

(Zuo You Jiao Zhou) 左右交肘

When your opponent's right hand has grabbed your right wrist while his left arm is circling your neck, immediately use your left hand to grab his left wrist and push it forward to stop his circling (Figure 6-538). Next, grab his right wrist with your right hand and pull it to your right while pushing his left hand to his left with your left hand (Figure 6-539). Finally, push his right hand down while pulling his left arm upward to lock him in position (Figures 6-540 and 6-541).

Theory:

Misplacing the Bone (elbow) and Pressing the Tendons (upper-arm). To make the control effective, his left arm must be straight. In addition, his right forearm should be pressed against the tendons located on the rear side of his upper-arm.

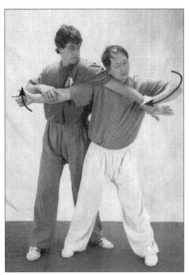

Figure 6–542

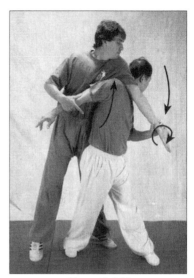

Figure 6–543

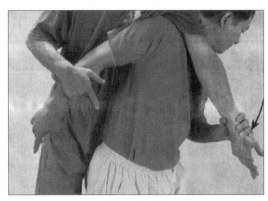

Figure 6–444

Technique #2: Shoulder Carries a Pole

(Jian Tiao Bian Dan) 肩挑扁擔

When your opponent has grabbed your right hand and is using his left arm to encircle your neck, immediately use your left hand to grab his left wrist and push it out (Figure 6-542). Immediately rotate his left hand until his palm is facing upward, while turning your body to your left and placing your right shoulder under his left upper-arm (Figure 6-543). Finally, use the leverage of your left hand and right shoulder to lock him upward (Figure 6-544).

Theory:

Misplacing the Bone (elbow) and Pressing the Tendon (upper-arm). If you notice your opponent is going to attack you with his right hand, you may jerk your power downward to increase the pain. You may also use your right elbow to strike his right chest or stomach area.

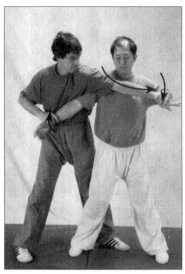 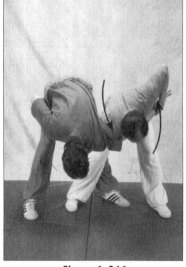 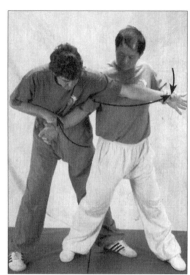

| *Figure 6–545* | *Figure 6–546* | *Figure 6–547* |

Technique #3: Two Children Worship the Buddha

(Shuang Tong Bai Fo) 雙童拜佛

Again, when your opponent's right hand has grabbed your right wrist and his left arm is circling your neck, use your left hand to grab his left wrist and push it forward (Figure 6-545). Immediately turn his left arm until his palm is facing forward, and then pull his left arm backward while pressing your right shoulder forward against his upper-arm's tendons (Figure 6-546).

Theory:

Misplacing the Bone (elbow and shoulder) and Pressing the Tendon (upper-arm). In this technique, the pain is generated from the control of his upper-arm's tendons. This technique is difficult to use for permanent control.

Technique #4: Luo Han Bows or Small Elbow Wrap

(Luo Han Xing Li or Xiao Chan Zhou) 羅漢行禮，小纏肘

When your opponent has grabbed your right wrist with his right hand and is circling his left arm around your neck, again use your left hand to grab his left wrist and push it away (Figure 6-547). Next, bend your right arm in to free your right wrist from his grabbing (Figure 6-548). Then, place your right forearm on his elbow and press it downward, while pulling his left wrist upward (Figure 6-549). Finally, pull his arm to your front to destroy his balance while sweeping your right leg backward to make him fall (Figure 6-550).

Theory:

Misplacing the Bone (elbow and shoulder). In order to make your opponent fall, after you have locked him, you should pull him to your front to destroy his balance while sweeping your left leg backward. Once your opponent is on the ground, if necessary you may rotate his arm toward his head and pop his shoulder out of joint.

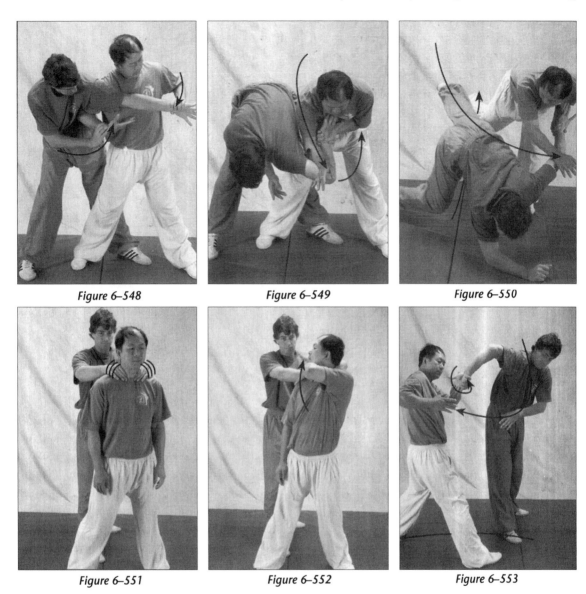

Figure 6–548

Figure 6–549

Figure 6–550

Figure 6–551

Figure 6–552

Figure 6–553

B. FROM BEHIND

I. TWO HANDS HOLD THE NECK

Technique #1: Send the Devil to Heaven

(Song Mo Shang Tian) 送魔上天

When your opponent's two hands are holding your neck from behind (Figure 6-551), turn your body and head to your right while grabbing his right hand with your left hand (Figure 6-552). Next, step your left leg backward while twisting his right arm and grabbing his wrist with both hands (Figure 6-553). Finally, step your right leg back and use your left hand to twist his right hand to lock his pinkie, while using your right hand to grab his fingers and bend them downward (Figure 6-554).

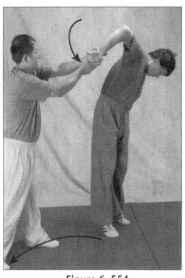
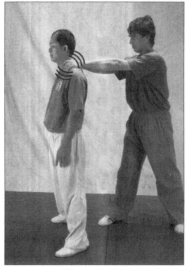
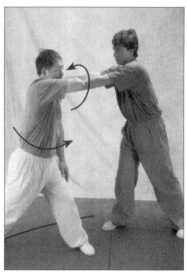

| Figure 6–554 | Figure 6–555 | Figure 6–556 |

Theory:

Dividing the Muscle/Tendon (wrist) and Misplacing the Bone (shoulder). The trick to making this technique effective is, when you have locked your opponent in the final position, you should emphasize more the pinkie's locking, which makes this technique more efficient and effective.

Technique #2: White Ape Worships the Buddha or Reverse Wrist Press

(Bai Yuan Bai Fo or Fan Ya Wan) 白猿拜佛 ，反壓腕

When your opponent's hands are on your neck (Figure 6-555), immediately step your right leg forward and turn your body to your left while using your right hand to grab his left wrist (Figure 6-556). Next, turn his left hand until his palm is facing upward, while also using your left hand to grab his wrist (Figure 6-557). Finally, step your left leg backward while pressing his wrist down until his elbow touches the floor (Figure 6-558).

Theory:

Dividing the Muscle/Tendon (wrist). When you bend his hand to control his wrist, you should use the power of both of your hands instead of just using thumbs. You may also twist his hand to your right and then press it down to generate pain.

Technique #3: White Tiger Turns Its Head or Upward Elbow Wrap

(Bai Hu Fan Shou or Shang Chan Zhou) 白虎返首 ，上纏肘

When your opponent's hands grab your neck from behind (Figure 6-559), immediately step your left leg forward, turning your body to your right while using your left hand to grab his right wrist (Figure 6-560). Next, twist his right hand with your left hand while placing your right hand on his forearm area (Figure 6-561). Then, step your left leg behind him while coiling your right hand to his elbow and pushing it upward (Figure 6-562). Finally, lock his right arm with your right hand and stomach area, while using your left hand to push his neck to his left to generate good leverage for his arm's locking (Figures 6-563 and 6-564).

Theory:

Dividing the Muscle/Tendon (wrist) and Misplacing the Bone (elbow). When you rotate both of your hands to lock your opponent up, you should use your entire body to direct the motion. Your rotational power can then be strong.

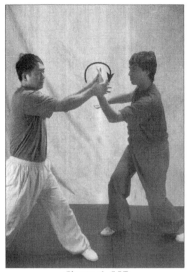

Figure 6–557

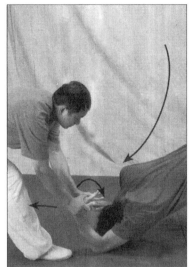

Figure 6–558

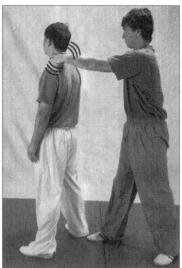

Figure 6–559

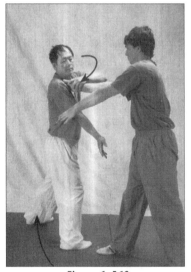

Figure 6–560

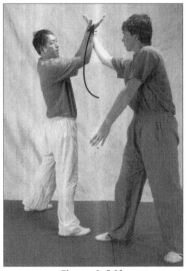

Figure 6–561

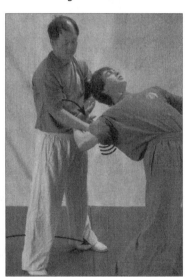

Figure 6–562

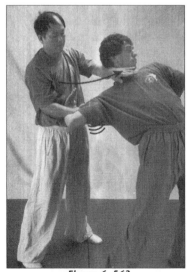

Figure 6–563

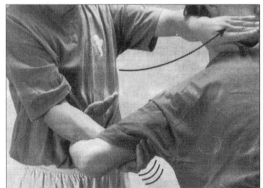

Figure 6–564

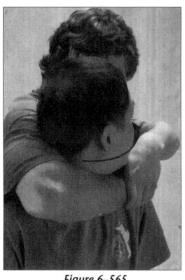
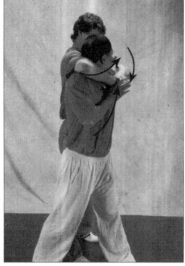
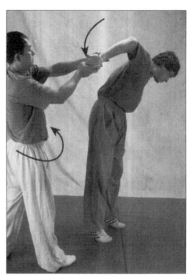

| Figure 6–565 | Figure 6–566 | Figure 6–567 |

II. THE ARM CIRCLES THE NECK

When your opponent uses his arm to encircle your neck from behind, you should immediately turn your head to the side to protect your throat (Figure 6-565). If you can, you should use one of your hands to grab his wrist and pull it outward to stop him from squeezing tighter.

Technique #1: Send the Devil to Heaven

(Song Mo Shang Tian) 送魔上天

When your opponent's right arm is circling your neck, immediately turn your head to your left while using both of your hands to grab his right wrist and push it outward (Figure 6-566). Next, step your left leg backward while using the body's rotating momentum to twist his wrist and pinkie and lock him upward (Figure 6-567).

Theory:
Dividing the Muscle/Tendon (wrist) and Misplacing the Bone (shoulder). The trick to making this technique effective is using your left hand to twist his hand-especially his pinkie-while using your right hand to grab his fingers and bend them downward.

Technique #2: Hand Grabs the Dragon Pearls

(Shou Zhua Long Zhu) 手抓龍珠

When your opponent uses his right arm to encircle your neck, again turn your head to your left, while using your right hand to grab his right wrist and pull it outward (Figure 6-568). Next, step your right leg to your right while using your left to grab his groin (Figure 6-569). This will force him to release his arm lock. If he does not let you go, simply increase your squeezing pressure. This may kill him. You may also strike his groin instead of grabbing it.

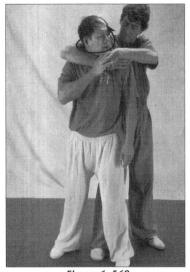
Figure 6-568

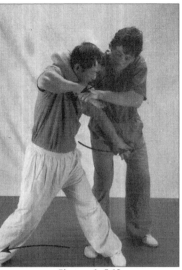
Figure 6-569

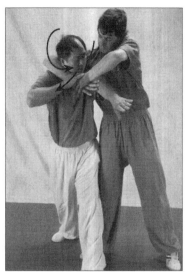
Figure 6-570

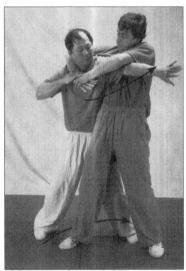
Figure 6-571

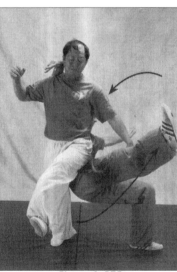
Figure 6-572

Theory:
Grabbing the Organ (testicles). In this technique, you may also use your left fist to strike his face or elbow to attack his solar plexus. Often, you may use the heel of your shoes to kick his shin or to step on his toes.

Technique #3: Arms Turn Over the Large Bear

(Bi Fan Da Xiong) 臂翻大熊

When your opponent uses his right arm to encircle your neck, again turn your head to your left and grab his right wrist with your right hand and pull it out (Figure 6-570). Next, circle your left arm on his upper chest while stepping your left leg behind his right leg (Figure 6-571). Finally, use the leverage of your left arm and leg to take him down (Figure 6-572).

Theory:
Taking Down. To make his technique effective, you must be strong. In addition, to prevent him from resisting, you should push his upper body backward. This will make him lose balance.

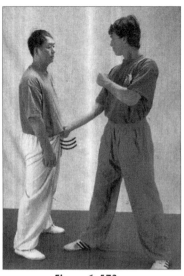

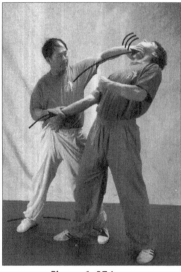

| *Figure 6–573* | *Figure 6–574* |

6-7. Qin Na Against Belt Grabbing

I. FROM THE FRONT

Technique #1: Crane Claw to Seal the Throat

(He Zhua Suo Hou) 鶴爪鎖喉

If your opponent grabs your belt with his right hand (Figure 6-573), immediately step your left leg behind his right leg, grabbing his right wrist with your right hand while using your left fingers to grab this throat (Figure 6-574).

Theory:

Sealing the Breath (throat). When you grab your opponent's throat, you should grab the top section of the throat. Once you have squeezed tight, you may seal his breath.

Technique #2: Arm Wraps Around the Dragon's Neck

(Bi Chan Long Jing) 臂纏龍頸

When your opponent grabs your belt with his right hand (Figure 6-575), again step your left leg behind his right leg, using your right hand to grab his right wrist while circling your left arm around his neck (Figure 6-576). Finally, lock his neck backward until his heels are off the ground (Figure 6-577).

Theory:

Sealing the Artery (neck) and Sealing the Breathing (throat). To prevent your opponent from struggling, you should lock his neck tightly until his face looks upward. You may kill your opponent if you lock him too long.

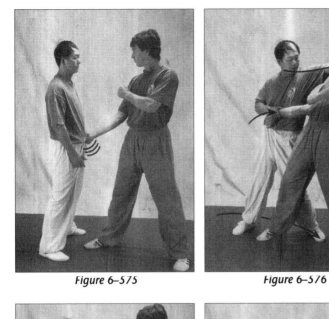

Figure 6–575

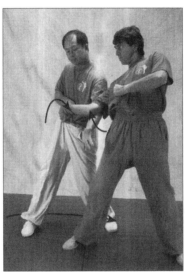

Figure 6–576

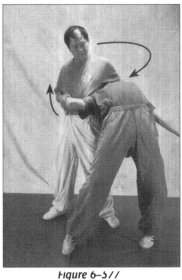

Figure 6–577

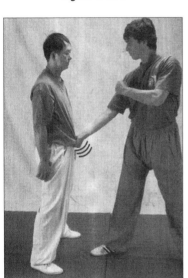

Figure 6–578

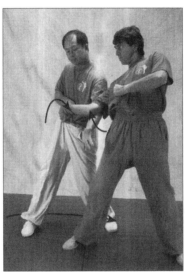

Figure 6–579

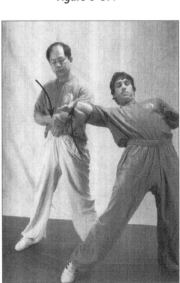

Figure 6–580

Technique #3: Feudal Lord Lifts the Tripod

(Ba Wang Tai Ding) 霸王抬鼎

When your opponent's right hand grabs your belt (Figure 6-578), immediately step your left leg behind his right leg, grabbing his right wrist with your right hand while pushing your let arm against his right elbow (Figure 6-579). Finally, lift up his right elbow with your left arm while still locking his right wrist with your right hand (Figure 6-580).

Theory:

Dividing the Muscle/Tendon (wrist) and Misplacing the Bone (elbow). The leverage generated from the left and the right hands is a very important key for the locking. Your right hand should twist his wrist strongly, while the left hand generates the pressure of bending.

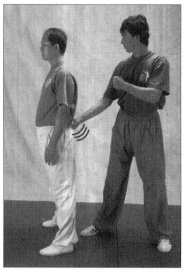

Figure 6–581

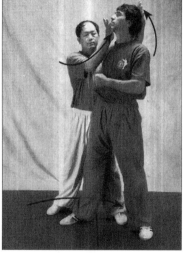

Figure 6–582

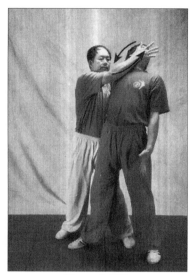

Figure 6–583

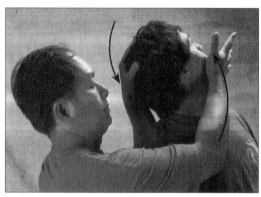

Figure 6–484

II. FROM BEHIND

Technique #1: Twist the Neck to Kill a Chicken

(Sha Ji Niu Jing) 殺雞扭頸

If your opponent grabs your belt from behind (Figure 6-581), step your left leg behind his right leg while placing your left hand behind his head and right hand on his chin (Figure 6-582). Finally, use the leverage of both of your hands to twist his neck to his left and upward (Figure 6-583). This can break his neck. If you do not want to break your opponent's neck, you may simply sweep your right leg backward to take him down.

Theory:

Misplacing the Bone (neck). The angle of twisting is very important. The angle of twisting should be sideways and upward (Figure 6-584). With a good angle, you may dislocate his neck joint easily.

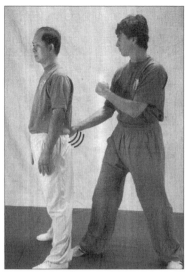

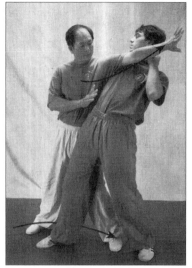

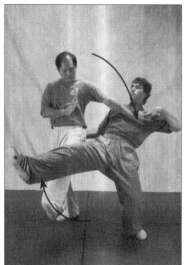

Figure 6-585   Figure 6-586   Figure 6-587

Technique #2: Arms Turn Over the Large Bear

(Bi Fan Da Xiong) 臂翻大熊

Again, when your opponent grabs your belt from behind (Figure 6-585), step your left leg behind his right leg while placing your left arm on his neck area and pushing his upper body backward (Figure 6-586). Then, using the leverage of your left arm and left leg, take him down to the ground (Figure 6-587).

Theory:

Taking Down. The leverage generated from your left leg sweeping and left arm pushing is very important. With practice, you will make your opponent fall easily.

Technique #3: Old Man Bows Politely

(Lao Han You Li) 老漢有禮

If your opponent grabs your belt from behind (Figure 6-588), first turn your body to your left and use your right hand to grab his right wrist while placing your left hand on his elbow (Figure 6-589). Next, push his elbow upward and then downward (Figure 6-590). Finally, bow and keep pushing his elbow until his left hand touches the ground (Figure 6-591).

Theory:

Misplacing the Bone (elbow). This technique will not be as effective if your opponent bends his elbow down and stiffens his arm. In this case, just punch his nose with your left hand.

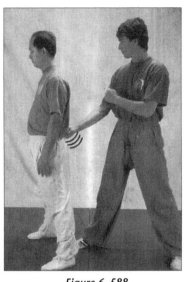

Figure 6–588

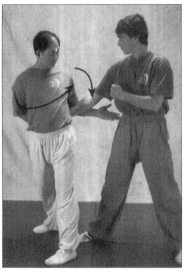

Figure 6–589

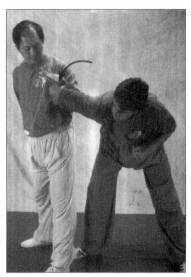

Figure 6–590

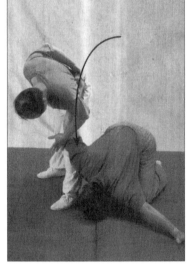

Figure 6–591

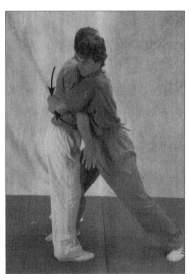

Figure 6–592

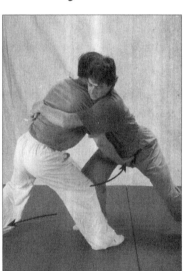

Figure 6–593

6-8. Qin Na Against Embracing

I. FROM THE FRONT

Technique #1: Hand Grabs the Dragon Pearls

(Shou Zhua Long Zhu) 手抓龍珠

When your opponent embraces your upper body with his both arms (Figure 6-592), simply expand both of your arms while stepping your left leg backward and using your right hand to grab his groin (Figure 6-593).

Theory:

Grabbing the Organ (testicles). When you are forcibly embraced, you may simply use both of your hands to hold his body while using your right knee to kick his groin. Although the above techniques are not classified under traditional Qin Na controlling theory, they are easy and effective. Therefore, we introduce this technique here.

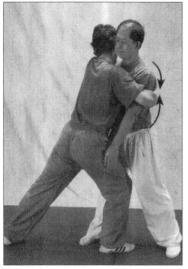

Figure 6–594

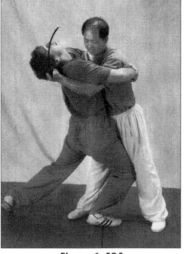

Figure 6–595

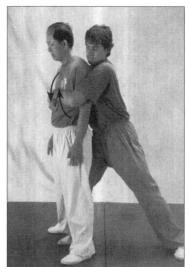

Figure 6–596

Technique #2: Hand Grabs the Hair

(Shou La Mao Fa) 手拉毛髮

When your opponent embraces your upper body with both of his arms (Figure 6-594), simply use both of your hands to grab his hair behind his head and pull them downward (Figure 6-595). Alternatively, you may also grab his ears and pull them downward.

Theory:

Pulling the Hair. Although this is not classified under traditional Qin Na controlling theory, it is easy and effective. Therefore, we introduce this technique here.

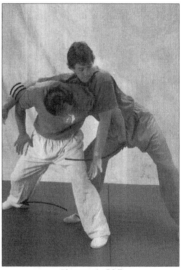

Figure 6–597

II. FROM BEHIND

Technique #1: Hand Grabs the Dragon Pearls

(Shou Zhua Long Zhu) 手抓龍珠

When your opponent embraces your upper body with both of his arms from behind (Figure 6-596), immediately step your right leg forward, expand both of your arms outward to loosen his embracing while using your left hand to grab his groin (Figure 6-597). This will force him to release you. Naturally, you may strike his groin instead of grabbing it.

Theory:

Grabbing the Groin. Although this technique is not classified under traditional Qin Na controlling theory, it is easy and effective. Therefore, we introduce this technique here.

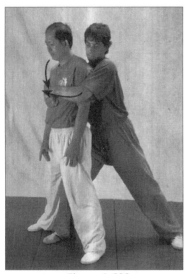

Figure 6–598

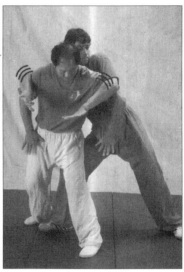

Figure 6–599

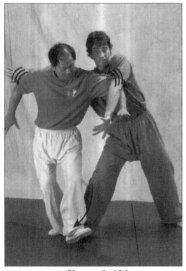

Figure 6–600

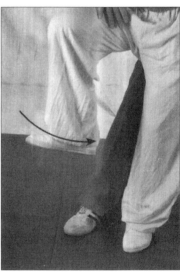

Figure 6–601

Technique #2: Foot Steps on Toes

(Jiao Ta Jiao Zhi) 腳踏腳指

When your opponent embraces your upper body with both of his arms from behind (Figure 6-598), immediately expand your both arms to loosen the embracing (Figure 6-599). Then, use your heel to stomp hard on his toes (Figure 6-600). This will cause great pain and provide you a chance to escape from his embracing. Naturally, you may also kick his shin to injure him (Figure 6-601).

Theory:

Stepping (Toes). Although this technique is not classified under traditional Qin Na controlling theory, it is easy and effective. Therefore, we introduce this technique here.

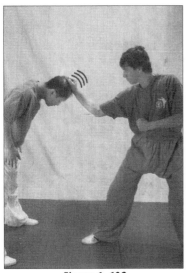
Figure 6–602

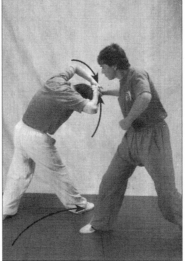
Figure 6–603

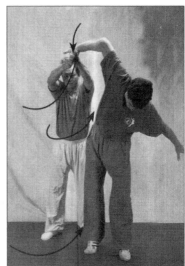
Figure 6–604

6-9. Qin Na Against Hair Grabbing

Qin Na against hair grabbing is not easy. The reason for this simply because, when your opponent has grabbed your hair, the only place you can reach easily is his wrist. Once your hair has been grabbed, you should try to get as close as possible to your opponent. This will allow you to attack him and at the same time ease his pulling pressure. In addition, once you have a chance, you should immediately grab his wrist with both of your hands. This will provide a good opportunity for your counter-action.

I. FROM THE FRONT

Technique #1: Send the Devil to Heaven

(Song Mo Shang Tian) 送魔上天

When your opponent grabs your hair with his right hand from the front (Figure 6-602), immediately step forward to release the tension on your hair, while also grabbing his wrist with both of your hands (Figure 6-603). Then, rotate your body to your left while twisting his right arm and locking him up (Figure 6-604). You should increase your twisting and bending pressure until his heels are off the ground.

Theory:

Dividing the Muscle/Tendon (wrist) and Misplacing the Bone (shoulder). The important point for executing this technique successfully is, when you have locked your opponent in the final position, you should emphasize more the pinkie's locking and his fingers' bending.

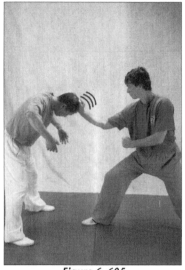
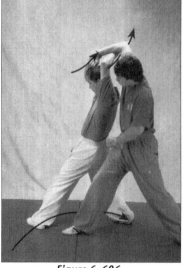
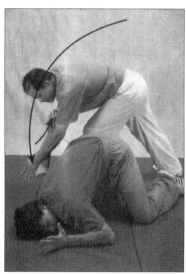

Figure 6–605   Figure 6–606   Figure 6–607

Technique #2: Large Python Turns Its Body

(Da Mang Fan Shen) 大蟒翻身

When your opponent grabs your hair with his right hand (Figure 6-605), step your right leg behind his right leg, rotate your body counterclockwise, and grab his wrist with your right hand while placing his elbow with your left forearm (Figure 6-606). Finally, use the leverage of your right hand and left arm to press him down to the ground (Figure 6-607).

Theory:
Misplacing the Bone (elbow and shoulder). In order to make the control effective, your opponent's arm should not be bent all the time. Naturally, since this Qin Na is a large circle Qin Na, your speed is very important.

Technique #3: Turn the Body and Pull Down

(Zhuan Shen La Dao) 轉身拉倒

When your opponent's right hand grabs your hair (Figure 6-608), immediately grab his wrist with both of your hands and start to rotate to your right (Figure 6-609). Next, spin your body clockwise while twisting his right arm (Figure 6-610). Finally, press his wrist and pull him down to the ground (Figure 6-611).

Theory:
Misplacing the Bone (elbow and shoulder) and Taking Down. In order to make the control effective, your opponent's arm should neither be straight nor bent too much. A correct angle to bending will offer you a good set up for your control (Figure 6-612).

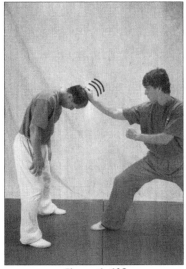

Figure 6–608

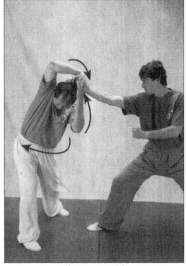

Figure 6–609

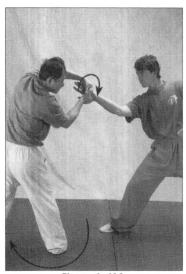

Figure 6–610

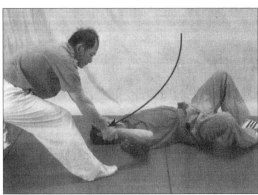

Figure 6–611

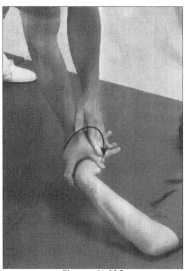

Figure 6–612

II. FROM BEHIND

Technique #1: Spiritual Dragon Spits the Pearl

(Shen Long Tu Zhu) 神龍吐珠

When your opponent grabs your hair from behind and pulls it down (Figure 6-613), first step your right leg backward, turn your body to your right, and grab his right wrist with your left hand while placing your right fingers on his throat (Figure 6-614). Next, use your right hand to grab his throat while still controlling his left wrist by twisting (Figure 6-615).

Theory:

Sealing the Breath (throat). When you grab the throat, you should grab the top section of the throat. When you squeeze until your thumb and index fingers are

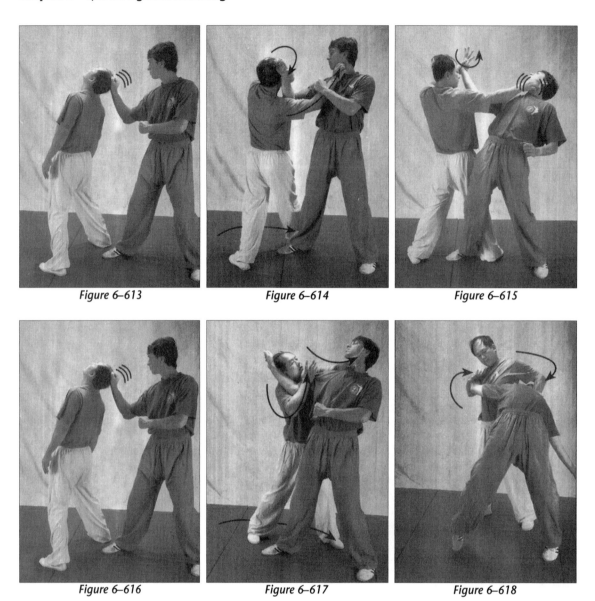

Figure 6-613   Figure 6-614   Figure 6-615

Figure 6-616   Figure 6-617   Figure 6-618

able to reach each other, you have crushed your opponent's esophagus. This will seal his breath and kill him. Therefore, you should not do so unless it is necessary.

Technique #2: Arm Wraps Around the Dragon's Neck

(Bi Chan Long Jing) 臂纏龍頸

When your opponent grabs your hair from behind and pulls it down (Figure 6-616), immediately spin your body clockwise, step your left leg behind his right leg, and lock his right arm with your right arm while circling your left arm to his neck (Figure 6-617). Finally, circle your left arm around his neck while still locking his right arm (Figure 6-618).

Theory:

Sealing the Artery (neck) and Sealing the Breathing (throat). To prevent your opponent from struggling, you should lock his neck tightly until his heels are off the ground. You may kill your opponent if you use too much power.

▪ Chapter 7 ▪

OFFENSIVE QIN NA

TECHNIQUES

7-1. Introduction

You should know that, compared with strikes and kicks, Qin Na techniques are relatively much harder to use offensively. This is especially true if your opponent is an experienced martial artist. The reason for this is simply that, compared with striking, which is fast and simple, Qin Na is more complicated and takes a longer time. Generally, an effective attacking Qin Na requires great speed and high skill.

Because of this, unless there is a special reason, a martial artist normally will not use Qin Na for offense. For example, you may like to seize or control your opponent, but without the intention of harming him. Because of this, attacking Qin Na techniques have commonly been used by the Chinese police and guards since ancient times.

There are not very many attacking Qin Na. However, if you play a trick and cause your opponent to extend his hand either for attacking or blocking, then you will have available many techniques which have been discussed earlier. In this chapter, we will only introduce some of the direct attacking Qin Na techniques for your reference.

7-2. Attacking Qin Na Techniques

In this section, we will introduce the attacking Qin Na by dividing the two possibilities: attack from the front and attack from behind.

I. FROM THE FRONT

Technique #1: Wild Chicken Spreads Its Wings

(Ye Ji Zhan Chi) 野雞展翅

In this technique, first step your right leg beside your opponent's right leg and use your right hand to grab his right wrist (Figure 7-1). Next, step your left leg to your left, while also grabbing his wrist with both hands and circle his arm upward (Figure 7-2).

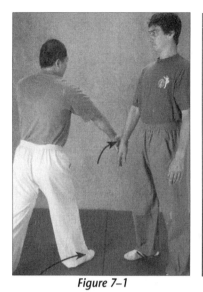

Figure 7–1

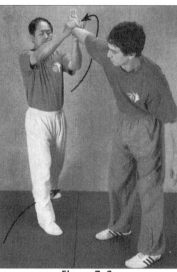

Figure 7–2

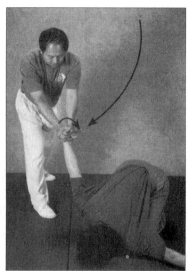

Figure 7–3

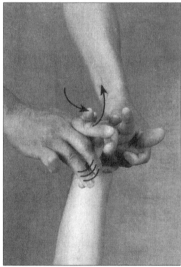

Figure 7–4

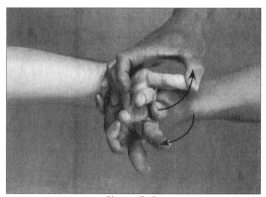

Figure 7–5

Finally, press his hand forward and downward to force him down (Figure 7-3). You should press him down until his face touches the ground.

Occasionally, you will find someone who is double jointed, which makes your technique ineffective. Once you have noticed this, immediately sandwich his pinkie between your right thumb and index finger while hooking his ring finger with your other three fingers. Bend his pinkie backward while using your thumb to press the base joint of his pinkie to generate pain (Figure 7-4). Alternatively, you may simply use your thumb to bend back his pinkie to generate pain (Figure 7-5).

Theory:

Dividing the Muscle/Tendon (wrist), Misplacing the Bone (pinkie in optional technique). When you grab, you are using the entirety of both of your hands to grab, and when you turn your opponent's hand clockwise, you should use your entire body instead of just using arms. When you press your opponent down, the power is generated from the leverage of your pinkie and thumb area. Keep trying until the most effective angle and leverage are found.

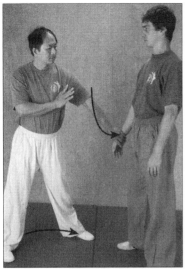

Figure 7–6

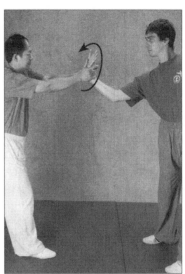

Figure 7–7

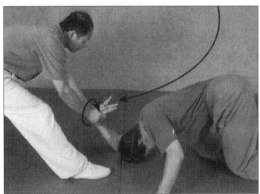

Figure 7–8

Technique #2: White Ape Worships the Buddha or Reverse Wrist Press

(Bai Yuan Bai Fo or Fan Ya Wan) 白猿拜佛，反壓腕

In this technique, first step your left leg beside your opponent's right leg and use your left hand to grab his right hand (Figure 7-6). Next, step your left leg back and turn your left hand counterclockwise while also using your right hand to grab his right wrist (Figure 7-7). Finally, use both of your hands to press his hand forward and downward (Figure 7-8). You should press him down until his elbow touches the ground. When you press him down, you may twist his hand to the side slightly and therefore generate more pressure on his pinkie tendon. This can generate more pain.

Theory:

Dividing the Muscle/Tendon (wrist and pinkie). To make the control effective you must generate good leverage between your thumbs and pinkie. Once you have locked the hand, press downward with the entirety of both of your hands instead of just the thumbs.

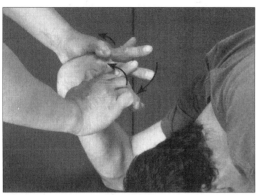

Figure 7–9

Technique #3: Fingers Lock the Dragon's Tail or Turning Finger Dividing

(Zhi Suo Long Wei or Zhuan Fen Zhi) 指鎖龍尾，轉分指

In the last technique, right after you have turned your opponent's right hand, immediately use your right hand to split his ring finger and pinkie, then twist his fingers and use your right thumb to press the base joint of his pinkie (Figure 7-9). You should press him down until his elbow touches the floor.

Theory:

Dividing the Muscle/Tendon and Misplacing the Bone (ring finger and pinkie). In this technique, you should not release your left hand control on your opponent's right wrist until he is completely controlled to the ground, .

Technique #4: Send the Devil to Heaven

(Song Mo Shang Tian) 送魔上天

In this technique, first step your left leg to your opponent's right hand side while using your right hand to grab his right wrist (Figure 7-10). Next, step your right leg behind his right leg and grab his right wrist with both of your hands, while turning your body to your left and then circling his right arm upward (Figure 7-11). Continue to rotate your body and at the same time use your left hand to twist his hand, while using your right hand to grab his fingers and bend them downward (Figure 7-12). You should increase your twisting and bending pressure until your opponent's heels are off the ground.

Theory:

Dividing the Muscle/Tendon (wrist) and Misplacing the Bone (shoulder). The important key point of applying this technique is, when you have locked your opponent in the final position, you should emphasize the pinkie lock, which is more efficient and effective.

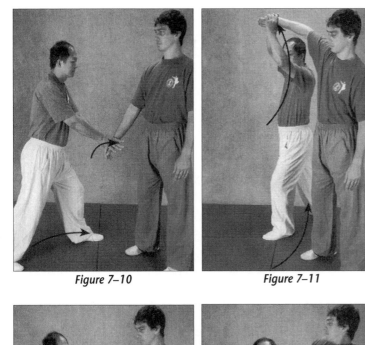
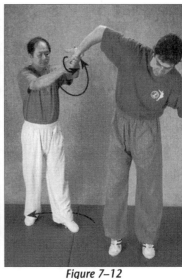

| Figure 7–10 | Figure 7–11 | Figure 7–12 |

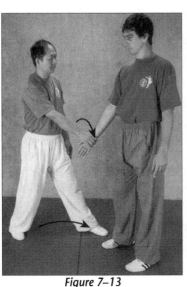
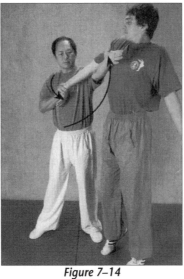
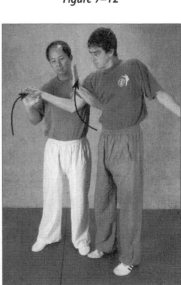

| Figure 7–13 | Figure 7–14 | Figure 7–15 |

Technique #5: Feudal Lord Invites to Dinner

(Ba Wang Qing Ke) 霸王請客

In this technique, first use your right hand to grab your opponent's right wrist while stepping in your left leg to his right hand side (Figure 7-13). Next, use your left forearm to press upward against his right elbow, while pushing his wrist down with your right hand to lock it up (Figure 7-14). Then, bend your left arm to control his right arm and lift your right hand to bend his right arm (Figure 7-15). Finally, use both of your hands to press his hand down to lock his wrist (Figure 7-16). You should increase your locking power until his heels are off the ground. In order to prevent him from biting your fingers, simply use your left hand to control the wrist while using your right hand to pull his hair toward you. If you find that your opponent is double jointed, you should immediately push his pinkie backward and lock it (Figure 7-17).

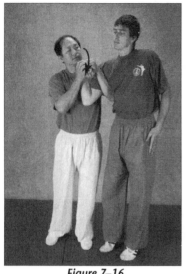
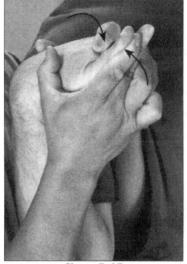
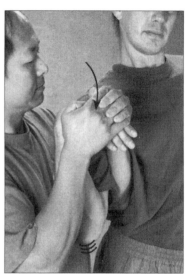

Figure 7–16 *Figure 7–17* *Figure 7–18*

Theory:

Dividing the Muscle/Tendon (wrist). When you step in your left leg, in order to prevent your opponent from striking you with his right elbow, you must use your left forearm to lock his elbow upward. When you lock his arm, the leverage of locking is generated from both of your hands held against your chest (Figure 7-18).

Technique #6: Arm Wraps Around the Dragon's Neck

(Bi Chan Long Jing) 臂纏龍頸

When you apply this technique, first step your right leg in beside your opponent's right leg while also using your right hand to grab his right wrist (Figure 7-19). Next, step your left leg to his right hand side and lock his right arm against your chest (Figure 7-20). Finally, circle your left arm around his neck and lock it up there (Figure 7-21).

Theory:

Sealing the Artery (neck). When you step in your left leg, in order to prevent your opponent from striking you with his right elbow, you must pull his right arm backward against your chest to lock him.

Technique #7: Feudal Lord Pushes the Caldron

(Ba Wang Tui Ding) 霸王推鼎

In this technique, first use your left hand to hook and push your opponent's right arm away while stepping your left leg to his right hand side (Figure 7-22). Next, place your left hand on his sacrum and right hand on his chin (Figure 7-23). Finally, use the leverage of the two hands to push him off balance (Figure 7-24).

Theory:

Taking Down. When you execute this technique, your position is very important. Without a good position, your opponent can strike you with his left hand.

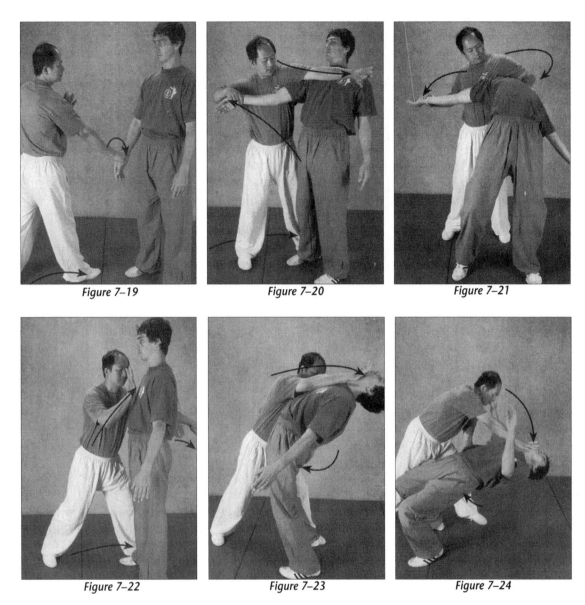

Figure 7–19

Figure 7–20

Figure 7–21

Figure 7–22

Figure 7–23

Figure 7–24

II. FROM BEHIND

Technique #1: Feudal Lord Invites to Dinner

(Ba Wang Qing Ke) 霸王請客

If you are behind your opponent and wish to control him, first use your right hand to grab his right wrist (Figure 7-25). Next, place your left forearm against his elbow while pushing his right wrist down (Figure 7-26). Then, bend your left arm to control his right arm and use your right hand to bend his right arm, and finally use both of your hands to press his hand downward (Figure 7-27). You should increase your locking power until his heels are off the ground. In order to prevent him from biting your fingers, you may simply use your left hand to control the wrist while using your right hand to pull his hair toward you.

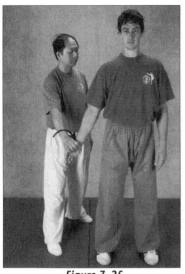

Figure 7–25

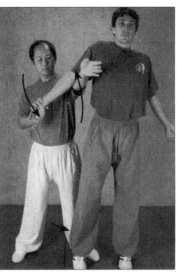

Figure 7–26

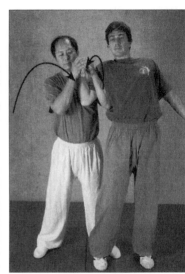

Figure 7–27

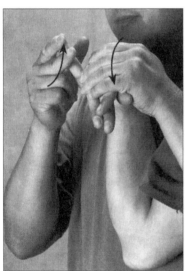

Figure 7–28

Theory:
Dividing the Muscle/Tendon (wrist). When you step in your left leg, in order to prevent your opponent from striking you with his right elbow, you must use your left forearm to lock his elbow upward. If you realize that your opponent is double jointed, you should immediately push his pinkie backward and lock it (Figure 7-28).

Technique #2: Upper Hook Dividing

(Shang Diao Fen) 上刁分

When you approach your opponent from behind, use your right hand to grab his left ring finger and pinkie while rotating them to generate pain in the base of fingers (Figure 7-29). As you do this, also use your index finger to control the orientation of his palm. Next, use your left hand to move his right elbow against your right front chest and finally, press his ring finger and pinkie downward to lock him up (Figures 7-30 and 7-31).

Theory:
Dividing the Muscle/Tendon (between ring and middle fingers). Before you lock his arm in front of your chest, you should control his elbow and prevent it from striking you. To do this, simply circle his ring finger and pinkie to the side (Figure 7-32).

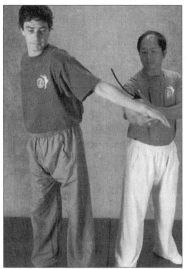
Figure 7–29

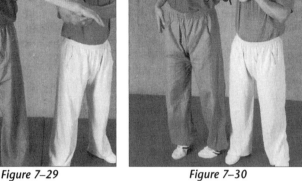
Figure 7–30

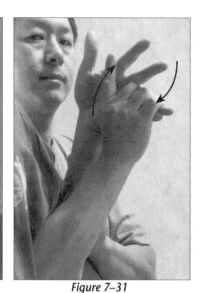
Figure 7–31

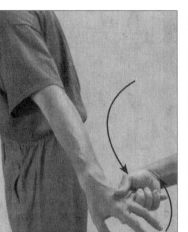
Figure 7–32

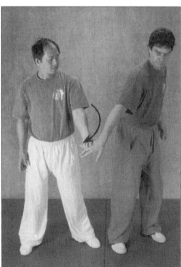
Figure 7–33

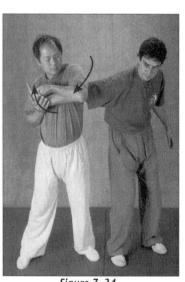
Figure 7–34

Technique #3: Lower Hook Dividing

(Xia Diao Fen) 下 刁 分

In this technique, first use your left hand to grab your opponent's ring finger and pinkie (Figure 7-33), place your left elbow on the top of his left elbow (Figure 7-34). Next, use your left elbow to push in his elbow to make it bend (Figure 7-35). Finally, use the leverage of your left hand and elbow to lock him down to the ground (Figure 7-36). To make the control more effective, you should use your right hand to press your opponent's fingers to generate more pain (Figure 7-37).

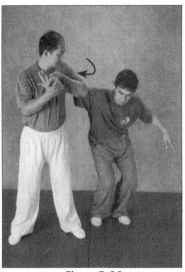

Figure 7–35

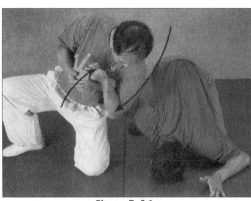

Figure 7–36

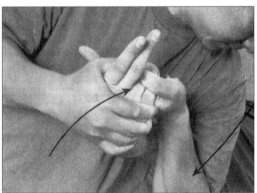

Figure 7–37

Theory:

Dividing the Muscle/Tendon (between ring and middle fingers). In order to control your opponent's wrist efficiently, his arm should be bent. If you bend your left knee and touch it to the ground, it will give you more space for control.

Technique #4: Walk With Me

(Yu Wo Tong Xing) 與我同行

When you approach your opponent from behind, stay on his right hand side. First, use your right hand to grab his right hand and twist it clockwise (Figure 7-38). Next, lift his right hand up to bend his elbow and immediately use your left hand to grab his hand (Figure 7-39). Finally, lock his arm in front of your left chest (Figure 7-40). You may use your right hand to bend any of finger backward to control him more effectively. In order to prevent him from attacking you with his left hand, you may also use your right hand to grab his hair and pull it toward you.

Theory:

Dividing the Muscle/Tendon (wrist). In order to make the control effective, you should use more pressure near his pinkie area.

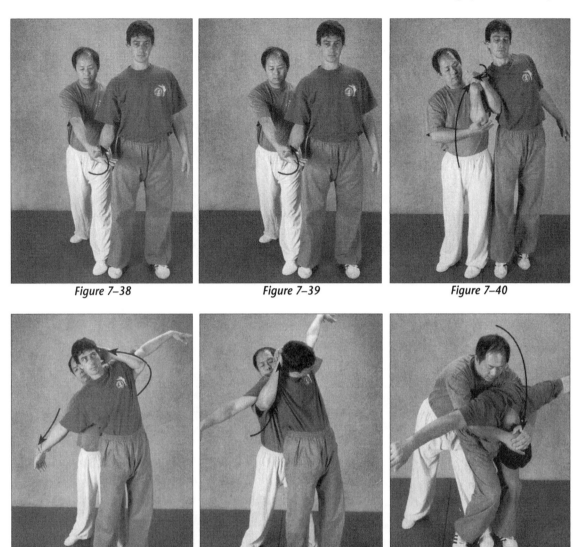

Figure 7–38   Figure 7–39   Figure 7–40

Figure 7–41   Figure 7–42   Figure 7–43

Technique #5: Force the Bow

(Qiang Po Ju Gong) 強迫鞠躬

When you approach your opponent from behind, use your right hand to grab his right hand while inserting your left hand under his left armpit and reach the back of his neck (Figure 7-41). Next, place both of your hands behind his neck (Figure 7-42) and finally, press his head down (Figure 7-43).

Theory:

Misplacing the Bone (neck). If you do not lock your opponent's neck properly, he may simply lift up his both arms and drop his body to get away. To prevent him from doing so, you must press his head hard forward.

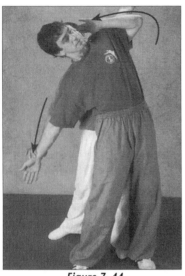

Figure 7–44

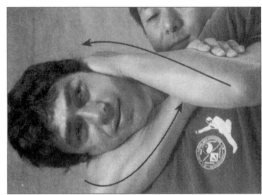

Figure 7–45

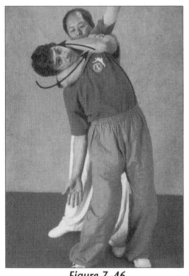

Figure 7–46

Technique #6: Single Arm to Seal the throat

(Dan Bi Suo Hou) 單臂鎖喉

In this technique, again use your right hand to grab your opponent's right wrist while inserting your left hand under your opponent's left armpit and reach the back side of his head (Figure 7-44). Immediately release your right hand, circle his neck and grab your left fore-arm (Figure 7-45). Finally, increase your squeezing power to seal his breathing (Figure 7-46).

Theory:

Sealing the Breathing. In order to prevent him from escaping, your right hand's locking is very important.

Technique #7: Pressing Shoulder with Single Finger and Extending the Neck for Water

(Yi Zhi Ding Jiang and Yin Jing Qiu Shui) 一指頂肩，引頸求水

First, use your right hand to grab your opponent's right wrist and push it upward to keep it bent (Figure 7-47). Next, insert your left arm under his right arm and reach the back side of his upper-arm (Figure 7-48). Finally, lock his arm behind his back and use your index finger to press the *Jianneiling* cavity (M-UE-48)(Figure 7-49). This will cause sig-

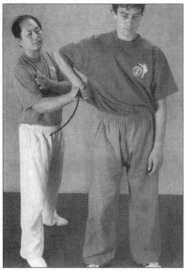

Figure 7–47

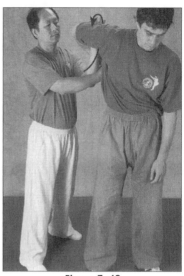

Figure 7–48

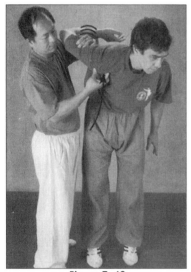

Figure 7–49

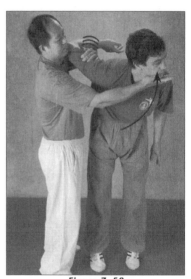

Figure 7–50

nificant pain in the shoulder area. You should increase the pressure on your index finger until your opponent's heels leave the floor. Alternatively, you may use your right hand to push his chin upward (Figure 7-50). This will also produce great pain.

Theory:

Misplacing the Bone (shoulder), and Cavity Press (*Jianneiling* Cavity). When you use your left arm to lock your opponent's right arm and lift it upward, you generate a strain on his right shoulder's tendons and ligaments. This action also exposes his *Jianneiling* cavity for your cavity press attack. Without an accurate locking position for the shoulder, the cavity press will not be effective.

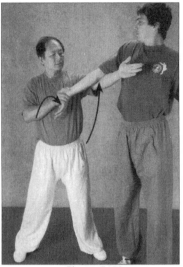

Figure 7–51

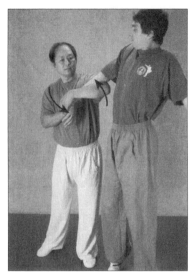

Figure 7–52

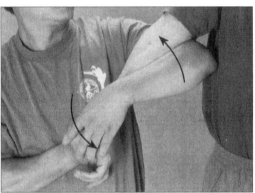

Figure 7–53

Technique #8: Hands Prop a Large Beam or Prop Up Elbow

(Shou Ban Da Liang or Shang Jia Zhou) 手扳大樑，上架肘

In this technique, again use your right hand to grab your opponent's right wrist while pressing your left forearm upward to his right elbow and keep his arm straight (Figure 7-51). Then, bend your left arm and use the leverage generated from your left hand and elbow to lock his arm upward (Figure 7-52).

Theory:

Misplacing the Bone (elbow). You may also use this technique when you are facing your opponent. The leverage generated from your left elbow and both hands is the key to locking (Figure 7-53).

Technique #9: Forward Wrist Press

(Qian Ya Wan) 前壓腕

This technique can be used either from the front or the rear of your opponent. First, use your right hand to grab your opponent's right wrist and then immediately bend it upward (Figure 7-54). Immediately place your left hand on his elbow and finally squeeze both hands against his wrist and elbow (Figure 7-55).

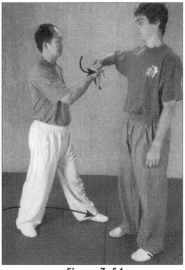

Figure 7–54

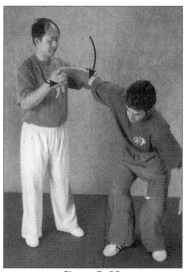

Figure 7–55

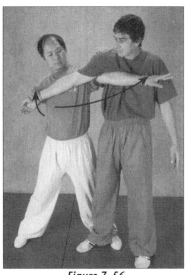

Figure 7–56

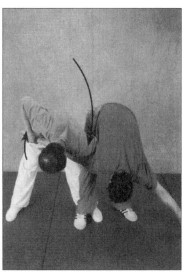

Figure 7–57

Theory:

Dividing the Muscle/ Tendon (wrist). When you squeeze your right hand, you should place your pressure on the base of his fingers. This will offer you better leverage to execute this technique.

Technique #10: Two Children Worship the Buddha

(Shuang Tong Bai Fo) 雙童拜佛

In this technique, use your right hand to grab his right wrist while inserting your left arm under his armpit (Figure 7-56). Next, bow your body forward while pulling your right hand backward while thrusting your left shoulder against his right shoulder to lock him (Figure 7-57).

Theory:

Dividing the Muscle/Tendon (wrist). In this technique, the pain is generated from your left shoulder and your right hand. This technique can only control your opponent temporarily.

■ Chapter 8 ■

CONCLUSION

Now, at the end of this book, I would like to remind you of a few important things. First, you should again recognize that Qin Na is only a part of Chinese martial arts. It has existed in every Chinese martial style. No independent "Qin Na style" has ever existed. Therefore, you should understand that, in order to perfect your Chinese martial arts skills, it will not be enough only to learn Qin Na. Qin Na techniques must be applied together with Shuai Jiao (Chinese wrestling) and skillful striking, then this art can be manifested to its greatest benefit. It is also because of this reason that Qin Na techniques can be adopted in any martial style.

Second, as mentioned before, there are probably more than 700 Qin Na techniques which have been developed in the last few thousand years in China. This book has offered you only some of the ones with which I am familiar. However, you should understand that even though there are so many techniques, they are all based on the same few principles and roots. Once you have grasped these essential keys, you will be able to grow and develop continuously. Remember, as long as you are humble, patient, and perseverant, with pondering and continued experience you will become a truly proficient Qin Na master.

Third, when you learn Qin Na, merely remembering the techniques is not enough. You must spend a great deal of time pondering and practicing. Only then can the techniques be executed skillfully.

Fourth, at the beginning, you may learn only the external techniques. However, as time passes, you should gradually apply internal Qi, through your own mental control, to make the technique more effective. The key to entering the doorway from the external to the internal is through reading and participating in seminars. You may refer to the books: *The Root of Chinese Chi Kung* by YMAA.

Finally, you should remember, when you practice with your partner, to prevent injury from occurring. Do not apply a great deal of power to your playmate. However, when the situation occurs that you must use power to handle the situation more efficiently, then you must apply martial jerking power (Jin). Through correct body movement and Qi coordination, the manifestation of power can be devastatingly penetrating and harmful. Therefore, when you practice Qin Na with Jin power with your partner, you must be very careful. To grasp the key to Jin training, read the book: *Advanced Yang Style Tai Chi Chuan* by YMAA. Alternatively, you may join the seminars YMAA offers.

Remember, a truly wise man will not doubt himself and will not be confused by others. Build up your confidence and remain humble. Someday, you will realize that you have left those others far, far behind you.

■ **Appendix A**■

NAMES OF QIN NA TECHNIQUES

▪ Appendix B ▪

TRANSLATION AND GLOSSARY OF CHINESE TERMS

Baguazhang 八卦掌

Means "Eight Trigram Palms." The name of one of the Chinese internal martial styles.

Ba Wang Qing Ke 霸王請客

Federal Lord Invites for Dinner. Name of a traditional Qin Na technique.

Bai He 白鶴

Means "White Crane." One of the Chinese southern martial styles.

Bi 閉

Means "close" or "seal."

Bi Qi 閉氣

Qi here means "air." It means oxygen we inhale. Therefore Bi Qi means to "seal the oxygen supply" or "seal the breath."

Bo Xue Jing Shi 博學敬師

Humble Study and Respecting One's Teacher.

Cai 採

Plucking.

Chai (Sai) 釵

A kind of hairpin for ancient Chinese women. Later, it was derived into a kind of southern Chinese weapon.

Chang Chuan (Changquan) 長拳

Means "Long Range Fist." Chang Chuan includes all northern Chinese long range martial styles.

Chang Xiang-San 張詳三

A well known Chinese martial artist in Taiwan.

Changquan (Chang Chuan) 長拳

Means "Long Range Fist." Changquan includes all northern Chinese long range martial styles.

Cheng Gin-Gsao 曾金灶

Dr. Yang Jwing-Ming's White Crane master.

Chi (Qi) 氣

The energy pervading the universe, including the energy circulating in the human body.

Chi Kung (Qigong) 氣功

The Gongfu of Qi, which means the study of Qi.

Chin (Qin) 擒

Means 'to catch" or "to seize."

Chin Na (Qin Na) 擒拿

Literally means "grab control." A component of Chinese martial arts which emphasizes grabbing techniques, to control your opponent's joints, in conjunction with attacking certain acupuncture cavities.

Chize (L-5) 尺澤

Name of an acupuncture cavity. It belongs to the Lung channel.

Chongqing City 重慶市

A city in Sichuan province.

Chuan Fu Cheng Gao 船夫撐篙

The Boat Man Pushes His Oar. Traditional name of a Qin Na technique.

Cuo Gu 錯骨

Cuo means "to misplace" or "to disorder" and Gu is "bone." Therefore, Cuo Gu means "to misplace the bone or joint."

Cuo Gu Shou 錯骨手

Misplacing the Bone Hands (techniques). Early name of Qin Na.

Dan Chan Si Wan 單纏絲腕

Single Wrapping Wrist. Traditional name of a Qin Na technique.

Dian 點

Means "to point" or "to press."

Dian Mai 點脈

Mai means "the blood vessel" (Xue Mai) or "the Qi channel" (Qi Mai). Dian Mai means "to press the blood vessel or Qi channel."

Dian Xue 點穴

Dian means "to point and exert pressure" and Xue means "the cavities." Dian Xue refers to those Qin Na techniques which specialize in attacking acupuncture cavities to immobilize or kill an opponent.

Diao 刁

Hooking.

Dim Mak 點脈

Cantonese of "Dian Mai."

Du Mai 督脈

Usually translated Governing Vessel. One of the eight extraordinary vessels.

Duan Mai 斷脈

Duan means "to break" and Mai means "the blood vessel." Duan Mai means "to seal or to break the blood vessel."

Emei 峨嵋

Name of a mountain in Sichuan province, China.

Fen Jin 分筋

Fen means "to divide" and Jin means "muscles/tendons." Fen Jin means "to divide the muscles/tendons."

Fen Jin Shou 分筋手

Dividing Tendon Hands (techniques). Early name of Qin Na.

Gongfu (Kung Fu) 功夫

Means "energy-time." Anything which will take time and energy to learn or to accomplish is called Gongfu.

Gung Li Chuan 功力拳

The name of barehand sequence in Chinese Long Fist martial arts.

Guoshu 國術

Abbreviation of "Zhongguo Wushu," which means "Chinese Martial Techniques."

Han Ching-Tang 韓慶堂

A well known Chinese martial artist, especially in Taiwan in the last forty years. Master Han is also Dr. Yang Jwing-Ming's Long Fist grandmaster.

Hei Hu Tao Xin 黑虎掏心

Black Tiger Digs the Heart. Traditional name of a Qin Na technique.

Huang Ying Che Chi 黃鷹掣翅

Yellow Eagle Pulls Its Wings. Traditional name of a Qin Na technique.

Jiache (S-6) 頰車

Name of an acupuncture cavity. It belongs to the Stomach channel.

Jianneiling (M-UE-48) 肩內陵

Name of an acupuncture cavity. A special point.

Jin 勁

Chinese martial power. A combination of "Li" (muscular power) and "Qi."

Jin Shao-Feng 金紹峰

Master Yang Jwing-Ming's White Crane grandmaster.

Kao Tao 高濤

Master Yang Jwing-Ming's first Taijiquan master.

Kong Qi 空氣

Air.

Kou 扣

Wrapping.

Kou Zhi Shou 扣子手

Locking Hands (techniques). Early name of Qin Na.

Kung Fu (Gongfu) 功夫

Means "energy-time." Anything which will take time and energy to learn or to accomplish is called Kung Fu.

Lao Lu E Ti 老驢扼蹄

Old Mule Holds Its feet. Traditional name of a Qin Na technique.

Le 将

Pulling.

Li Mao-Ching 李茂清

Master Yang Jwing-Ming's Long Fist master.

Liang Dexing (Jeffrey D. S, Liang) 梁德馨

Master Liang Shou-Yu's uncle, currently residing in Seattle, Washington.

Liang Shou-Yu 梁守渝

A well known Chinese martial arts and Qigong master. Currently resides in Vancouver, Canada.

Lien Bu Chuan 連步拳

One of the Long Fist barehand sequences.

Liu He Ba Fa 六合八法

One of the Chinese internal martial arts, its techniques are combined from Taijiquan, Xingyi, and Baguazhang.

Liu Jin-Sheng 劉錦昇

Grandmaster Han Ching-Tang's classmate.

Na 拿

Means "to hold" or "to grab."

Na Xue 拿穴

Means "to grab the cavity."

Na Xue 拿血

Means "to grab the blood vessel."

Nanking Central Guoshu Institute 南京中央國術館

A national martial arts institute organized by Chinese government in 1928.

Qi (Chi) 氣

Chinese term for universal energy. A current popular model is that the Qi circulating in the human body is bio-electric in nature.

Qi Mai 氣脈

Means "Qi channels."

Qian Cheng Li Rang 謙誠禮讓

Humble and Polite.

Qigong (Chi Kung) 氣功

The Gongfu of Qi, which means the study of Qi.

Qin (Chin) 擒

Means 'to catch" or "to seize."

Qin Na (Chin Na) 擒拿

Literally means "grab control." A component of Chinese martial arts which emphasizes grabbing techniques, to control your opponent's joints, in conjunction with attacking certain acupuncture cavities.

Qin Na Shu 擒拿術

Qin Na Techniques.

Qin Shi 親師

Literally means "close or love teacher."

Qin Xiong 擒兇

To catch the murderer.

Qing dynasty 清朝

A dynasty in Chinese history (1644-1912 A.D.).

Qu Zhi Yi Suan 曲指一算

Bend the Finger to Count. A traditional name of a Qin Na technique.

Quchi (LI-11) 曲池

Name of an acupuncture cavity. It belongs to the Large Intestine channel.

Ren Mai 任脈

Conceptional Vessel. One of the Eight Extraordinary Vessels.

Sai (Chai) 釵

A kind of hairpin for ancient Chinese women. Later, it was derived into a kind of southern Chinese weapon.

Shaohai (H-3) 少海

Name of an acupuncture cavity. It belongs to the Heart channel.

Shaolin 少林

Young woods. Name of Shaolin Temple.

Shaolin Temple 少林寺

A monastery located in Henan province, China. The Shaolin Temple is well known because of its martial arts training.

Shi Qin Zhi Xiao 侍親至孝

Show the great feelings of love and respect to one's parents.

Shuai Jiao 摔交

Chinese wrestling. Part of Chinese martial arts.

Shuang Chan Si Wan 雙纏絲腕

Double Wrapping Wrist. Traditional name of a Qin Na technique.

Sichuan province 四川省

A province in China.

Suo 鎖

Locking.

Taiji 太極

Means "grand ultimate." It is this force which generates two poles, Yin and Yang.

Taijiquan (Tai Chi Chuan) 太極拳

A Chinese internal martial style which based on the theory of Taiji (grand ultimate).

Taipei 台北

The capital city of Taiwan located on the north of Taiwan.

Taipei Xian 台北縣

The county on the north of Taiwan.

Taiwan 台灣

An island to the south-east of mainland China. Also known as "Formosa."

Taiwan University 台灣大學

A well known university located on the north Taiwan.

Taiyang (M-HN-9) 太陽

Name of an acupuncture cavity. A special point.

Taizuquan 太祖拳

A style of Chinese external martial arts.

Tamkang 淡江

Name of a University in Taiwan.

Tamkang College Guoshu Club 淡江國術社

A Chinese martial arts club founded by Dr. Yang when he was studying in Tamkang College.

Tiantu (Co-22) 天突

Name of an acupuncture cavity. It belongs to the Conception vessel.

Tui Na 推拿

Means "to push and grab." A category of Chinese massages for healing and injury treatment.

Wai Dan Chi Kung (Wai Dan Qigong) 外丹氣功

External Elixir Qigong. In Wai Dan Qigong, a practitioner will generate Qi to the limbs, and then allow the Qi flow inward to nourish the internal organs.

Wilson Chen 陳威伸

Master Yang Jwing-Ming's friend.

Wushu 武術

Literally, "martial techniques."

Wuyi 武藝

Literally, "martial arts."

Xingyi 形意

An abbreviation of Xingyiquan.

Xingyiquan (Hsing Yi Chuan) 形意拳

One of the best known Chinese internal martial styles created by Marshal Yue Fei during Chinese Song dynasty (1103-1142 A.D.).

Xinzhu Xian 新竹縣

Birth place of Dr. Yang Jwing-Ming in Taiwan.

Xue Mai 血脈

Means "blood vessels."

Yang Jwing-Ming 楊俊敏

Author of this book.

Yang Mei-Ling 楊美玲

Master Yang Jwing-Ming's wife.

Zhejiang province 浙江省

A province on the south east of China.

Zhong Hua Guoshu Promoting Committee, Republic of China 中華國術進修會

A Chinese martial arts organization in Taiwan.

Zhua 抓

Means "to grasp" or "to grab."

Zhua Jin 抓筋

Means "to grab the tendons."

Zhua Xue 抓穴

Means "to grab the cavity."

Zhuang Shi Bei Hu 壯士背虎

The Hero Carries the Tiger. Traditional name of a Qin Na technique.

Zhui Yuan 追源

Literally "trace back its origin." It implies the appreciation or the respect the original source.

Zi Wu Liu Zhu 子午流注

Zi refers to the period around midnight (11:00 PM - 1:00 AM), and Wu refers to midday (11:00 AM - 1:00 PM). Jiu Zhu means the flowing tendency. Therefore: a schedule of the Qi circulation showing which channel has the predominant Qi flow at any particular time, and where the predominant Qi flow is in the Conception and Governing vessels.

■ Index ■

BOOKS FROM YMAA

more products available from...
YMAA Publication Center, Inc. 楊氏東方文化出版中心
1-800-669-8892 • ymaa@aol.com • www.ymaa.com

VIDEOS FROM YMAA

ADVANCED PRACTICAL CHIN NA — 1	T0061
ADVANCED PRACTICAL CHIN NA — 2	T007X
COMP. APPLICATIONS OF SHAOLIN CHIN NA 1	T386
COMP. APPLICATIONS OF SHAOLIN CHIN NA 2	T394
EIGHT SIMPLE QIGONG EXERCISES FOR HEALTH 2ND ED.	T54X
NORTHERN SHAOLIN SWORD — SAN CAI JIAN & ITS APPLICATIONS	T051
NORTHERN SHAOLIN SWORD — KUN WU JIAN & ITS APPLICATIONS	T06X
NORTHERN SHAOLIN SWORD — QI MEN JIAN & ITS APPLICATIONS	T078
QIGONG: 15 MINUTES TO HEALTH	T140
SHAOLIN LONG FIST KUNG FU — YI LU MEI FU & ER LU MAI FU	T256
SHAOLIN LONG FIST KUNG FU — SHI ZI TANG	T264
SHAOLIN LONG FIST KUNG FU — XIAO HU YAN	T604
SHAOLIN WHITE CRANE GONG FU — BASIC TRAINING 3	T0185
SIMPLIFIED TAI CHI CHUAN — 24 & 48	T329
SUN STYLE TAIJIQUAN	T469
TAI CHI CHUAN & APPLICATIONS — 24 & 4	T485
TAIJI CHIN NA IN DEPTH — 1	T0282
TAIJI CHIN NA IN DEPTH — 2	T0290
TAIJI CHIN NA IN DEPTH — 3	T0304
TAIJI CHIN NA IN DEPTH — 4	T0312
TAIJI WRESTLING — 1	T0371
TAIJI WRESTLING — 2	T038X
TAIJI YIN & YANG SYMBOL STICKING HANDS–YANG TAIJI TRAINING	T580
TAIJI YIN & YANG SYMBOL STICKING HANDS–YIN TAIJI TRAINING	T0177
WILD GOOSE QIGONG	T949
WU STYLE TAIJIQUAN	T477
XINGYIQUAN — 12 ANIMAL FORM	T310

DVDS FROM YMAA

ANALYSIS OF SHAOLIN CHIN NA	D0231
BAGUAZHANG 1,2, & 3 —EMEI BAGUAZHANG	D0649
CHEN STYLE TAIJIQUAN	D0819
CHIN NA IN DEPTH COURSES 1 — 4	D602
CHIN NA IN DEPTH COURSES 5 — 8	D610
CHIN NA IN DEPTH COURSES 9 — 12	D629
EIGHT SIMPLE QIGONG EXERCISES FOR HEALTH	D0037
FIVE ANIMAL SPORTS	D1106
THE ESSENCE OF TAIJI QIGONG	D0215
QIGONG MASSAGE—FUNDAMENTAL TECHNIQUES FOR HEALTH AND RELAXATION	D0592
SHAOLIN KUNG FU FUNDAMENTAL TRAINING 1&2	D0436
SHAOLIN LONG FIST KUNG FU — BASIC SEQUENCES	D661
SHAOLIN SABER — BASIC SEQUENCES	D0616
SHAOLIN STAFF — BASIC SEQUENCES	D0920
SHAOLIN WHITE CRANE GONG FU BASIC TRAINING 1&2	D599
SIMPLE QIGONG EXERCISES FOR ARTHRITIS RELIEF	D0890
SIMPLE QIGONG EXERCISES FOR BACK PAIN RELIEF	D0883
SIMPLIFIED TAI CHI CHUAN	D0630
SUNRISE TAI CHI	D0274
SUNSET TAI CHI	D0760
TAI CHI CONNECTIONS	D0444
TAI CHI ENERGY PATTERNS	D0525
TAI CHI FIGHTING SET—TWO PERSON MATCHING SET	D0509
TAIJI BALL QIGONG COURSES 1&2—16 CIRCLING AND 16 ROTATING PATTERNS	D0517
TAIJI BALL QIGONG COURSES 3&4—16 PATTERNS OF WRAP-COILING & APPLICATIONS	D0777
TAIJI MARTIAL APPLICATIONS — 37 POSTURES	D1057
TAIJI PUSHING HANDS 1&2—YANG STYLE SINGLE AND DOUBLE PUSHING HANDS	D0495
TAIJI PUSHING HANDS 3&4—MOVING SINGLE AND DOUBLE PUSHING HANDS	D0681
TAIJI SABER — THE COMPLETE FORM, QIGONG & APPLICATIONS	D1026
TAIJI & SHAOLIN STAFF - FUNDAMENTAL TRAINING	D0906
TAIJI YIN YANG STICKING HANDS	D1040
TAIJIQUAN CLASSICAL YANG STYLE	D645
TAIJI SWORD, CLASSICAL YANG STYLE	D0452
UNDERSTANDING QIGONG 1 — WHAT IS QI? • HUMAN QI CIRCULATORY SYSTEM	D069X
UNDERSTANDING QIGONG 2 — KEY POINTS • QIGONG BREATHING	D0418
UNDERSTANDING QIGONG 3 — EMBRYONIC BREATHING	D0555
UNDERSTANDING QIGONG 4 — FOUR SEASONS QIGONG	D0562
UNDERSTANDING QIGONG 5 — SMALL CIRCULATION	D0753
UNDERSTANDING QIGONG 6 — MARTIAL QIGONG BREATHING	D0913
WHITE CRANE HARD & SOFT QIGONG	D637

more products available from...

YMAA Publication Center, Inc. 楊氏東方文化出版中心

1-800-669-8892 • ymaa@aol.com • www.ymaa.com